WESTMINSTER PUBLIC LIBRARY

D0482763

Praise f[...]

turned on

"A witty discussion of the indirect role sex plays across political, economic, religious, and cultural landscapes...marinated in provocative assertions that are certain to instigate debate and productive discussion."

—*Kirkus Reviews*

"Ross Benes's smart and enjoyable book takes us on a fascinating odyssey through the hidden ways that humanity's endless struggle with sex influences the entirely unsexual aspects of our daily lives. The secret history of graham crackers, the rise of pelvic massages by sheepish doctors, the story of military-sanctioned brothels—all are narrated with wit and unexpected insight."

—Ogi Ogas, coauthor of *A Billion Wicked Thoughts: What the World's Largest Experiment Reveals about Human Desire*

"*Turned On* is an entertaining and well-researched exploration of the unintended consequences of our sexual misapprehensions and mythologies. Benes reminds us at every turn how persistent and pervasive is the parallax between what's true about human sexuality and what we insist on believing about it."

—Rachel Maines, author of *The Technology of Orgasm*

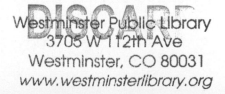

DISCARD

Westminster Public Library
3705 W 112th Ave
Westminster, CO 80031
www.westminsterlibrary.org

"This is a no-nonsense, honest, factual, and clearly exposed dialogue about human sexuality. The social constructs and interesting historical developments that shape attitudes toward masturbation, homosexuality, religious influences, and scandals all come under intelligent consideration. The text is infused with sociological and psychological wisdom without ever being dogmatic and certainly never boring."

—Richard Sipe, author of *A Secret World: Sexuality and the Search for Celibacy and Sex, Priests, and Power: Anatomy of a Crisis*

"Benes has combined history, epidemiology, anthropology, neuroscience, and whatever it takes to produce a well-written, engaging, clever, highly informative book. *Turned On* is a welcome respite from the usual partisan bickering and moralizing that this subject usually evokes."

—Edward C. Green, former director of the Harvard AIDS Prevention Project

"The topic of sex elicits intense moral and political sentiments, so it's especially important to approach it in a clear-headed way. This book does an excellent job with that—the only preaching you'll find here is in favor of a more rational understanding of sex. Far more wide-ranging than most books about sex, it surveys the diverse and counterintuitive ways in which sex impacts society. Engaging and honest, you'll be surprised by how much you learn."

—Michael Price, Brunel University psychology professor and *Psychology Today* contributor

"A thought-provoking read on a subject that would otherwise seem to have been overworked already."

—Daniel Halperin, coauthor of *Tinderbox*, former senior HIV prevention advisor at USAID and former faculty member of Harvard School of Public Health

"Benes winnows out many surprising motivations behind familiar products and also shows how, for everyone from cereal-makers to pharmaceutical companies, sometimes the best-laid plans lead to marvelous tangential results. Conversational, approachable, and credible, Benes delivers story after story that will surprise you and challenge your assumptions. Once you have read this book, I doubt you will ever eat a weasel again."

—Patchen Barss, author of *The Erotic Engine*

"In this fascinating work, buttressed with massive research from impeccable sources, Benes shows how sex and the perception of sex affect so many aspects of cultures—from why we eat corn flakes to the economic influence of gay communities and more."

—Richard Kimbrough, author of *History Mysteries*

turned on

A Mind-Blowing Investigation into How Sex Has Shaped Our World

Ross Benes

Foreword by A. J. Jacobs

Previously titled *The Sex Effect*

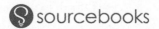 sourcebooks

Copyright © 2017, 2018 by Ross Benes
Cover and internal design © 2018 by Sourcebooks, Inc.
Cover design by Lucy Kim
Cover image © Larry Washburn/Getty Images

Sourcebooks and the colophon are registered trademarks of Sourcebooks, Inc.

All rights reserved. No part of this book may be reproduced in any form or by any electronic or mechanical means including information storage and retrieval systems—except in the case of brief quotations embodied in critical articles or reviews—without permission in writing from its publisher, Sourcebooks, Inc.

This publication is designed to provide accurate and authoritative information in regard to the subject matter covered. It is sold with the understanding that the publisher is not engaged in rendering legal, accounting, or other professional service. If legal advice or other expert assistance is required, the services of a competent professional person should be sought.—*From a Declaration of Principles Jointly Adopted by a Committee of the American Bar Association and a Committee of Publishers and Associations*

This book is not intended as a substitute for medical advice from a qualified physician. The intent of this book is to provide accurate general information in regard to the subject matter covered. If medical advice or other expert help is needed, the services of an appropriate medical professional should be sought.

All brand names and product names used in this book are trademarks, registered trademarks, or trade names of their respective holders. Sourcebooks, Inc., is not associated with any product or vendor in this book.

Published by Sourcebooks, Inc.
P.O. Box 4410, Naperville, Illinois 60567-4410
(630) 961-3900
Fax: (630) 961-2168
sourcebooks.com

Originally published in 2017 as *The Sex Effect* by Sourcebooks, Inc.

Library of Congress Cataloging-in-Publication Data

Names: Benes, Ross, author.
Title: Turned on : a mind-blowing investigation into how sex has shaped our world / Ross Benes.
Description: Naperville : Sourcebooks, [2017] | Includes bibliographical references.
Identifiers: LCCN 2016032655 | (paperback : alk. paper)
Subjects: LCSH: Sex--History--21st century. | Sex customs. | Sex instruction. | Sex--Religious aspects--Catholic Church. | Religion and civil society.
Classification: LCC HQ21 .B436 2017 | DDC 306.7--dc23 LC record available at https://lccn.loc.gov/2016032655

Printed and bound in the United States of America.
VP 10 9 8 7 6 5 4 3 2 1

For Eddie, the best damn friend a boy could ever have.

contents

foreword

The human sex drive is powerful and complicated, and it leads to all sorts of unintended consequences. For instance, in the late twentieth century, Ron Benes and Sue Benes mated, which resulted in a baby named Ross Benes, who would grow up to be a talented journalist, and, much to their surprise, write a book about sex.

Sorry to bring your parents' bedroom life into this, Ross. But I'm not sorry your parents procreated.

Ross produced a book that is fascinating and original. It's also wide-ranging—Ross talks about the impact sex has had on everything from hipster neighborhoods to politics, from modern warfare to breakfast. (In case you didn't know, corn flakes were invented in the nineteenth century as a way to reduce teenage boys' masturbation habits. They were spectacularly ineffective in that department, but they are still delicious.)

The book is also provocative—as any book on sex should be. You may not agree with all of Ross's conclusions (I took issue with a couple myself!), but you will absolutely enjoy the journey. If I were to pitch the book in an elevator, I'd say it's *Freakonomics* without pants. Then I'd probably be escorted off the elevator by security.

One word of advice when reading this book: Don't skip the footnotes. Some of the most interesting information and insights can be found in Ross's small type. Noel Coward once said that "having to read footnotes resembles having to go downstairs to answer the door while in the midst of making love." An appropriately carnal metaphor. But in this case, the trip downstairs is worth it. Your partner will be waiting for you when you return.

I first met Ross when he was working at *Esquire* magazine, where I was an editor. He was a fountain of ideas. He talked fast and read voraciously. And he's written some wonderful pieces both for *Esquire* and for other publications.

He wrote about his experience at a silent retreat—which was a brave endeavor, since he is the most talkative person I know. He wrote about Scientology, which is also a brave endeavor, because the Scientologists harass journalists for even typing the word "Scientology." He has also written about wrestling and his love for orange Hi-C.

But this book about sex is his most interesting work yet.

I hope you enjoy it as much as I did, if not as much as the act itself.

—A. J. Jacobs, *New York Times* bestselling
author of *Drop Dead Healthy*, *The Year of
Living Biblically*, and *The Know-It-All*

introduction

For all the time we spend thinking about it, talking about it, and engaging in it, sex still arouses contention and confusion for many people. From exhibitionists who advocate free love to celibate religious leaders who condemn promiscuity, and everyone in between, sex evokes a powerful reaction across cultures and societies. The emotional response that often follows one of our most primal behaviors has severely distorted the public's understanding of the most basic statistics, trends, and behaviors related to sexuality—everything from what percentage of the population is gay to how often people divorce.

As you'll see in the following pages, many of the ideas our society holds to be self-evident about monogamy, affairs, divorce, rape, porn, abstinence, STDs, contraception, fertility rates, and reproductive technologies are often far from the empirical truth. Many of these misconceptions about human sexuality occur because sex inevitably incites emotion. And emotion lends itself to politicizing, where statistics are interpreted according to the ethics of whatever group a person identifies with. Other misconceptions likely arise from simple ignorance and fear. And many people also hold misconceptions stemming from the fact that good data gets lost in the vast and, incidentally, misleading informational overload our culture spews. From celebrities selling gossip to pastors warning of the "homosexual agenda" to sex tips in glossy magazines, there is an unending amount of conflicting information that makes it difficult to spot accurate and reliable facts.

Sex occupies a significant spot in our civilization, as both a want and a need. Biologically, we need sexual reproduction for our species to survive. Advertisers manipulate the natural human urge to procreate and condition us to desire sex even more by branding our favorite nonsexual products (such as beer, body spray, and food) with sexual images, and by constantly sending subliminal messages that sex can be obtained by purchasing a particular product. Add in religious and cultural taboos relating to sexual behavior, and you get a forbidden-fruit syndrome that makes discussing, analyzing, and having sex an alluring and forbidden act often regarded with simultaneous shame and elation. The stigma surrounding sex makes any rational analysis of sexual behavior nearly impossible outside institutional contexts because of the overwhelming amount of bias that many researchers, commentators, and theorists allow to cloud their perceptions, which leaves most of us in the dark about how sex actually functions in our society.

But our attitudes and beliefs about sex itself are not what

is most interesting about it. Scores of books, magazines, and movies have already investigated the battle between our bodies and our ideologies. Understanding the direct impact of sex on our society is very important, but most of the conversations we're currently having on this topic focus on the obvious. It's already clear that sex is all around, causing people to perpetually act irrationally, from politicians risking strategically built careers for a quick tryst, to johns soliciting prostitutes during AIDS epidemics. These behaviors seem baffling at first glance, but it makes sense for sex to be at least occasionally unreasonable, because irrational sex has evolutionarily benefitted the survival of *homo sapiens*. To some degree, humans still retain the tendencies of their ancient ancestors, who were subconsciously compelled to pass on their "selfish genes," even though it often wasn't in their best personal interest to do so.[1]

Throughout history, people have had children despite lacking the resources to support themselves, let alone provide a high quality of life for their offspring. Today, there are Western teens and young adults who have children earlier than they planned because evolution has predisposed them to reach their peak fertility years during the "adolescent" stage that contemporary society has constructed.[2] These people were driven by a biological tendency to procreate, because natural selection favors projecting genes into the future over the well-being of an individual's health, sanity, and bank account.[3] As Helen Epstein commented in a report about AIDS in Africa, "If sex were an entirely rational process, the species would probably have died out long ago."[4] While the irrational aspect of sex gets a lot of attention, what's actually most fascinating about sex is what has been *left out* of the conversation—the hidden (but powerful) influences sex imposes on our everyday lives—and, conversely, the ways our sexual behavior shape the world around us.

Sex's largest impact in our society doesn't come from things the average person would recognize as overtly sexual: sex workers turning tricks, contraceptives, or instant porn access. Rather, sex's greatest effects can be seen in innocuous, seemingly nonsexual aspects of our everyday lives. The power of sex can also provide political, religious, and business leaders social capital that allows them to gain power. In this book, you'll see how sex indirectly influences society through inadvertently affecting things such as how easily we purchase products online, crime rates, and how people eat breakfast. You'll also see the other side of the coin—how nonsexual aspects of society indirectly influence how people have sex, because past political edicts have conditioned people to stick to one spouse, pro-natalist policies subtly nudge people to have more children, and the marketing of biomedical products has led people to engage in riskier sex. You'll find that the hidden relationships between sex and political, economic, and religious institutions can shape behaviors ranging from how much income families save to how people rely on others from different religious faiths.

This book is about the impact of those relationships, as investigated by an everyday observer rather than a researcher-consultant, politician, moral reformer, or corporate entity already invested in the business of sex. Because human behavior is incredibly complex, and has millions of co-occurring variables, it's difficult to draw hard-and-fast conclusions about how and why sex works in our society. There will be no "three rules of the sex effect" or "seven habits of successful couples" principles here. In reality, the investigation of human sexuality's role in society is a multidisciplinary study full of uncertainty and surprise. Think of this book not as a guidebook written by a "sexpert," but as a conversation starter meant to inspire dialogue and uncover the hidden relationships between our sexuality and the world around us.

———

Part of the dialogue we're trying to initiate revolves around examining the miscalculations of ideologues. As you'll see, when people in power try to restrict sexual influences, they can create whirlpools of disastrous, unexpected outcomes. But there are other times that deferring to "sex-positive," politically correct approaches ends up dumping gas on the flame. Conservative or liberal, Democrat or Republican, Puritan or free lover, devout or agnostic—it doesn't matter. At some point every group displays improbable logical fallacies when differentiating between its perception of sex and the realities of the world we live in. Each group has, in some ways, blinded itself with its respective ideologies, resulting in unintended sexual and societal consequences.

The point of this book isn't to talk about how good or bad sex is, or how, when, and why people should be having it. The point is to get everyday people thinking about what factors *really* drive sexual decisions and how human behavior is shaped by their consequences, as viewed through political, economic, and cultural lenses. We'll also look at the opposite angle—how society influences our sex lives—to inspire discussions about how political, economic, and religious policies affect human sexuality. Ideally, this book will get people talking about what makes humans do what they do. And if nothing else, readers will experience eating corn flakes in a whole new way.

PART I

POLITICS

what's love got to do with it?

n Western society, it's assumed that most adults will eventually find a partner they love, and will marry them with the intent of staying together for the rest of their lives and with the goal of remaining sexually faithful throughout the relationship. What's often unrealized about this commonplace ideal of sticking with one spouse is that it was likely introduced into human society through calculated political strategy—which originally came about as a consequence of war, not love. The ubiquity of monogamy in our society, and its perceived superiority over other marriage models, stems from the decisions of powerful leaders and revolutionary social changes, not natural human instinct.

The construct of monogamy is a powerful force in our society, having been shown to reduce crime and motivate fathers to invest more time and resources in their children. But humans are not necessarily naturally inclined to be monogamous, and they constantly battle sexual jealousy. The perceived societal value of monogamous marriage shows how calculated political decisions can last well beyond their original contexts while still maintaining their influence on human behavior, and how laws can shift humans away from our animalistic instincts.

A Very Brief Summary of Monogamy's Long and Convoluted History

The marriage system of any particular society is ultimately tied to what's proscribed by its political structure. Because prehistory involves a lot of gaps and projections, it's difficult to trace the exact evolution of monogamy throughout the world. But we'll briefly break down monogamy's timeline.

Although enforced monogamy has been common in Western society for a few thousand years, it's only within the last few hundred years that most of the world's *population* has lived in "monogamous cultures."[1]* Even though many people practice monogamy today, it was the legal norm in only about

---

*   According to John Witte Jr., most of this shift occurred when Japan, Thailand, Nepal, China, and India (with exceptions for Muslims) prohibited polygamy.

15 percent of the roughly 1,200 *cultures* the *Ethnographic Atlas Codebook* analyzed from 1962 to 1980.[2]

And these are modern stats. The further back you trace mating and marriage practices, the less common enforced monogamy appears to be. There is also a lot of nuance in humanity's history with monogamy—as words like "spouse," "partner," "mate," and "marriage" have much different connotations depending on what time period they refer to. The level of commitment and the legal status of "polygamous" partners also tend to vary by culture. But for simplicity's sake, *polygamy* and its related terms here will just mean someone, usually a man, having more than one regular committed partner (i.e., polygyny). Technically, *polygyny* is defined as one man in relationships with multiple women, while *polyandry* is defined as one woman in relationships with multiple men. And there are times when what researchers refer to as polygamy more resembles modern polyamory or promiscuity. To avoid confusion, and to prevent this chapter from having an academic appendix of nuanced linguistic changes every time a new culture or time frame is mentioned, "polygamy" will function as a catchall for non-monogamy here.

Around 200,000 BC, hunter-gatherers lived in mildly polygamous societies, according to historian Kyle Harper. Men who had "wives" had about three on average, leaving other men partnerless.[3†] After another 190,000 years of

---

† Some researchers believe that even in these ancient societies that permitted polygamy, most marriages were still monogamous, because it was difficult for most men to acquire enough resources to attract and support multiple wives. Michael

foraging, hunter-gatherers realized that instead of wandering around to find food, they could plant crops and domesticate animals, allowing for a more stable, stationary livelihood. This led to the invention of agriculture, known as the Neolithic Revolution.[4]

The act of creating settlements allowed humans to accumulate new levels of wealth. Along with the benefits of agriculture came property rights, as the ownership of land became paramount for anyone wishing to gain higher status. Eventually, humans began having fewer children and investing more resources in the kids they had. Property rights and the idea of having fewer children to give each child a better quality of life led to rules and codes that bound men, women, and their property together. With land ownership, marriage became more important for inheritance purposes, and it tied couples together in new social and legal ways. Another major effect of land accumulation was the development of enormous income disparity and extreme cases of polygamy. The men with the most wealth and power ended up with the most wives, while men with the least clout often ended up with just one wife or no wife at all.[5]

The prevalence of these nonmonogamous societies may have something to do with the fact that the evolutionary benefits of having multiple sexual partners are clear, as having sex with multiple partners gives people a better chance of

---

Price writes, "Polygyny was the idealized state of marriage in the world of the past, something that the majority of men aspired to but that only a minority could achieve."

producing healthy and successful offspring who will continue to pass their genes along.[6] Generally, males are wired to spread their seed as widely as possible to increase the number of likely offspring.[7]* They prefer many trysts with young, fertile women. Females tend to be more selective, as they want the best genes and resources for their limited offspring.[8] They are more likely to select a wealthy spouse who can provide for their child, but are also prone to copulating with a handsome man with superior genes right before ovulation.[9]† In some species, the inclination to seek the best genes, regardless of how many partners an individual may already have, leads to alpha males running a monopoly on female mates. Which is *somewhat* reminiscent of rulers such as King Solomon controlling personal harems.

From here, according to Harper, the evolution of monogamy worldwide didn't change much until democracy was invented in Greece around sixth century BC.[10] At the heart of the concept of democracy is the belief that every person's vote matters and everyone should participate, even if only indirectly, in government. As democratic ideals began

---

*   Males also accumulated more wealth so they could attract more women. As to why that is, Lynn Saxon writes, "The sex which invests most in parenting any offspring is a limited reproductive resource competed for by the sex which invests the least."

†   Men also prefer women's odors near ovulation, which is when women are most likely to conceive. During ovulation, women report a stronger desire to cheat and less likelihood to use a condom during sex. Women also report they feel more attractive when they are at the most fertile stage of their cycle. They also put on more makeup and wear skimpier clothes during this time.

spreading from government into people's personal lives, it
made sense, then, that every man entitled to a vote should
be entitled to a woman, too.[11] Within just a few generations
of Homer's *Iliad*, monogamy became the preferred marriage
practice in Greek society. According to Stanford historian
Walter Scheidel, "Monogamy was regarded as quintessen-
tially 'Greek'" in the ancient world.[12]

Because researchers speculate most marriages in history
were monogamous (even if monogamy wasn't what was
desired by most men or enforced by most cultures), it's worth
noting the Greeks didn't "invent" pair-bonding with a single
sexual partner.[13] However, by outlawing polygamy, Greek
lawmakers began a slow conditioning process that shaped
modern mating. Over time, the social conditioning initially
brought on by Greco-Roman rules led to the paired, gradual
phenomena of the increasing unacceptability of having multiple long-term sexual partners and the increasing common-
ness of sticking with a single partner, to the point that most
Westerners now default toward one partner without much
questioning of this practice.[14] While democracy may have
played a role in Greco-Roman culture's outlawing polygamy
and enforcing legal monogamy, the reasons leaders pushed for
their followers to legally bind themselves to one spouse show
that the story of monogamy is much more than an equality-
based feel-good tale. Rather, monogamy was likely enforced
because it gave leaders political leverage.

HEY JEALOUSY

As evolutionary biologist David Barash notes in the *Chronicle of Higher Education*, "Just as multiple sexual partners can *increase* the fitness of a philanderer, the same behavior on the part of one's partner can *reduce* the other's fitness. Hence, sexual jealousy is a very widespread and fitness-enhancing trait, as is a roving eye (along with, occasionally, other body parts)."[15] By "fitness," Barash is referring to the evolutionary concept of an organism's ability to see its genes carried on by future generations. Barash indicates that sexual jealousy developed so animals and humans could ensure they were raising their own offspring and not the child of some wandering philanderer.

To better understand modern humans' pesky jealous quirks, you need to understand the ancient environment in which human brains evolved. Evolutionary psychologists refer to this setting as the environment of evolutionary adaptedness (EEA). It is in this ancient context that humans became subconsciously focused on having the highest number of surviving offspring.

But some evolutionary adaptations developed in the EEA have outlived their usefulness. A common example is how humans developed a taste for sugary food in an environment where fruit existed and candy didn't.[16] Eating sweet ripe fruit was good for the diet. But sweet foods were rare, and finding them was a difficult task, which meant it was in people's best interests to load up on scarce sugary substances when they came across them. But now, humans have an urge to eat lots of sugar in an environment filled with processed foods and high-fructose corn syrup, which present new dietary challenges our ancestors never faced. Overindulging in this tendency for sweets can lead to obesity, high blood pressure, tooth decay, and eventually death. Similarly, overindulgence in the inherited desire for males to spread their seed can also cause discolored, rotting infections that can eventually lead to death.

So even though many couples plan to never have children, they still get angry over infidelity. This jealous impulse comes from past reproductive strategies—but being familiar with our ancestors' EEA will be of little practical concern to a wife who catches her husband screwing his secretary, or a husband who catches his wife with her yoga instructor.

Research from David Buss, an evolutionary psychologist who specializes in mate selection research, shows that each gender evolved to react to jealously differently. When imagining sexual unfaithfulness, men get sweaty and their heart rates jump more than the Dow Jones after a market boom. Men react to emotional infidelity as well, but not to the same magnitude. For women, the results are reversed. Envisioning emotional infidelity causes more distress than sexual unfaithfulness.[17] The reasons go back to evolution.

Ancient males feared their wives would get pregnant by a rival male, so sex with strange men wasn't to be tolerated. Males who became obsessed over their wives' social and sexual habits made sure their women weren't getting impregnated by other men, which gave the genes of these jealous males a better chance of projecting themselves into future generations. Females feared their men would desert them and move on to giving other women their resources. Women whose jealousy brought them to shield their men from becoming emotionally involved with other women helped ensure that their man's resources wouldn't be spent elsewhere, which gave these women's offspring a better chance at survival. People with these jealous tendencies had better chances of passing on their genes, and over time, those with a genetic predisposition toward gender-specific jealousy were more likely to successfully spawn offspring that would survive into adulthood and to see their genes live on.[18] Women don't enjoy their men sleeping around, nor do men enjoy their women emotionally bonding with other men behind their back. But in general, for evolutionary reasons, males react more strongly to sexual infidelity and females to emotional infidelity.

Do as the Romans Do

It's likely that Greece influenced the Romans to adopt monogamy and embed it into their culture.[19]* The "ancient

---

*   Greeks and Romans did occasionally allow polygamy in a few exceptional cases. Athenian officials allowed it after the Peloponnesian War killed most of the city's men, necessitating repopulation efforts. Some rulers in Macedonia and the Aegean Islands practiced polygamy as well.

law" of Rome defined "lawful marriage" as "the union of a man and a woman, a partnership for the whole of life, involving divine as well as human law."[20] According to ancient Roman jurist Gaius, "[A] woman cannot marry two men, nor can a man have two wives." Polygamy was considered "nefarious," and a man who tried to obtain multiple wives was "considered to have neither a wife nor children." If a man had multiples wives, the wives were to be viewed as "harlots," while his children were "spurious bastards conceived through promiscuous intercourse."[21]

By the third century CE, Roman officials formally criminalized polygamy, imposing punishments on polygamists and their accomplices while blocking children from second spouses from claiming inheritance. An imperial edict stated that "anyone under Roman rule who has two wives will be branded with infamy." In Rome, "infamy" was a social stigma that meant a person was blocked from holding public office or other positions of authority and had several rights taken away from them.[22] By the sixth century CE, Emperor Justinian said polygamy was "contrary to nature." Under Justinian's rule, the state began seizing one-quarter of the property of known polygamists.[23] These anti-polygamy laws limited the amount of women that wealthy men could monopolize, which effectively gave poor men access to women who previously were unobtainable.

Though the Roman system allowed many poor men a chance to obtain a lifelong mate for the first time, let's not get carried away and conclude that Caesar deeply cared about constituents' sex lives.[24]* Monogamy in Rome wasn't of the "soul mate" variety today's romantic comedies sell lonely moviegoers. Ancient Roman society may have upheld monogamy as a legal ideal, but sexual promiscuity was still common in the culture. Romans had lots of sex with people other than their spouses, particularly with slaves and prostitutes.[25] Roman monogamy was little more than a legal code founded on political calculation—and that political calculation was rooted in militaristic expansion.[26]

Greco-Roman leaders were ambitious military conquerors. They wanted to gain new land to build their vast empire while preventing uprisings in their newly conquered territories. According to evolutionary psychologist Michael Price, Greco-Roman leaders' survival depended on maintaining large, controlled, and well-supplied armies:

> The ancient Greco-Roman and medieval European leaders who embraced anti-polygyny laws were heavily invested in the business of war, and their own social status and indeed survival often depended on their ability to maintain large, well-funded armies. And the imposition of monogamy produced bigger,

---

* John Witte Jr. notes that Julius Caesar was infamous for philandering, and that he "ordered that a special law be passed 'allowing him, with the hope of leaving issue, to take any wife he chose, and as many of them as he pleased.' His contemporaries, however, charged him with 'unnatural lewdness and adultery,' and little evidently came of his efforts. Julius Caesar's successor, the first Roman emperor, Caesar Augustus (63 BCE–14 CE) enacted sweeping reforms of Roman law, including the laws of marriage and family life, with monogamy again at the foundation."

better armies, because monogamous groups can grow larger than polygynous ones.

Why can monogamous groups grow larger? Because men want wives, and if you need a lot of men on your team, you must offer them something that they want. In monogamous groups, unlike polygynous ones, high-status males cannot hoard large numbers of women for themselves. The more equal distribution of women in monogamous groups means that more men can acquire wives, and fewer men have to leave the group to search for wives elsewhere. And the larger the group, the more men there are to fight in battles and to pay taxes for the funding of wars. Socially imposed monogamy, therefore, emerged in the West as a reciprocal arrangement in which elite males allowed lower-ranking males to marry, in exchange for their military service and tax contributions.[27]*

As the Romans expanded their empire, they instilled their culture, laws, and beliefs—including that of monogamy—in the populations of their conquered territories.[28] Of course, Roman influence isn't solely responsible for why monogamy became the norm among modern civilizations or why Westerners today believe it's their duty to stay with a single spouse for life. After all, Rome fell about 1,500

---

*   It has been hypothesized that access to consistent sex had the effect of both satisfying and distracting sexually frustrated lower-ranking men, which reduced the probability that they would start revolutions to overthrow the elite.

years ago—but not before it influenced the world's most popular religion.[29†]

The Two Will Become One

Prior to Rome's adoption of monogamy, Judeo-Christian tradition allowed for polygamy, as evidenced by some important Old Testament figures. Jacob, for example, had two wives and two concubines, David had at least six wives with even more concubines, and King Solomon had seven hundred wives with three hundred concubines. But unlike Judaism, Christianity developed in a society that enforced legal monogamy.

It was the laws of Roman society that influenced the religion, which consequently influenced how Christians had sex. The religion didn't invent monogamy and impose it on the society it grew up in, although it is easy to conceptualize it that way, given that Christian sexual ethics are often perceived as restrictive, while ancient Roman society is presented as sexually decadent.[30‡] In the fifth century, St. Augustine, who

---

†   According to Witte, Christians adopted several practices from Roman law, such as the marriage and family structures discussed in this chapter. "They also taught the faithful to pay their taxes, to register their properties, and to obey the Roman rulers up to the limits of Christian conscience and commandment," Witte writes. Harper notes that winebibbing, which influenced how Christians distribute the Eucharist, was also a Roman practice Christians adopted.

‡   Witte writes, "The reality was that real polygamy was simply not a major topic of the canon law of the church. Instead, the first-millennium church looked to the state and its criminal laws to continue to prohibit and punish real polygamy as it

is arguably more responsible for shaping Christian sexual ethics than any other person in history, acknowledged Rome's influence on Christian sexual teaching when he wrote, "Now indeed in our time, and keeping with Roman custom, it is no longer allowed to take another wife, so as to have more than one wife living."[31] Augustine also reasoned that Old Testament polygamists committed no offense against "nature" or "custom," because polygamy "was no crime when it was the custom; and it is a crime now, because it is no longer the custom."[32] This suggests that the mating systems Judeo-Christian leaders found tolerable were influenced by the legal norms in the societies they inhabited.[33]

Although Christian apologists were influenced by Roman monogamy, they also added their own rules to regulating sexuality. According to John Witte Jr., a scholar of law and religion, early Christian apologists were

> pressing for a monogamous union that was more egalitarian, more exclusive, and more enduring. Roman law forced parties to choose between a concubine and a wife; they could not have both. Christianity denounced concubinage altogether, requiring Christians either to marry or to remain single. Roman law maintained a sexual double standard, forbidding wives to commit adultery but allowing husbands to indulge with impunity in sex

---

had since antiquity." He also noted, "It was the law of the state, not the law of the church, that prohibited real polygamy, and it did so with growing severity."

with prostitutes and slaves. Christianity denounced extramarital sex altogether, and called Christian husbands and wives alike to remain faithful to each other exclusively.[34]

It may be surprising to today's Christians that ancient social contexts based on Greco-Roman politics, rather than theological teachings, were what originally drove Christian doctrine to adopt monogamy as the only acceptable marriage practice.[35] Christianity's phenomenal spread allowed it to promote its own version of monogamy—one that emphasized fidelity and discouraged divorce—in places the Roman Empire never could have reached. And because Christianity survived the fall of Rome, it continued to keep the monogamy ideal vibrant after the great empire's dissolution.[36]

But just because monogamy is culturally conditioned, rather than a natural human instinct, doesn't mean it can't produce positive side effects. Arguments that denounce monogamy because it is "unnatural" put individual people's desires on a pedestal while ignoring how monogamy affects society at large. In reality, it's these large-scale societal reasons that led leaders to implement monogamy in the first place.[37]

═══ SEXUAL CONDITIONING ═══

The decision of whether to practice monogamy or polygamy isn't the only sexual behavior guided by social norms. Whom we want to marry (or at least have sex with) is also influenced by our surroundings. As marketers are well aware, the physical traits humans find sexually attractive are as much conditioned as they are innate. For centuries, people in different cultures have used various methods to make themselves "more attractive" according to their respective societies' standards.

According to A. J. Jacobs's *The Know-It-All*, Mayan Indians found crossed eyes attractive, so they hung objects between babies' eyes to cause the condition; Padaung women increase their sex appeal by stretching their necks with fifteen-inch brass neck rings that pull the vertebrae into the neck; and modern Asian women now undergo eyelid surgery to make their eyes appear more rounded and Western. Meanwhile, breasts have seen it all. They were compressed in seventeenth-century Spain, are often distended in Paraguay, and are inflated to obscene sizes in California today.[38]

Finding thin, tan-skinned women attractive is a modern Western ideal. Previously, pudginess was prized, as it symbolized wealth, because few people could afford enough food to become fat.[39] Even today, there are places where pudginess is the cultural ideal, as seen in the wife-fattening farms of Mauritania, where obesity is a sign of wealth and attractiveness.[40] But in modern America, cheap Big Gulps and supersized meals equate fatness with laziness and poor health. In many Western countries, women frequent tanning salons to get a good fake bake to entice potential suitors. In the East, Chinese and Korean women carry umbrellas with them on sunny days, and some will wear ski masks to the beach, because they want to avoid becoming tan like peasant workers.[41] Some Asian women also apply skin cream to make themselves appear lighter.[42]

And it's not just the ladies hoping to reach subjective standards of physical attractiveness. The internet is full of products for enlarging penises, and some men even undergo surgery for this today, even though the ancient Greeks found small penises more aesthetically pleasing.[43] Between history, cultures, and marketing, is there really such a thing as "default" or "normal" human attraction?

Monogamy's Social Benefits

When early Christians began spreading the virtues of monogamy, the social benefits of the marital practice at the time were clear. Lifelong marriages rooted in fidelity encouraged men to weigh the major responsibility of raising children against a few minutes of sexual pleasure, which was important in cultures without accessible or effective birth control.[44] Regarding the institution of inseparable monogamous unions into Christianity, historian John Boswell notes the Bible's authors did not intend

to explain or legislate on the whole range of human affections, and they made no pretense of providing moral guidance on all forms of love. They simply answered troublesome questions about heterosexual marriage submitted to them by persons attempting to establish a new sexual morality in societies where there were no social services for the widowed or orphaned; no legal guarantees of protection for unwed mothers or alimony for divorcees; no effective means of birth control except abstinence, abortion, or abandonment of unwanted children.[45]

Although lifelong unions originally provided crucial social safety nets that were otherwise unavailable to women, that's no longer the case. Western women now have more legal rights, more choice in sexual partners, more economic power, and more reliable ways to control fertility. Also, people live much longer (and their bodies physically mature at younger ages) than they did when modern monogamy was originally constructed. These factors make lifelong monogamy appear unrealistic, unnecessary, and undesirable for many people, relegating monogamy to the punchline of corny jokes in which single people razz their married friends about their "boring" sex lives and how they've given up sexual freedom in favor of being tethered to a ball and chain. While monogamy may seem restrictive, predictable, and dull to many people, focusing on one partner can contribute to powerful sociological phenomena—and many of these effects are actually quite pleasant. Let's start with sex.

Despite the common perception that being officially unattached equates to a hot sex life, it's actually the single people who could use some help in the bedroom. People who go from relationship to relationship or engage in casual sex and stay single report fewer instances of intercourse than those in long-term exclusive relationships.[46] Their sexual satisfaction is also lower than that of long-term monogamous couples.[47]

Monogamous men may also be delighted to learn that, despite a potential reduction in total lifetime sexual partners, males are the biggest winners in monogamous marriage.* Married men get into less legal trouble compared to their single counterparts. Married men begin to disregard antisocial behavior in favor of their family. They drink less, fight less, and commit crimes less frequently than single men.[48] And because monogamy allows more men to marry by ensuring that no single man keeps two or three (or ten) women for himself, and because married men commit fewer crimes, it then should reason that monogamy prevents some men from committing crimes and landing in jail, lowering the overall crime rate.[49†]

A study published in a journal run by the Royal Society,

---

* Well, the well-to-do men will experience a slight reduction in partners. Men with fewer resources may actually see their number of partners increase from zero to one. With polygamy, it was high risk, high reward, because whenever a man hoarded scores of women, that left loads of other men single and lonely. Polygamy is like investing in a junk bond, in that you are more likely to default and get nothing in return. However, if you do get a return, it's likely to beat the market average. Monogamy is like investing in an indexed mutual fund. You are less likely to lose your investment, but your rewards won't trump everyone else's. Rather, they will come consistently, slowly, and over time.

† This correlation could also mean that women choose men who are less likely to fight and get thrown in jail. And that marriage doesn't necessarily domesticate men, but rather that domesticated men are more likely to be selected as partners by women. Like most social things, it's probably a bit of both. Instead of viewing this as correlation versus causation, maybe it'd be more appropriate to view each factor as a contribution.

a prestigious British scholarly organization, found that, throughout history, societies that enforce monogamy have historically had lower crime rates than societies that allow men more than one wife. In a data set of 157 countries, the researchers found that the more people practicing polygamy within a country, the higher the percentage of unmarried men. In turn, a higher percentage of unmarried men correlated with higher rates of rape and murder.[50]* Along with reducing instances of rape and murder, legal monogamy was also found to reduce assault, theft, and fraud.[51]

Monogamy also encourages men to spend fewer resources on obtaining more women, and more resources on providing for their offspring, which "increases savings, child investment, and economic productivity," according to the study's authors. The study's authors also theorized that monogamy decreases gender inequality and reduces child abuse.[52] Similarly, after examining the marital systems of more than 170 countries and controlling for GDP and sex ratios, a pair of researchers in the *Emory Law Journal* concluded, "Polygynous structures increase violence toward women and children, decrease civil rights and political liberties in the state more broadly, and increase the allocation of resources in society toward weapons procurement. Polygyny exerts economic, physical, and political consequences for societies in which such practices remain prevalent."[53]

---

*   According to historian David Herlihy, Christianity's teachings on monogamy led to a more even distribution of women, which, "surely reduced abductions and rapes of women and probably calmed the endemic violence of early medieval life."

Michael Price suggests it isn't coincidence that while only a minority of the world's societies have imposed monogamy, the most powerful societies the world has produced can be found in this monogamous minority. He notes that polygamy often leads to more conflict and less cooperation between citizens. Countries such as Japan and China abolished polygamy relatively recently, not because they wanted to become more Christian, but because in the monogamist marital structure they saw a way to mimic Western economic prowess. Price writes:

> The entire historical record suggests that monogamy has spread because of the political dominance of monogamous societies. This spread has occurred in two main ways: when leaders have observed the power of monogamous societies and proceeded to abolish polygyny among their own subjects, typically in efforts to stay competitive with or form alliances with monogamous societies; and when leaders of monogamous societies have conquered polygynous populations and proceeded to impose monogamy.[54]

The theory here is that monogamy has spread because it holds political advantages over polygamy. Although monogamy has power to influence social behaviors unrelated to sex, such as crime rates, it still took a lot of effort from political and religious leaders to force people to stick to one partner. Monogamy facilitates group-level benefits, but at the individual level, it is difficult for many people, because having sex with only one person clashes with evolutionary tendencies to seek sex with multiple partners. In this way, the desires of the individual can clash with the goals of society, turning how many sexual partners a person can obtain into an externality.

One, the Loneliest Number?

Monogamy is interesting from a social-science point of view because it produces conflict. The idea of committing to just *one* sexual partner for the rest of one's life can pit biology, ethics, and social norms against each other. So often, the popular debates about monogamy focus on the individual and psychological levels. Affairs, divorces, and one-night stands are condemned by people who believe monogamy is the "natural" and preferred state of human sexuality, and shrugged off by people who believe monogamy is an "unnatural" cultural imposition fostering conditioned jealousy. Opponents of monogamy like to focus on our "natural" desire for multiple partners, while proponents of monogamy focus on how "natural" sexual jealousy appears.

Using monogamy's alleged innateness or non-innateness for personal political capital—say, to demand authority from religious adherents or to sell glamorous lifestyle guides to the sexually adventurous—quickly turns into futile moralizing. These "sex-negative" and "sex-positive" disputes usually ignore monogamy's collective societal effect. They ignore the sociological impact brought on by conditioning millions of people to stick to one sexual partner. Historical, ethnographical, and biological research together indicate that the tendency of

Westerners to yearn for *one* soul mate is a conditioned behavior that became popular because political leaders prohibited polygamy in favor of socially beneficial monogamy. In this, we see that how most Westerners have sex is influenced by past politics. In turn, this sexual ethic affects the political economy, which is probably why, over time, more countries have adopted monogamy.

The point here isn't to argue whether monogamy is more "moral" or more practical than other mating systems. The point is to examine how, through subtle implementation of laws and ethics, ancient political strategies radically changed how people have sex and raise families. The status quo of marriages today proves that societal institutions can be quite effective at dictating sexual custom to the masses, because the marriage institution Westerners are familiar with was created out of war, not love. The emotions many couples experience— from irrational jealousy when their lover glances at someone else, to exuberance over the thought of being the only one their partner cums for—are the unintended consequences of ancient policies colliding with evolutionary tendencies, which make up many modern people's sexual realities.

=2=

all the presidents' women

BREAKING DOWN THE PREDICTABLE
PHENOMENA OF POLITICIAN SEX SCANDALS

E ven before the U.S. declared independence, its leaders' sex lives were shaping the country. From the founding fathers through JFK and Clinton, American politicians have indulged in extramarital affairs with slaves, movie stars, sisters-in-law, and interns. Today, the amount of cable news coverage and tabloid magazine articles on political scandals might make it appear as if the occurrence of affairs is on the rise, but high-powered political sex affairs have always been part of the American tradition. The only thing that has changed is public perception, which is largely due to changes in media coverage. It might seem irrational to have an affair while in office, because politicians have so little to gain but so much to lose. But psychological research shows why it isn't unusual for a powerful person to risk their reputation for a quick tryst.[1]*

Profiling the Political Personality

In a famous *Simpsons* episode, anchorman Kent Brockman may have been onto something when introducing an upcoming TV special about politician sex: "Tonight, *Eye on Springfield* takes a look at the secret affairs of Kennedy, Eisenhower, Bush, and Clinton. Did fooling around on their wives make them great? We'll find out next, when we play 'Hail to the Cheat.'"[2]

Brockman's question—whether great presidents are more likely to be adulterous—is interesting, but unanswerable. For one thing, the media zeitgeist has changed so much throughout American history that it's pretty difficult to

---

*　It's fitting that the biological phenomenon where mammals show heightened sexual interest in new partners is named after a president. "The Coolidge Effect" comes from a joke about President Calvin Coolidge. Allegedly, Mrs. Coolidge noticed a rooster mating furiously. She asked the farmhand how often the rooster had sex. When the man said dozens of times daily, Mrs. Coolidge said, "Tell that to the president." The president then asked the man, "Same hen every time?" When the man said, "No, it's a different hen each time," the president said, "Tell that to Mrs. Coolidge."

But the best joke about Calvin Coolidge comes from Jon Stewart's *America (The Book)*: "Coolidge still ranks as the quietest president of all time. Famously, a woman once approached him saying, 'I bet my friend I could get you to say more than two words,' to which Coolidge wittily replied, 'Fuck you.'"

compare *known* affairs of presidents to see whether "good presidents" have more affairs than "bad presidents," as that involves lots of arbitrary judgment and small samples. Although we can't exactly test whether cheating affects a politician's performance, what we do know is that Alexander Hamilton, Thomas Jefferson, Franklin Roosevelt, John Kennedy, Martin Luther King Jr., and Bill Clinton are great and influential leaders who each committed sexual indiscretions.[3] Given that the potential costs of these affairs were so much greater than the potential benefits they provided these powerful men, it's worth examining why they risked public shame for private orgasm.

Personality psychology suggests that great leaders are risk takers who are highly confident and assertive.[4] They believe they know better than others what is best for them. These traits overlap with narcissism. And research shows narcissists tend to get into positions of power and authority,[5] and are also sexually aggressive.[6] Once they've gained powerful positions, these types of people tend to become *more* narcissistic.[7] All of these tendencies make politicians more prone to taking sexual risks.[8]

Psychologists have defined risk takers as people with the "lack of ability to inhibit an automatic or prepotent response or to self-regulate one's behavior, resulting in limited delay of gratification and risky decision making."[9] The risks these people take can be influenced by subconscious tendencies, because risk takers are prone to have different brain chemistries than non–risk takers. For example, they generally have lower levels of monoamine oxidase A (MAOA), which regulates dopamine, the neurotransmitter that controls pleasure in the brain.[10] Because there's less regulation of the brain's pleasure center, people with less MAOA take more risks and put themselves in more unpredictable situations seeking sensation. [11]

Marvin Zuckerman, professor emeritus of psychology at the University of Delaware, pioneered the study of sensation seeking, which he describes as a "trait defined by the *seeking* of varied, novel, complex, and *intense* sensations and experiences, and the willingness to take physical, social, *legal*, and *financial* risks for the sake of such experience."[12] Through studies comparing identical and fraternal twins, Zuckerman and other researchers found sensation seeking was about 60 percent genetic, which is quite high, given that most personality traits are about 30 to 50 percent genetic.[13] Other researchers have built off this work and found that high sensation seekers are more likely to cheat on their romantic partners.[14] Sensation seekers often are high-energy and high-functioning people who—because of their biological makeup, which can be reinforced by their social settings and conditioned outcomes—become easily assertive, aggressive, and sexually aroused in their quests for excitement and pleasure.[15] The thrills they seek can range from pursuing public power to soliciting risky sex. As Columbia University historian David Eisenbach and *Hustler* publisher Larry Flynt note in *One Nation under Sex: How the Private Lives of Presidents, First Ladies, and Their Lovers Changed the Course of American History*:

The same man who hungers for adoring crowds hanging on his every word will also tend to seek the thrill of extramarital sex. Combine this psychological tendency with the manifold sexual opportunities open to even the lowliest politician, and what do you think is going to happen? Ironically, the same biochemical drive that impels a politician to dedicate his life to winning the presidency will also get him impeached over sex with an intern.[16]

There might also be genetic links between risk-taking and sexual infidelity. A study from Binghamton University found that the presence of a certain dopamine receptor influenced people's likelihood of cheating on their partners. People with this receptor were more likely to have a history of uncommitted sex and infidelity.[17] "The motivation seems to stem from a system of pleasure and reward, which is where the release of dopamine comes in," said Justin Garcia, the study's lead author. "In cases of uncommitted sex, the risks are high, the rewards substantial, and the motivation variable—all elements that ensure a dopamine 'rush.'"[18]

While genes aren't deterministic, they do create predispositions. Having or lacking a dopamine receptor won't *cause* someone to act in a certain way, but it can make them *more inclined* to do so. People with this particular gene can choose to not cheat on their partners. And there are people without the gene who still cheat. But, regardless, the presence of the gene is linked to greater odds of cheating.

These studies hint that people's natures—and not just

their social conditions, opportunities, or environment—can contribute to their vulnerability toward infidelity, and that some people may just be more likely to cheat than others. While there's no way for us to know what kind of brain chemistry our former presidents had, or which ones had genes that *may* have made them more likely to be unfaithful, through anecdotally examining the most famous presidents who have had known affairs, we see a group of confident, assertive, and risk-taking individuals with lots of power and resources. It's a group of people from whom, quite frankly, affairs should be expected. Because the traits that make them attractive leaders and more likely to pursue office in the first place—wealth, good looks, confidence, charisma, assertiveness, risk-taking—also make them desirable sex partners. Once in office, the power they attain makes them even more desirable. As former U.S. Secretary of State Henry Kissinger put it, "Power is the ultimate aphrodisiac."[19]

Given that politicians possess traits that make them more likely to pursue extramarital sex, why are people so surprised whenever a prominent public figure's affair hits the airwaves? Even though politicians sell themselves as well-intentioned social reformers, most people don't look to them for moral guidance, and many people assume politicians are inherently dishonest. So what explains this disconnect between people's expectations (that politicians will remain faithful to their spouses) and the reality (that many politicians aren't faithful to their spouses) is that technology led to increased information access at the same time that journalists began publishing more investigative pieces exposing the secrets of leaders, which together led to a huge increase in the amount of public information about politicians' sexual affairs. Though they no longer extend such courtesy, for many decades, journalists protected the secrets of our country's leaders in exchange for better access to sources. That practice conditioned many Americans to think sexual affairs from prominent leaders were rare. It distracted people from realizing that political leaders have always had affairs, and that tendency isn't likely to change.

Despite how prominently they are reported, politician's sex scandals don't directly affect domestic or international policies. However, public perception of a president's personal life *can* affect how efficiently an administration carries out its goals. And the public perception of these sexual adventures has been shaped by the media, depending on what has been acceptable to publish during particular time frames. It's this fluctuation in information release that has dictated how moral and effective much of the public still believes particular presidents were in office. So let's examine the most famous American political sexual affairs, and how the media affected their impact on the American public.

Founding Fornicators

The founding fathers were remarkable men: inventors, politicians, generals, authors, bankers, publishers, and brewers, among other things. Men such as Thomas Jefferson and

Alexander Hamilton are examples of man at his best, and their accomplishments still remain incredibly influential in law, economics, and politics today. But sexually and socially deviant behaviors also accompanied their brilliance.

Alexander Hamilton's affair with Maria Reynolds, a married woman, was one of the first major American political sex scandals. America's first secretary of the treasury was so enamored with this woman that he paid her husband, James Reynolds, to keep the relationship secret.[20] In the end, though, Hamilton's sexual peccadillo was eventually exposed by a zealous pamphleteer named James Callender.

Pamphlets were a forerunner to newspapers that allowed people to broadcast their written opinions. According to historian Homer Calkin, "Most pamphlets were written to appeal to some certain emotion or to some particular group of people. Patriotic, religious, and economic motives often formed the theme of a pamphleteer."[21] The writing found in these pamphlets was often extremely ideological, because political parties and people with financial power used pamphlets as propaganda tools. It wasn't unusual for writers such as Callender to get hired to attack the pamphlet publisher's enemies.[22]* Though pamphleteering eventually gave way to modern journalism, Callender and his contemporaries were more like angry bloggers than nonpartisan journalists.[23]

Callender's expose on Hamilton pleased Hamilton's

---

*   Politicians such as Hamilton would also attack enemies by writing the screeds themselves under pseudonyms.

nemesis, Thomas Jefferson, so much that Jefferson hired Callender to target more of his political enemies, including John Adams, hoping Callender would find more smoking guns.[24]* But Callender and Jefferson eventually had a falling-out, leading Callender to shift the target of his aggressive pamphlets to Jefferson himself, according to Flynt and Eisenbach.[25]

Callender revealed that forty-year-old Jefferson had had a relationship and sired children with his teenaged slave, Sally Hemings.[26]† To make things even worse, Hemings also was the half-sister to Jefferson's late wife. But in the early 1800s, people cared much more about a white man screwing

---

* As noted in *One Nation under Sex*: "Throughout history we have seen how politicians have used sex to destroy their political enemies. Thomas Jefferson exposed Alexander Hamilton's affair with Maria Reynolds to foil his plans to modernize the banking system and industrialize the economy. Joe McCarthy went after pinks and pansies in the Truman administration to halt 20 years of Democratic rule in the White House. J. Edgar Hoover collected dirt on every powerful person in America and tried to destroy Martin Luther King Jr. In our own time, Newt Gingrich and the House Republicans sabotaged Bill Clinton's presidency with a futile impeachment fight about Monica Lewinsky. In each of these historical examples, the accusers were eventually exposed for being guilty of their own sexual indiscretions."

† Before he became president, Jefferson made sexual advances on Betsy Walker, the wife of his friend. And years later after Jefferson's wife died, it's alleged he had a fling with a married woman, Maria Cosway. If the allegations behind these relationships are true, then, unlike the relationship with Hemings, they would involve adultery. However, the press during Jefferson's time and the press today seem content to ignore these women and focus on the sexual relationship Jefferson had with Hemings.

his black slave than they did about an old man robbing his sister-in-law's cradle. Even though Hemings was three-fourths white and Jefferson was no longer married, there was no avoiding a PR disaster with a president having children with a slave.[27]

Jefferson's affair became open to public scrutiny because of the media ethic at the time. The printed press during this era discussed political parties and candidates with over-the-top headlines and sensational stories, including an 1828 *Cincinnati Gazette* story about Andrew Jackson that screamed, "General Jackson's mother was a COMMON PROSTITUTE, brought to this country by British soldiers! She afterward married a MULATTO MAN with whom she had several children, of which General JACKSON IS ONE!!!"[28]

But media coverage of politicians' personal issues later changed. During the Great Depression, World Wars, and the Cold War, journalists ditched desperate attempts to expose leaders in favor of concealing their indiscretions so they could gain better access to government sources. Basically, journalists would look the other way and not report on the sexual lives of elected officials in exchange for insider tips and invitations to events, which journalists hoped would help them land big scoops.[29] It is because of the change in media coverage, and not the actual sexual behavior of politicians, that until recently, many modern presidential sex scandals remained unknown until after the presidents had left office. And the biggest beneficiary of this shift in the media climate was Franklin Roosevelt.

Old Secrets of the New Deal

By the time FDR became president, journalists tended to portray politicians favorably, keeping their secrets hidden in exchange for information access. Historians also theorize that journalists protected politician's personal lives during this time as a matter of national security.[30] With the uncertainty brought on by the Great Depression and World War II, journalists protected presidents from scandals, which could have shifted the nation's attention while worsening people's confidence in their commander in chief.[31]* Journalists were so good at concealing FDR's personal life that millions of Americans didn't realize he was paralyzed until after his death. Even today, very few photos exist of FDR in a wheelchair.[32]

In concealing FDR's personal life, journalists prevented the public from learning about FDR's sexual relationships. Many Americans *still* are unaware that FDR had numerous affairs and that his wife was possibly bisexual, if not a full-blown lesbian.[33]† According to Joseph Persico's *Franklin and Lucy: Mrs. Rutherford and the Other Remarkable Women in Roosevelt's Life*, which details FDR's affairs, journalists in

---

*   "The Cold War also fostered a hands-off approach to the president's sex life because a scandal involving the commander in chief would have threatened the national security and been considered treasonous," Eisenbach and Flynt write.

†   People sometimes like to bring up that FDR and Eleanor were "cousins." In reality, they were distantly related. Put simply, they would not have seen each other at Christmas, anniversaries, or family graduations. If someone really wants to go to the fifth degree, then at some point everyone is related. And if the story of Adam and Eve is true, then every sexual act between humans is incest. It's all just varying degrees.

support of FDR prevented other reporters from photograph-
ing the president in his wheelchair. If someone tried to photo-
graph the president so as to show his disability, journalists
would block their view or knock their camera to the ground.
In newspapers, cartoonists portrayed FDR as a strong super-
hero. If ever cameras began rolling when he was lifted out
of his wheelchair, FDR said things like, "No movies of me
getting out of the machine, boys."[34]

FDR had at least one affair before he even became president, maintaining an ongoing relationship with Lucy Mercer,
who was a secretary for his wife Eleanor.[35] After Eleanor found
out, she threatened to leave him if he kept seeing Lucy. FDR
was tempted to get a divorce.[36†] He loved Lucy and didn't want
to give her up, but his mentors and family told him a divorce
would kill his political career. His mother threatened to cut
off him from the family's finances should he leave Eleanor.[37]
From that point on, the couple stayed together more as political partners than as a loving husband and wife. This is how
the Mercer affair altered the couple's dynamic, according to
FDR's son Elliot:

> Through the entire rest of their lives, they never did
> have a husband-and-wife relationship, but...they
> struck up a partnership agreement. This partnership
> was to last all the way through their life; it became
> a very close and very intimate partnership of great

---

†   Ronald Reagan and Donald Trump are the only U.S. presidents who have had a
    divorce.

affection—never in a physical sense, but in a tremen-
dously mental sense.[38]

FDR continued seeing Mercer throughout his presidency,
even though he had promised to end the relationship. He
also pursued other women freely despite his paralysis. FDR's
friend asked Roosevelt's doctor, "Is the president potent?" The
doctor replied, "It's only his legs that are paralyzed."[39]

Allowing FDR to focus on other women freed Eleanor
from having to attend to her husband sexually. She became
a political figure in her own right while exploring her own
sexuality. Eleanor stood up for racial and gender equality
during a very racist and sexist period in the U.S. She was
the first First Lady to hold her own press conferences, write
newspaper columns, and challenge her spouse publicly.[40] Even
after FDR's death, she remained an important political figure,
most notably as a delegate and the first chair of the United
Nations Commission on Human Rights. And several historians believe she also had a relationship with a butch lesbian
newspaper correspondent, Lorena Hickok.[41]

FDR and Eleanor helped lead the U.S. through perhaps
its most trying time. Their relationship *appeared* rock solid
to Americans as the country battled through the Great
Depression and WWII. Because of the media climate at the
time, their power dynamic and political potential weren't
overridden by scandalous media accounts of their personal
lives. In contrast to what a modern president could face if
caught having an affair, FDR's affairs didn't lead to constant
public criticism or drawn-out trials. Instead, Roosevelt had

his affairs and focused his time and energy on getting America through economic catastrophe and war.

====== **THE RAINBOW HOUSE** ======

There has never been an *openly* homosexual American president. However, the history of presidents' sex lives may not be entirely straight. Some news outlets proclaimed Barack Obama as America's "first gay president" because he has been supportive of LGBT rights during his second term in office. *Newsweek* even ran a ridiculous cover with Obama sporting a rainbow halo with the caption, "The First Gay President."[42] But many people don't know that there *may* in fact have been an actual gay president about 150 years before Obama—James Buchanan.[43]

Buchanan was the only American president to never marry, but he lived with former Vice President William Rufus King for more than a decade. King, by the way, is America's only bachelor vice president. They both were single for life at a time when only *3 percent* of men stayed single lifelong.[44] They were also inseparable. Andrew Jackson called the couple "Miss Nancy" and "Aunt Fancy."[45] When King moved to Paris to become ambassador to France, Buchanan wrote him this broken-hearted letter:

> I am now "solitary and alone," having no companion in the house with me. I have gone a wooing

> *to several gentlemen, but have not succeeded with any one of them. I feel that it is not good for man to be alone; and should not be astonished to find myself married to some old maid who can nurse me when I am sick, provide good dinners for me when I am well, and not expect from me any very ardent or romantic affection.*[46]

> But far from being a gay icon, Buchanan is regarded as one of the worst presidents in American history, largely because he encouraged secessionists on the brink of Civil War.[47]

The Camelot

When asked which presidents have had affairs, most Americans easily recall John Kennedy with Marilyn Monroe and Bill Clinton with Monica Lewinsky. But it's not often discussed that both of these men had other affairs, nor that they both dealt with very different public responses to their affairs due to changes in media coverage.

JFK's sex life is straight Casanova. Some of his affairs, like the one with Marilyn Monroe, are very well documented and generally accepted as fact. Others, like the weird love pentagon between JFK, his brother RFK, his wife Jackie,* Jackie's

---

*   Jackie had her own romps in the park. While much of America was dismayed that she married foreign tycoon Ari Onassis, Jackie also allegedly got off with RFK and stars like Marlon Brando, who may have made her an offer she couldn't refuse.

sister Lee Radziwill, and Jackie's second husband Aristotle Onassis, are so out there it's tough to tell what is real history and what is tabloid soap-opera material.[48][†] But it is confirmed that JFK had sex with teenage interns and aging celebrities, as well as many women in between. "I get a migraine headache if I don't get a strange piece of ass every day," Mr. President once told Lyndon Johnson's aide Bobby Baker.[49]

Despite all that we now know about JFK's affairs, he never had a public sex scandal while in office—and the reason comes back to the media, not his actual behavior. According to a Hollywood Associated Press writer who helped keep the JFK-Monroe affair out of the press, "Before Watergate, reporters just didn't go into that sort of thing. I'd have to have been under the bed in order to put it on the wire for the AP."[50] Like FDR, JFK benefitted from a comfortable relationship with the press in which secrets stayed hidden in exchange for access.

Not long after JFK was assassinated, President Lyndon Johnson increased America's involvement in the Vietnam War, an action that led to years of antigovernment protests. Fewer than ten years after JFK's death, the presidency faced the greatest scandal in its history with Watergate, which led to President Richard Nixon's resignation and bred distrust in the American public toward its government. With Vietnam,

---

†   Aside from sharing women with his brother, JFK also is alleged to have shared movie star Marlene Dietrich with his father. Also, Hollywood stars, hookers, interns, secretaries, and women of just about any occupation or age were included in JFK's sex life.

thousands of young American men, who were disproportionately working class, were sent to die in a war the U.S. had entered because of its misguided obsession with communism. With Watergate, there was a major corruption scandal by a sitting president hoping to thwart his opponent. These events made journalists more aware of their duties to inform the public of current events.

Reporters reverted to exposing political secrets. Woodward and Bernstein became stars after Watergate. Other reporters yearned for that recognition. By the time Bill Clinton took office, 24/7 news networks and the World Wide Web gave reporters tools to spread indiscretions faster. The world became more connected just as journalists became more exploitative.

THAT DAMN HOOVER

For nearly 50 years, FBI director J. Edgar Hoover controlled politicians by using surveillance to gather dirt on people who threatened his power and using that information to blackmail anyone who got in his way. After gathering information about the sexual affairs of powerful people, Hoover pressured people into doing what he wanted, a feat that was only possible because the press hadn't reported these stories and many Americans were likely to decry sexual peccadilloes.[51]

One of Hoover's most egregious power abuses came after he convinced Attorney General Robert Kennedy to begin surveillance on Martin Luther King Jr.

One of King's closest advisors, Stanley Levison, was one of the top financiers of the Communist Party USA in the 1950s. With communist paranoia looming large at the time, Hoover convinced RFK that communist ties made MLK a potential threat to national security.[52] Hoover was also driven to destroy King because King criticized the FBI's failure to uphold civil rights laws in the South, which led Hoover to call King "the most notorious liar in the country" at a 1964 news conference.[53]

Using surveillance, Hoover learned that the preacher and civil rights crusader was having extra-marital sex. FBI agents Hoover sent to spy on King recorded King saying things such as, "I'm fucking for God!" and "I'm not a negro tonight!" King's reply to a friend who told him to refrain from adulterous sex was, "I'm away from home twenty-five to twenty-seven days a month. Fucking is a form of anxiety reduction."[54] (Regarding MLK's affairs, President Lyndon Johnson said, "Goddammit, if you could only hear what that hypocritical preacher does sexually.")[55] Using the affair as leverage, Hoover sent King a threatening letter, which included the following:

> You are no clergyman and you know it. I repeat
> you are a colossal fraud and an evil, vicious one
> at that... Your "honorary" degrees, your Nobel
> Prize (what a grim farce) and other awards will
> not save you. King, I repeat you are done...
> There is but one way out for you. You better take

it before your filthy, abnormal fraudulent self is bared to the nation.[56]

While Hoover was accustomed to threatening people with exposure of their sexual secrets, the biggest secret may the one Hoover kept to himself. Though it hasn't been definitively proven, a lot of evidence suggests Hoover was a closeted homosexual who had a gay relationship with FBI Associate Director Clyde Tolson. After meeting Tolson, he instantly gave him a job, and within a few years Tolson vaulted to the top of the Bureau. The two were lifelong bachelors during an age when the vast majority of men were married by their mid-twenties. They went on vacations together. Tolson inherited Hoover's estate. And he resigned from the FBI after Hoover's death and remained a recluse for the rest of his life.[57] The circumstances surrounding Hoover and Tolson's relationship suggest that the two were lovers. Or that, coincidentally, the Bureau's top positions happened to be simultaneously held by men interested in each other and disinterested in dating women.

Slick Willie

During Clinton's presidency, the economy boomed. Crime rates dropped,[58] as did unemployment.[59] Although there were conflicts, the '90s were relatively peaceful for America's armed forces. But all of those accomplishments received much less attention than Bill Clinton's most noted act in office. Nothing got people talking like Monica Lewinsky's blow jobs.

Lewinsky, then twenty-two, was a recent college graduate interning at the White House. During her time at the White House, she began a sexual relationship with President Clinton that lasted from 1995 to 1997.[60] For more than a year after the scandal broke in 1998, Clinton's relationship with Lewinsky remained the top story on cable news networks. When a grand jury asked why Clinton told his aides, with respect to Lewinsky, "[T]here's nothing going on between us," Clinton said he hadn't lied and responded, "It depends on what the meaning of the word 'is' is."[61] He eventually admitted that Lewinsky had performed oral sex on him, but his confession took many months and resulted in jury testimonies and his impeachment by the House of Representatives. Although he was saved by an acquittal from the Senate, Lewinsky's blow jobs nearly cost Clinton his job. Despite leading a booming economy and having a solid approval rating, Clinton's biggest career stain wasn't a failed policy or an unpopular war. It was what he puddled on Lewinsky's blue dress, and his ensuing denial.

Clinton lived in a much different era than JFK or FDR. In exposing the president, Matt Drudge, the man who broke the Lewinsky story, wasn't acting in a manner atypical for members of the media at the time. Any journalist would have loved to get that tip. Running that story didn't make Drudge a villain—it made him a major media figure. In the past, photographers who revealed FDR's disability got their cameras broken. Now, reporters that break stories on presidential affairs become celebrities.

All of these changes in the media worsened the public's perception of Clinton's affairs, which in turn worsened many people's perception of his presidency. In an earlier era, his affair with Lewinsky would have been kept quiet. But because it happened in the 1990s, it defined much of his legacy. Having to fight impeachment and battle years' worth of public scrutiny took much of Clinton's time and energy throughout his second term in office. This wasn't without consequence, according to authors of *One Nation under Sex*:

> The same month Clinton was impeached, he received a classified report, dated December 4, 1998, titled "Bin Laden preparing to Hijack U.S. Aircraft and Other Attacks." While the Lewinsky affair consumed America in the winter of 1998, Osama Bin Laden approved the attacks that would kill 3,000 people on September 11, 2001.
>
> For decades to come, historians will ask whether the Monica Lewinsky scandal made 9/11 possible. The scandal certainly was a major distraction to the president. [...] Ultimately, we ordinary Americans are to blame for allowing our leaders and ourselves to become diverted by a sexual sideshow rather than focusing on the mounting threat to American lives.[62]*

---

* Lewis Merletti, head of the Secret Service, said, "What they should have been investigating was terrorism. Chasing down Monica Lewinsky. A lot of good that did for us."

Bill Clinton had other affairs that were reported on, and it's certainly possible he's had sexual indiscretions that were hidden from the public view that were not as consensual as his encounters with Lewinsky. But it's his affair with Lewinsky in particular that became one of the biggest stories of the decade. Now that Clinton is out of office and convenient to shun, many liberals have recently paraded a faux moral authority by accosting him for Lewinsky twenty years after the fact even though they stood by Clinton at the time of the scandal. The most sanctimonious commentators use Lewinsky as a historical revisionist device to advance their own agenda at a time when serious sexual assault charges are being levied against many powerful men, including several Republican politicians. There are power dynamics at play whenever a president has adulterous sex, but few of the people claiming to be sympathetic to the suffering of Lewinsky— who was taken advantage of by politicians on both sides of the aisle, the press, Linda Tripp, and others—consider Lewinsky's own personal agency, which makes their calls for action seem like mere political opportunism. About twenty years after the scandal first surfaced, Lewinsky wrote: "Sure, my boss took advantage of me, but I will always remain firm on this point: it was a consensual relationship. Any 'abuse' came in the aftermath, when I was made a scapegoat in order to protect his powerful position."[63]

Clinton's affairs weren't the first of their kind. They were merely a new addition to an American tradition. Prior to 1776 and on through today, American politicians have had countless sexcapades at various levels of government and in all regions of the country. But the American public still reacts in fury, as if each successive political sex affair were a novel event.

A Farewell Address

Based on what they see on the news each night, people might believe crime is on the rise, war and disease are more prominent than ever, politicians are having more affairs, and the world is simply going to hell in a handbasket. But carefully examining data and reality rather than media-driven perception will lead people to realize that it is the media coverage of these events, not the events themselves, that has changed. That's why people must look beyond the news to get their facts, and examine changes in reporting and shifting mores so they can better evaluate the information they're presented.

It is difficult to trace direct links between the sex lives of politicians and economic outcomes, international relations, military success, or any other important field, but politicians' affairs do matter because of the reactions they provoke in constituents and political enemies. And the best way to limit the influence of sex scandals is for the public to quit obsessing over them—as long as there's consent, that is. This might seem hypocritical, given that this chapter is about presidents' sex lives. But hear this out.

This chapter is devoted to showing how human psychology shows us that it's not unlikely for our elected officials to indulge in sexual escapades, and how the media's behavior, and not the politicians' actual sexual behavior, dictates public perception. It's worth studying, rather than sensationalizing, politician sex affairs, because analytically thinking them through shows that sexual affairs aren't aberrations of political systems. In many cases, they are characteristic of the type of person that reaches the highest political levels. It matters how the public perceives political sex scandals because these regularly occurring peccadillos have immense power to distract the public from important domestic and international issues that actually affect people's lives. Obsessing over what presidents do in the bedroom only diverts our attention, adding politician sex to sports, celeb news, and reality TV as topics that distract people from social policies. But the difference between things such as reality TV and politician sex is that fluffy reality shows don't get confused with the effectiveness of political policy, or invade "hard news" programs and politics-based websites. Unfortunately, because of our preoccupation with our leaders' sex lives, when people want to become more educated on the policies and organizations that will shape the structure of American institutions, the channels they turn to are becoming infested with gossipy personal details that in reality are divorced from the impact of political proceedings.

When the next political affair inevitably occurs, it will get a ton of attention. Pundits will act surprised. Subscribers of *Us Weekly* might pay attention to "hard news" for the first time in months, "shocked" by what said politician did. Callers to radio shows will express outrage. And the cycle will never end, as a new scandal will likely surface shortly thereafter.

The responsibility for the continuation of this cycle must fall on the public, because media is a business (and one that is currently struggling). Media outlets are going to promote what gets them viewers, and thus money. Affairs take so much airtime because they bring good ratings. The influence of these affairs will only be curbed once Americans stop relentlessly seeking mere gossip. If people want a better media, they need to practice better viewing habits.

Politicians aren't people to get a beer with, and their personal lives should not cross over into the public's perception of their effectiveness. Although they kiss babies and make fancy speeches, the men and women who lead our country are often narcissistic risk seekers. They are leaders who get things done by influencing people and decisions. Once society quits obsessing over their *consensual* sexual transgressions and begins looking at their actual effectiveness in office, there might be progress toward a better-informed public who elects more effective leaders. The only thing perplexing about a powerful person using their traits and resources to obtain sex is that people are surprised whenever it happens.

=3=

tragedy of the condoms

WHY WESTERN BIOMEDICAL APPROACHES HAVE FAILED TO STOP AIDS EPIDEMICS IN AFRICA

When a reporter pointed out that the Catholic Church's stance against condoms is "often considered unrealistic and ineffective" in the fight against AIDS, Pope Benedict XVI responded, "If there is no human dimension, if Africans do not help [reduce HIV transmission through responsible behavior], the problem cannot be overcome by the distribution of prophylactics: on the contrary, they increase it."[1] As usual, the media was outraged by the pope's conservative stance. The *New York Times* said the pope "deserves no credence when he distorts scientific findings about the value of condoms in slowing the spread of the AIDS virus."[2] The *Guardian's* headline read, "Pope's anti-condom message is sabotage in fight against AIDS."[3] Many people questioned how, in this day and age, the pope could discourage condom usage in good conscience. With AIDS spreading in Africa, it is absolutely crazy to criticize condoms as a defense against the virus, they reasoned. But what's even crazier is that the pope was right.

Uganda's Homegrown Solution to HIV

Edward Green is an anthropologist who has worked on a plethora of AIDS projects, from leading Harvard's AIDS Prevention Research Project to serving on the Presidential Advisory Council on HIV/AIDS. Green is also a self-described radical leftist and agnostic, *and* the one who pointed out that the pope was right about the ineffectiveness of condoms in Africa and that we need to rethink our approach to AIDS prevention on that continent.[4]

To back up the pope's reasoning, Green points out that from 1991 to 2004, Uganda cut its HIV prevalence by about two-thirds, from 15 percent of all adults to 5 percent of all adults, in the most successful campaign ever waged against AIDS in Africa—a campaign that didn't, in fact, focus primarily on condom use.[5] Under President Yoweri Museveni, Uganda began a social awareness campaign in the mid-1980s that was gradually phased out in the 1990s as outside donor money came in. Instead of focusing on condoms, which is what so many other AIDS prevention campaigns have done, Uganda's fight against AIDS emphasized the importance of limiting sexual partners. From 1989 to 1995, the number of Ugandan women reporting having had casual sex (sex outside a committed relationship) in the past year dropped from 16 percent to 6 percent, while the percentage of men having casual sex declined from 35 percent to 15 percent.[6] Instances of premarital sex declined as well. In people aged fifteen to twenty-four, reported premarital sex for females declined from 53 percent to 16 percent, and for males it declined from 60 percent to 23 percent.[7]

The success Uganda had in reducing HIV rates led the United States Agency for International Development (USAID) to eventually adopt an "ABC" model to combat AIDS, where "A = abstinence or delay of sexual activity; B = be faithful (including partner reduction and avoiding high-risk partners); C = condom use, particularly for high risk sex."[8] According to Sam Okware, the former director of Uganda's national AIDS Control Program, getting people to restrict their sex activity was accomplished by driving "fear into the people" by emphasizing to them "Practice ABC or D," with "D" meaning death.[9] AIDS groups were able to spread the theme "Beware of AIDS. AIDS Kills," by displaying posters and billboards throughout Uganda that featured images of skulls, coffins, and grim reapers. Other posters emphasized fidelity, promoting themes such as "Zero Grazing" and "Love Faithfully."[10] A poster popular in this campaign featured a man driving a truck through town while ignoring women who were running after him, trying to get his attention. The ad suggested that the best way to fight AIDS was for people to reduce their number of sexual partners and stay faithful. It read, "Thank God I Said NO to AIDS… I Am Driving Straight Home to My Wife."[11]

Ads found throughout the rest of Africa, where many countries were witnessing increases in their HIV rates, sent quite different messages, implying that condoms were the ideal way to fight the virus. "The fight against AIDS has become like a battle against lung cancer in which resources were devoted mainly to chemotherapy and surgery while little useful was done to curb smoking," write Daniel Halperin (former senior HIV prevention and behavior change advisor for USAID) and Craig Timberg (former Johannesburg bureau chief for the *Washington Post*) in their book *Tinderbox: How the West Sparked the AIDS Epidemic and How the World Can Finally Overcome It.* "The result is ever more infections, and ever larger demands for expensive treatment dependent on the continued largesse of foreign donors."[12] The foreign-donor priorities Halperin and Timberg refer to are displayed in materials such as a comic book funded by the Ford Foundation that chronicled crime fighters "Captain Condom" and "Lady Latex" and their "War with the Army of Sex Diseases," where they battled foes like "Sergeant Syphilis" and "Admiral AIDS."[13]*

According to a study tracking Uganda's AIDS-fighting

---

*   The most interesting part of this educational comic is when an illustrated man, Reggie, is about to have sex with his girlfriend. Reggie exclaims, "Yeah, this freak body is ripe!" As they begin caressing, his girlfriend replies, "Ooh! This honey is hot!" Then Lady Latex pops in and tells the woman to use a condom because Reggie has a dirty dick. Reggie replies, "Are you people cock-blockers or something? GET OUT OF HERE!" His girlfriend, realizing Reggie lied about having syphilis, storms out of the room. Reggie, now by himself with his right arm lodged inside his waistband, says, "Damn! My thing was ready to roll and now she's rolling out! Guess I better take their advice and pay that clinic a visit!"

strategies, "There were somber radio messages accompanied by the slow beating of a drum and a stern, raspy voice of an old man talking about AIDS in the manner of announcing funerals." A support group for people with HIV started sending people infected with AIDS to local communities and schools so healthy Ugandans could personally witness what it's like to live with the disease. One Ugandan AIDS educator told researchers: "When you see [people infected with AIDS] looking sick and emaciated, this seems to scare people into behavior change." When later asked in surveys why they changed their sexual behavior, the most common responses among Ugandans included "fear of AIDS." One Ugandan man's response read, "Look at me. I'm a living example. I went to visit [a support group for HIV victims] as a young man and I saw all those sick and emaciated and dying people. I decided to abstain, and I did this until I was married."[14] Many researchers have credited these grassroots campaigns as the catalyst that drove Ugandans to take fewer sexual risks (such as lowering their number of sexual partners), which in turn led to reductions in HIV rates.[15] While the amount of ongoing and casual sexual partners people have is a major determinant in how HIV spreads, it's worth examining the role of several other factors alleged to reduce HIV.

Condoms' Role

While the Ugandan government was fighting AIDS with behavior change messages, condom use increased as well. When surveys were taken in 1989, condoms hadn't yet been introduced to most places in Uganda, and only about 1 percent of adults reported *ever* having used a condom. By 1995, the amount of people to *ever* use a condom increased to 6 percent of women and 16 percent of men.[16] Condoms likely helped reduce HIV transmission for certain populations, particularly for people having sex outside of a committed relationship.[17]* However, condoms were being used by less than a sixth of the adult Ugandan population, which isn't a large enough percentage to explain the incredible drop in HIV rates.

In addition, the number of new HIV infections had already been declining in the late '80s and early '90s, before condoms were available in many places in Uganda.[18]† The lack of available condoms during Uganda's early success in lowering AIDS rates indicates that these astounding results weren't *primarily* achieved through condom distribution and promotion. Rather, a focus on fidelity and reducing sexual partners likely contributed heavily to the dramatic change. Mathematical models have also shown that Uganda's significant reduction in HIV was only possible through reductions in "sexual risk behaviour."[19]

Museveni emphasized his country's stance against relying

---

*   Condom use was virtually nonexistent in Uganda until AIDS-related groups began sending condoms to the country in the early 1990s. Condom use slowly caught on, and by 1995, among people who reported having casual sex in the last year, 20 percent of women and 36 percent of men reported using a condom the last time they had sex with a non-regular partner.

†   There is often at least a five-year time lag between changes in new HIV infections and overall changes in HIV prevalence in a population. Most of this comes from the lag between infection and mortality.

on condoms when he stated, "We are being told that only a thin piece of rubber stands between us and the death of our continent. I feel that condoms have a role to play as a means of protection, especially in couples who are HIV-positive, but they cannot become the main means of stemming the tide of AIDS."[20]

But Uganda's fight against AIDS through emphasis on fidelity and delaying sexual behavior began to unravel once Western advisers came along and waged war against AIDS in Africa using the same methods they had used in the U.S. throughout the 1980s and 1990s, which was to prevent HIV through increased condom usage and to fight infections with drug cocktails.[21]

The way HIV spreads in Africa is much different from how it spread in the U.S. In the U.S., and in most of the rest of the world, AIDS epidemics were usually heavily concentrated in specific communities—sex workers, gay men, and injecting drug users. In several African countries, AIDS is generalized throughout the continent, and much of the entire population is at high risk. In Africa, the disease spreads primarily through heterosexual sex, which is why the sexual and mating cultures of these nations must be examined when determining the most effective HIV prevention strategies.[22]

But rather than emphasizing behavior change built around the context of cultural mating habits, Western organizations have deferred to promoting condoms as a first line of defense against HIV. Which makes sense, given that many of these organizations (e.g., Population Services International, Marie Stopes International, the United Nations Population Fund (UNFPA)) were created during the 1960s and 1970s, when *The Population Bomb* sold millions of copies to people who feared that a "population explosion" could bring the end of the world as we know it.[23] The Joint United Nations Programme on HIV/ AIDS (UNAIDS) shows its population-control influence when it claims condoms are an extremely important tool in preventing HIV because "Condoms have helped to reduce HIV transmission and curtailed the broader spread of HIV in settings where the epidemic is concentrated in specific populations."[24] UNAIDS's claim that condoms prevent HIV from spreading to broader populations is echoed on the website for the President's Emergency Plan for AIDS Relief (PEPFAR), which says that condoms "can prevent concentrated epidemics from maturing into generalized epidemics."[25]

Although the theory that condoms help prevent concentrated epidemics from escalating into generalized epidemics makes intuitive sense, there is little evidence that condoms are needed to prevent the spread of HIV from one risk group to another group, because different subtypes of the virus tend to circulate in different risk groups.[26] For example, in South Africa in the 1990s, subtype B was most common among homosexuals, and subtype C was most common among heterosexuals, which indicates that HIV was primarily transmitted *within* each group of people, and that transmission *between* groups was rare.[27] If transmission between subgroups remains rare, then stirring up fear of a concentrated epidemic easily spreading to the population at large is alarmist. But even if we overlook these subtype squabbles and take at face value UNAIDS's and PEPFAR's claims that condoms are preventing HIV from spreading across risk groups, the major point that the strategies of these groups fail to address is that in generalized epidemics, in which HIV affects large percentages of the general population, condoms have been ineffective at lowering infection rates.[28]

The people working for the government agencies to fight AIDS are intelligent, and surely most of them have genuine intentions when they promote condoms. But with the amount of money flowing through the AIDS industry, there's little incentive for many groups to stray from biomedical approaches. The system in which Westerners supply condoms and drugs for Africans to rely and depend on has shown to be problematic in Uganda, where the "Love Faithfully" and "Zero Grazing" campaigns were shelved in favor of biomedical interventions once outside donors gained influence.[29] From 2004 to 2011, during which time the U.S. spent $1.7 billion[30] in Uganda to combat AIDS, HIV prevalence in Uganda increased about 14 percent[31], and the number of *new* infections increased between 10 and 60 percent, depending on which metric you look at.[32]* But condom use remained pretty

---

*   New infections are much harder to measure than prevalence in the population. All estimates show an increase in new HIV infections in Uganda from 2004 to 2011, but the magnitude of the increase varies per report. From a pure rate standpoint, UNAIDS estimates that Uganda's HIV incidence (new infections) rate increased by about 30.5 percent from 2004 to 2011. If you look at the increase from a numbers standpoint, and not on a per-rate basis, the highest estimate comes from a 2015 UNAIDS report, which claims that new infections hovered around 100,000 in 2004 and shot past 160,000 by 2011. Although new infections

stable throughout that time frame.[33] Because the proportion of sex that was protected by condoms stayed consistent, and condoms are supposed to prevent HIV transmission, what brought on the new infections?

Part of the increase in prevalence may come from the fact that as access to antiretroviral drugs has increased, people infected with HIV live longer. However, several researchers have provided other reasons as to why AIDS declines reversed themselves in Uganda. As HIV rates ticked up again in Uganda, researchers noted "recent increases in some HIV-related risk behaviors" and concluded "prevention efforts should be reinvigorated to address this, otherwise the past success in the HIV fight will be reversed."[34]* Although Uganda's population witnessed reductions in risky sexual behavior throughout the 1990s—by 1995, only 10 percent of men and 1 percent of women reported having multiple sex partners—this trend began to reverse itself in the 2000s. By 2000, the number of people having

have declined since 2011 (more recent UNAIDS reports estimate Uganda had roughly 140,000 new infections in 2013 and 2014) UNAIDS optimistically projects that new infections in Uganda will fall back to 100,000 by 2020.

*   Epstein believes the end of the Lord's Resistance Army insurgency in northern Uganda contributed to increased sexual networking and HIV transmission in the 2000s. She writes, "It is likely that war, rather than exacerbating the spread of HIV, can break up the sexual networks that sustain the spread of the virus. HIV infection rates tend to be higher in peaceful, prosperous countries such as Botswana and South Africa, and lower in such war-torn countries as the Congo and Somalia. The HIV rate soared in Mozambique when the civil war ended there in 1992, and the HIV rate fell in the Democratic Republic of Congo during the civil war between 1997 and 2003."

two or more sexual partners in the past year rose to 2 percent of women and 24 percent of men. In 2004, these figures increased again, to 4 percent of women and 29 percent of men.[35] While risky sex practices didn't change much from 2004 to 2011 (and in some cases declined *slightly*),[36] it's important to remember there's roughly a five-year lag between changes in behavior (and new infections) and changes in the overall HIV prevalence in the population.[37] It's possible the increases in risky sex seen around 2004 have contributed to the increased HIV rates seen in more recent years.

Some researchers have attributed these increases in risky behavior to Uganda changing its AIDS-fighting strategies to rely more on promoting HIV testing and condoms than on encouraging a reduction of ongoing sexual partners. In 2012, Ugandans told researchers that three-fourths of the "primary messages" they heard regarding HIV prevention involved condoms or getting tested for HIV. Only 15 percent of these messages involved the promotion of fidelity or delaying sexual contact. More than 60 percent of survey respondents said getting tested or using condoms was their highest priority in avoiding AIDS, while only 25 percent reported sticking to one sexual partner as a main priority.[38] Condom promotion has worked elsewhere in the world, where AIDS was mostly concentrated within specific subgroups. And condoms were effective in Africa as a *backup* solution for those who insisted on straying. However, as a first line of defense, condoms have been unsuccessful in Africa's generalized epidemics.

Aside from condoms, another factor many people advocate will reduce AIDS is education. But is education actually effective in altering HIV transmission in Africa?

The Education Effect

Some AIDS activists and commentators believe AIDS is a disease of poverty, and that the best way to fight AIDS in to increase education in poverty-stricken areas.[39] Intuitively, that sounds very logical, progressive, and humane. However, the effect of education on AIDS prevention isn't straightforward.

Reducing educational inequality and poverty is a worthwhile goal in its own right, but several of the most well-to-do countries in Africa (such as South Africa and Botswana) have higher HIV rates than the poorest nations on the continent. And even within the population of several individual countries, citizens with more wealth can be found to be more often infected with HIV than the poorer members of their communities.[40]* It's possible that providing more work skills

---

*   In the beginning of Africa's epidemic, wealthier and more educated people tended to have a greater likelihood of being HIV positive. Researchers reasoned that the wealthiest people, particularly wealthy men, could afford to support more concurrent sexual partners, which increased their chances of getting infected. But more recently, several African countries have been showing that people with secondary education are less likely to have HIV than people with only primary education. However, people with no education still report the lowest rates, which confounds a clear relationship between HIV and education. It may be that those with no education have the lowest HIV rates because uneducated people tend to live in

training and formal education opportunities in the sub-Saharan region could give migrant workers a better chance of employment outside the South African mines, which are notorious for having high rates of HIV transmission because miners hire sex workers and pursue concurrent relationships while stationed away from their families. [41] But as of now, it's somewhat theoretical that education will bring workers out of the mines, or that reducing the HIV rate among migrant workers and their partners will have a significant impact on generalized epidemics. So far, increasing education attainment for its own sake typically appears ineffective in reducing HIV transmission. However, *sex* education might prove to be beneficial in the fight against AIDS.

Sex education could potentially lower risky sex behaviors by better informing people of the risks they are taking. In some countries there is a lot of room for improvement in this area. In South Africa, about one-fourth of adults believe that they will likely contract HIV. But only about 4 percent of respondents reported they believed they would get HIV from having multiple sexual partners. A much larger proportion of respondents, about one-third, did *not* believe that having fewer sexual partners could

---

rural areas, which are much less stricken by HIV than cities. A clear relationship between HIV and education is further muddled because there remain other national surveys that continue to show HIV increases with each additional level of education. Education and wealth aren't exactly synonymous, but they often go together. When taken together, the relationship between HIV rates and wealth and education is pretty unclear, and tends to conflict with assumed sociological theory.

reduce their HIV risk, even though multiple concurrent partnerships accounted for an estimated three-fourths of new HIV infections in South Africa in the 1990s.[42] And it has been projected that if all concurrent partnerships had ended in 2010, South Africa would see a 39 percent reduction in its number of new HIV infections by 2020.[43]

Case studies show that some sex education intervention programs contribute to delayed sexual behavior, declines in unwanted pregnancy, and less risky sexual behavior in general.[44]* In Africa, sex education programs could potentially affect HIV transmission rates by informing people of the risks of having multiple overlapping sexual partners and by promoting condoms to those who absolutely insist on

---

* The effects of sex education aren't quite as crystal clear as sex education proponents claim. In a meta-analysis of 83 studies, Douglas Kirby and colleagues claimed that "[sex education] programs were effective across a wide variety of countries, cultures, and groups of youth." However, they found that most sex education programs did not have an impact in reducing biological indicators such as STD transmission or teen pregnancy. They also used an intervention program from Tanzania as evidence that sex ed programs can reduce risky sex for more than three years. However, in the Tanzania program they prop up, females in the intervention group ended up having *more* gonorrhea and chlamydia than those in the control group. For many years, Kirby was one of the world's biggest proponents of sex education and his research was used to justify these programs' effectiveness. However, many of his papers were published while he was employed by ETR Associates, a nonprofit dedicated to promoting sexual education and science-based health programs, which—although Kirby never hid this in any way and always disclosed it in his papers—could nonetheless be viewed as a subtle conflict of interest.

having multiple concurrent partners. To promote the "ABC" model isn't to be anti-condom. It just means placing emphasis on "A" and "B" instead of automatically deferring to "C." In Africa, sex ed's greatest potential in fighting AIDS lies in informing people about the dangers of "sexual webs."

Sex in Webs

In many African cultures, people have more overlapping sexual partners than Westerners do. Instead of going from a relationship with one person to a relationship with another person, which is called serial monogamy and is how most Westerners date, Africans tend to maintain relationships with several partners *at the same time*.[45] Having multiple partners creates a sexual web within communities that exponentially increases how quickly viruses are spread.

In the mid-1990s, virologist Christopher Hudson, statistician-sociologist Martina Morris, and epidemiologist Mirjam Kretzschmar concluded that in terms of disease transmission, having multiple concurrent partners is more problematic than having multiple partners spread over time, because HIV is most transmissible in its early stages and there is more virus in the system near the time of infection. The amount of virus later declines after antibodies are developed in the body, but then skyrockets years later when the victim develops AIDS.[46]

As an article in the *Lancet* puts it, "Therefore, as soon as one person in a network of concurrent relationships contracts HIV, everyone else in the network is placed at risk. By contrast, serial monogamy traps the virus within a single relationship for months or years."[47] A person who has several ongoing partners at the time of infection simply has the potential to spread the virus much more quickly than someone with only one sexual partner at a time (even if a serially monogamous person jumps from relationship to relationship).

This theory led Helen Epstein, journalist and author of *The Invisible Cure: Why We Are Losing the Fight Against AIDS in Africa*, to conclude that although the convention of monogamous romantic love is "responsible for many Western ills, including divorce and the neurotic pursuit, through painful serial relationships, of an ideal conjugal love that may not exist," it might have "helped spare the West a heterosexual AIDS epidemic on the scale of Africa's."[48] Another problem that sexual concurrency exacerbates is there are few to no symptoms in the early stages of HIV infection. People rarely feel sick when they are at their most infectious stage, and they can even test HIV-negative during this time, compounding the problem further. So when the virus is at its more transmissible levels, people with multiple ongoing partners may be giving HIV to several people without even realizing they have it.[49]

There's lots of research that indicates concurrency is a major determinant of Africa's HIV rates.[50]* Edward Green writes, "It's those ongoing relationships that drive Africa's

* While Africans tend to have more concurrent partners than Westerners, they do not have more lifetime sexual partners, and some studies show Africans have fewer lifetime partners than people in the West. The notion that Africans are hypersexualized is not backed by data.

worst epidemics."[51] But concurrency isn't the only cultural variable influencing HIV transmission in Africa. Let's examine two other factors that contribute to these epidemics.

Intergenerational Sex and Circumcision

After concurrent partnerships, Green believes male circumcision is the most important factor influencing Africa's HIV rates. He created a formula, $E = MC2$, where E = epidemic and MC = multiple concurrent (partners) and (lack of) male circumcision.[52] The formula indicates that a change in concurrency or circumcision will drastically alter an epidemic. Or as Halperin and Timberg write:

> In places where AIDS was fundamentally a disease contracted and spread through heterosexual relationships, both relatively high rates of multiple sex partners and low rates of circumcision needed to exist for a major, sustained epidemic to take hold. Take away either element of the tinderbox and the spread of HIV would slow. Take away both, and the flame of the epidemic would falter and eventually fizzle out.[53]

Green, Halperin, and Timberg are no longer on the fringe with their theories. The World Health Organization (WHO) recommends circumcision, claiming it can reduce HIV risk by about 60 percent.[54] And unlike treatment drugs, circumcision is quite cheap, estimated to cost about $40 per person.[55] But what makes circumcision so effective?

The foreskin of an uncut penis is much softer and thinner than the skin on the penis shaft, which makes the foreskin more prone to tearing during sex. When the foreskin tears, it can let the virus into the man's bloodstream, and it also can endanger the man's partner if man's exposed blood contains the virus. There's also a moist environment under the foreskin that allows viruses to survive longer.[56] One study even found that a larger foreskin area makes men more susceptible to HIV transmission.[57]

Another cultural factor that has helped keep HIV rates stubbornly higher in several African countries is intergenerational sex.[58]* Intergenerational sex allows the virus to transfer to new age cohorts. This phenomenon usually occurs when middle-aged "sugar daddies" in Africa financially support teenage girls in exchange for sex. If old men and young women refrained from having sex with each other and instead stuck to sex within their own age cohort, it's possible the epidemic would eventually nearly collapse as the infected older cohort died off. "Sugar daddies" transfer the epidemic to younger generations and allow it to continue.[59] Some countries, such as Botswana, have begun implementing "sugar daddy classes" in secondary schools to warn young women about the risks

---

* Untreated STDs are another sexual factor that's theorized to influence HIV rates. Untreated STDs increase the viral load in blood, semen, and vaginal fluids. A higher viral load means there is more HIV in a person's system, making it easier to transmit. While it makes sense in theory that untreated STDs could be a major factor influencing HIV transmission, most studies show that STD treatment doesn't have a significant effect in reducing HIV infections.

of having sex with older men, who tend to have *much* higher HIV rates than young men.[60]

Taken together, the factors discussed so far in this chapter show that what has worked best in lowering HIV rates in Africa—as seen in Uganda, Kenya, Zimbabwe, and in urban areas of Ethiopia, Rwanda, Malawi, Zambia, Burkina Faso, and Ivory Coast—is breaking up sexual networks through the promotion of fidelity and reduction of sexual partners. Practicing circumcision, delaying sexual activity, reducing intergenerational sex, and implementing sex education programs also hold potential and have contributed to reducing HIV transmission.[61] But promoting these behavioral factors over biomedical products can be political suicide.

Although no other African country has had as much success at reducing HIV rates as Uganda, HIV prevalence in Zimbabwe dropped from 29 percent in 1997 to 16 percent in 2007.[62] A group of researchers led by Halperin concluded that a reduction of sexual partners was likely the main contributor to Zimbabwe's success.[63] Regarding Zimbabwe's success in battling HIV, U.S. Global AIDS coordinator Mark Dybul stated, "Perhaps one of the most interesting things is that the greatest behavior change was in abstinence and fidelity. The relative change in condom use was not as remarkable."[64]

A day after Hilary Clinton became secretary of state in 2009, Dybul was fired, and critics came out of the woodwork accusing him of derailing AIDS efforts for being an advocate of the "religious right"—an interesting accusation to make against an openly gay doctor who treated AIDS patients in San Francisco before his political appointment.[65] Perhaps

Dybul could have kept his job had he more closely followed the script that researcher-consultants, AIDS donors, condom makers, and pharma companies provided him.

Script Writing

Large international organizations such as UNAIDS have relied on emotional stories and subtly deceptive tactics to nudge donors to support their cause. Through implanting misleading story lines and overestimating infection rates, they implied that AIDS would expand to general populations throughout the world because scores of helpless people were being sexually victimized. Despite all the money that trickled in, in many cases the only people who benefitted from these assertions were the people reporting the stories.

Elizabeth Pisani provides an interesting perspective on the politics behind these types of misleading AIDS narratives. She worked as a journalist for places such as *Reuters* and the *Economist* before becoming a consultant and epidemiologist who helped craft reports for powerful research groups such as UNAIDS and the Centers for Disease Control and Prevention (CDC). Some of these reports were written to intentionally mislead the public and the press in hopes of gaining funding for AIDS research. In her book *The Wisdom of Whores: Bureaucrats, Brothels, and the Business of AIDS,* Pisani provides several examples of how public perception of AIDS can be manipulated by those within powerful organizations. Here's an example from a UNAIDS report she helped put together that promotes the "innocent wives" narrative, implying that the virus spreads because helpless women are forced into sex by their promiscuous husbands: "The virus is firmly embedded in the general population, among women whose only risk behaviour is having sex with their own husbands."[66]

This broad generalization came from *one* small study examining women with STDs. Because the sample was made up of women with STDs attending STD clinics, there is a greater chance their husbands had visited prostitutes or been otherwise unfaithful, bringing an STD into the marriage, and their experiences didn't necessarily represent the "general population." But Pisani and her colleagues intentionally wrote the report to imply that HIV was harming scores of defenseless faithful Indian wives, which caused the virus to spread throughout the population. As she puts it:

> We weren't making anything up. But once we got the numbers, we were certainly presenting them in their worst light. We did it consciously. I think all of us at that time thought the beat-ups were more than justified, they were necessary. We were pretty certain that neither donors nor governments would care about HIV unless we could show them that it threatened the "general population."[67]

Pisani talks about relying on the "innocent wives and babies" story lines to persuade countries into donating money to AIDS research. Her team constructed emotional stories while pushing statistical validity to the side. In one instance, they implied that millions of Indonesian men buying sex could eventually equate to millions of infected wives, while actual estimates showed only about 16,000 women were *potentially* at risk in the scenario, because the prostitute-seeking men would have to both have a wife *and* test HIV-positive.[68]* Even though commercial sex was a major determinant in how HIV spread *in Indonesia*, Pisani's report doesn't acknowledge that many of these johns had neither a wife nor HIV.

Despite the statistical evidence to the contrary, the "innocent wives" narrative is backed by powerful anecdotes of women being wronged by devious, AIDS-infected men, concluding that the only way to fight AIDS is a reliance on condoms. Stories of discriminated-against innocent victims elicit strong emotions and open checkbooks, which AIDS groups, marketing firms, condom producers, and pharma companies need to keep the ball rolling. Even though HIV isn't spread *primarily* through "innocent wives," and nor is it a "disease of poverty" that's best curbed with more outside resources, it's within the interests of AIDS groups to sell these stories of victimhood and helplessness. Regarding how

---

*   The "innocent wives" story line doesn't hold empirical weight in Africa either. Research shows that South African women infect their husbands, as a result of extramarital affairs, just about as often as their husbands infect them. In couples where one partner has HIV and the other doesn't, women are the infected partner in 62 percent of couples in Kenya and Ivory Coast. In nine other African countries, women make up at least a third of the infected partners in these scenarios.

the international AIDS relief community has functioned this past decade, Halperin and Timberg write:

> More alarm, and more politically appealing victims, meant more programs, more staff, more money. [...] If AIDS was not just a public health problem but also a substantial development issue, the World Bank and the United Nations Development Program had a claim to rival the WHO's original one. If its list of victims included children, so did UNICEF. Soon UNAIDS became like a snowball tumbling downhill.[69]

Relying on sympathetic victims was an effective fundraising tactic for organizations Pisani worked for. Another common strategy to keep money pouring in has been to overstate the global AIDS threat.[70†] Which is something UNAIDS has historically done.[71]

Selling Doom

Through the late 1990s and early 2000s, it became clear AIDS wouldn't rampage through most of the world's general populations as some researchers had feared. Even though

---

† The authors of *Freakonomics* write that "advocates working for the cures of various tragic diseases" often use "a little creative lying" because lying "can draw attention, indignation, and—perhaps most important—the money and political capital to address the actual problem."

population-based surveys showed HIV rates declining, UNAIDS continued to warn the media that the epidemic was getting worse worldwide.[72] James Chin, former chief of surveillance for WHO's Global Programme on AIDS, told a reporter, "It's pure advocacy really... They keep cranking out numbers, that, when I look at them, you can't defend them."[73]

In a 1996 *Science* article, executive director of UNAIDS Peter Piot vaguely implied that one in three adults in Africa *and* Asia (which together make up about three-fourths of the world's population) could have AIDS, when he wrote about "heavily affected countries in Africa and Asia, where one out of three urban adults may be infected."[74] Giving a keynote lecture at an AIDS conference in Manila one year later, Piot warned that, "HIV will cut through Asian populations like a hot knife through cold butter!"[75] For years, Piot continued to issue similar dire statements based on exaggerated statistics. At a 2004 lecture at the Woodrow Wilson Center in Washington, DC, Piot said, "The situation we face in China, India, and Russia bears alarming similarities to the situation we faced twenty years ago in Africa. The virus in these populous countries is perilously close to a tipping point. If it reaches that point, it could transition from a series of concentrated outbreaks and hot spots into a generalized explosion across the entire population— spreading like a wildfire from there."[76]* When Piot made those assertions, most of Africa didn't have infection rates as high as he implied. And *nowhere* in Asia had rates anywhere close to

---

*   In defending the overestimated projections UNAIDS put out during his tenure, Piot told Timberg, "My job was really to make sure AIDS was taken seriously."

what Piot suggested. Why did Piot make such claims?[77][†] It may be because, as noted in the summary of another *Science* article he authored, he advocated that one of the "key challenges" in fighting AIDS involved "increasing human capacity and global funding."[78][‡] As Piot issued dire warnings about HIV spreading through the general populations of the world's most populous countries, annual global AIDS spending increased from $292 million in 1996 to $1.6 billion in 2001.[79]

Eventually, around 2007, UNAIDS acknowledged that new HIV infections had actually been declining worldwide for nearly a decade. There were not 42 million people with HIV, and the number was not rising, which is what UNAIDS had previously suggested. In fact, 33 million people worldwide were HIV-positive, and the number of people infected appeared stable, the organization admitted.[80] By the time UNAIDS admitted its error, $10 billion was being spent annually to fight AIDS around the world.[81] Piot writes in his

---

†   Piot has always denied a political connection to the overestimation in UNAIDS numbers. He's noted that the data that informed these reports disproportionately relied on pregnant women, urbanites, and young people, which are demographics generally more sexually active than the general population. To his credit, survey data and analyses improved over time, which allowed for UNAIDS to later make more accurate measurements. However, it took UNAIDS many years to make these adjustments, even after independent surveys showed its numbers to be too high. In one instance, in Zambia, UNAIDS actually increased its projected HIV rates after a large-scale survey implied UNAIDS numbers were much too high.

‡   Halperin and Timberg wrote that UNAIDS reports have a "signature mix of alarm sprinkled with a few uplifting stories and a declaration that only massive new funding could prevent the epidemic from getting even worse."

memoir, "In those days there was simply zero tolerance among some for anything other than advocating for more money, and while non-AIDS interest groups claimed that AIDS got too much money, they lobbied hard to get their issue included in AIDS budgets—often with success."[82]

Several researchers believe that the global decline in HIV infections during the 2000s had very little to do with the prevention programs that organizations such as UNAIDS sponsored. As already discussed, in several countries people began limiting their sexual partners, which had the effect of lowering HIV infections. Outside of these countries where people reduced their partners, much of the decrease in HIV infections was likely just part of the natural cycle epidemics follow. Regarding the global drop in HIV infections, an article in the *Lancet* concludes, "Most important surely are purely epidemiological phenomena—those most susceptible become infected first (because of sexual behaviour and networks) and the susceptible pool shrinks. Moreover, at some point the chain reaction derived from the infectiousness of newly infected people subsides."[83]* A similar phenomenon occurred when HIV rates declined among gay men in the U.S. in the 1980s. Gabriel Rotello, journalist and author of *Sexual Ecology*, writes, "It is possible that what we witnessed when new infections dropped was not the triumph of prevention, but the tragedy of saturation." He

---

*   The article adds, "There has also been important behavioural change, notably in Uganda, Kenya, and Zimbabwe."

adds, "From a population-wide perspective, the sudden drop in new infections seems not the result of the success of prevention, but of its tragic failure."[84]

The findings in the *Lancet* and from Rotello mimic the trajectory of many disease epidemics, which often begin slowly before climbing to a rapid peak, which is followed by a gradual decline after those most susceptible to the epidemic become infected. James Chin, the former WHO epidemic tracker, has written that organizations such as UNAIDS claim credit for drops in AIDS epidemics that are actually just natural declines expected in the course of an epidemic. Chin writes that UNAIDS was "riding to glory on the down slope of the epidemic curve."[85]

Since UNAIDS began declaring that HIV rates are actually declining, its narrative has shifted. As seen in a 2005 UNAIDS report, the organization used to imply it needed more money or this ever-growing epidemic would expand through much of the world's populations. It implied that to defeat AIDS, UNAIDS needed much more money to fix these countries' domestic and developmental problems:

> Several of the epidemics in Asia and Oceania are increasing, particularly in China, Papua New Guinea, and Viet Nam. There are also alarming signs that other countries—including Pakistan and Indonesia—could be on the verge of serious epidemics. [...] Only a handful of countries are making serious-enough efforts to introduce programmes

focusing on these risky behaviours on the scale required. [...] Bringing AIDS under control will require tackling with greater resolve the underlying factors that fuel these epidemics—including societal inequalities and injustices. It will require overcoming the still serious barriers to access that take the form of stigma, discrimination, gender inequality and other human rights violations. It will also require overcoming the new injustices created by AIDS, such as the orphaning of generations of children and the stripping of human and institutional capacities. These are extraordinary challenges that demand extraordinary responses.[86]

But UNAIDS now claims the number of new HIV infections has dropped significantly worldwide. In sub-Saharan Africa, where the majority of the world's HIV infections occur, it estimates new infections dropped almost 40 percent between 2001 (2.6 million) to 2012 (1.6 million).[87]* UNAIDS has admitted that HIV rates were actually *decreasing* at the time it released grim forecasts like those seen in the 2005 report quoted above.[88] The organization now implies that new infections of HIV have declined, not because of the natural course of the epidemic, as the *Lancet* authors claimed, but because of the massive amounts of money UNAIDS has spent fighting HIV. And that with more money, UNAIDS

---

*   Sub-Saharan Africa still accounted for 72 percent of new HIV infections during this time.

can eradicate the virus.[89†] The 2012 UNAIDS World AIDS Day Report states:

> The national declines in HIV incidence in populations shows that sustained investments and increased political leadership for the AIDS response are paying dividends. In particular, countries with a concurrent scale-up of HIV prevention and treatment programmes are seeing a drop in new HIV infections to record lows. [...] The historic slowdown indicates HIV prevention and treatment programmes are successfully reaching the people in need.[90]

The report doesn't mention that the declines in HIV transmission in countries such as Kenya and Ethiopia started occurring prior to the last ten years when lots of outside money started coming their way.[91†] It also doesn't mention

---

[†] A 2014 UNAIDS report states, "With the dramatic increase in HIV resources over the past decade, the world is closing in on the target of mobilizing US $22–24 billion annually by 2015, although even more funding will be required to end the AIDS epidemic by 2030." The report later uses guilt tripping to expand the point: "The cost of inaction will be huge—if countries do not scale up HIV prevention and treatment services rapidly by 2020, but instead continue with the existing coverage levels of services, they will lose the opportunity to save 21 million lives, and an additional 28 million people would be living with HIV by 2030. Instead of averting these deaths and new infections, continuation of current coverage levels will mean that the world will have to pay an additional US $24 billion every year for antiretroviral therapy by 2030."

[‡] Edward Green and Allison Ruark write, "In Africa as a whole, HIV incidence peaked in the late 1990s, soon followed by a decline in prevalence. These rates came down before ARVs were widely available."

that the biggest AIDS success story after 2001 occurred in a country, Zimbabwe, that received relatively little money from donors compared with other sub-Saharan African countries.[92] It doesn't mention that one of the countries receiving the most funds, Uganda, was the biggest AIDS success story the world had ever seen *until* lots of outside money came in. And ever since donor money has seeped into Uganda, the country's HIV rates have crept back up.[93] It doesn't mention that partner reduction has had a major contribution *everywhere* HIV rates have declined, not just in Africa, but also in Asia and the United States.[94]* Finally, it doesn't mention that most of the money they're advocating for will likely end up in the hands of American organizations that will spend it to maintain bureaucratic structures and promote ineffective prevention methods.[95]

Money, Money, Money

As bureaucratic structures expanded, USAID and other large funders began giving money to some of their contractors based on their ability to meet easily quantifiable goals—such

---

*   The report does mention that sexual behavior became safer in several countries with generalized epidemics. But it spends only two paragraphs of the report's forty-three pages doing so and claims, "Although population-level behaviour change has been shown to reduce the prevalence of HIV infection in several countries with generalized epidemics, linking behaviour change programming to specific HIV outcomes remains challenging." It's fine to be skeptical, but the report glosses over the difficulty in linking increased biomedical commodities to HIV outcomes and that the amount of outside intervention hasn't correlated well with changes in HIV transmission rates.

as delivering a particular number of condoms, for instance—
rather than score bidders on their ability to reach harder-to-
measure benchmarks, such as reducing new HIV infections.[96]
This focus led to lots of money being spent on condoms and
HIV medications to fight AIDS in Africa and an insistence
from AIDS lobbyists that their biomedical commodities be
used in favor of the homegrown behavior change initiatives
found in several African countries. Uganda's partner reduction program cost just about twenty-five cents per person
per year.[97] Circumcising a man cost about forty bucks per
person.[98] Both methods were found to be effective in slowing
HIV transmission.[99] Yet, when I Ialperin worked for USAID,
one of his superiors told him, "Don't talk about circumcision
anymore. Don't talk about ABC." Another screamed at him,
"I don't want to hear another fucking thing about ABC. We
do condoms!"[100]

Halperin's superior noted what's become a bureaucratic truism—as AIDS relief ballooned to an industry worth more than $20 billion a year, many Western
donors have structured their AIDS prevention programs around condom distribution.[101†] United Nations
Population Fund (UNFPA) data shows that the largest
Western donors collectively spent about $255 million per
year on condoms and contraception in developing countries
from 2005 to 2013.[102‡] About 60 percent of these funds were

---

†   According to a 2012 UNAIDS report, the U.S. accounts for roughly half of
international AIDS donations.

‡   This included the UNFPA itself and USAID, but didn't include the World Bank

directed toward sub-Saharan Africa.[103] Although a lot of money gets spent on condoms, much more gets spent on drug treatments. It's estimated that, in 2011, 6 percent of global HIV program funding went toward condoms, while more than 75 percent of funding went toward drug-related categories (such as treatment and mother-to-child transmission). The categories of behavior change and male circumcision, which have shown to be most effective at limiting the spread of HIV in generalized epidemics, received only 4 percent of funding *combined.*[104]

America's global HIV funding is part of the President's Emergency Plan for AIDS Relief (PEPFAR). Though the exact percentages vary each fiscal year, in general about 20 percent of PEPFAR funding is supposed to go toward prevention (which would include condoms), while a much larger chunk, 55 percent, goes toward treatment (which would include HIV drugs).[105]* President George W. Bush certainly didn't help calm critics' suspicions that American AIDS relief efforts were more invested in protecting Big Pharma than in reducing African HIV rates when he appointed the former CEO of pharmaceutical firm Eli Lilly

---

and in several reports did not include the Global Fund.

*   There is a very strong case to be made that treatment drugs are greatly needed, victims have a right to these drugs, and the drugs drastically improve victims' quality of life. The issue isn't that money is being spent on products to improve people's lives. It's that large organizations spread dishonest messages that biomedical products are the main key to prevention of transmission, even though real-world evidence shows that behavior change and circumcision programs are cheaper and more effective.

and Company, Randall Tobias, as the first person to head up PEPFAR and organize the distribution of its massive budget.[106] For the past six years, the U.S. has spent about $6.5 billion a year to combat AIDS internationally.[107]

But tracking this spending is quite a challenge, because it involves piecing together many organizations and levels of bureaucracy, and because PEPFAR doesn't publicly release many of its contracts in timely fashion or in an accessible way. It is difficult to ascertain exactly how much the U.S. government spends on HIV prevention and treatment products such as condoms and antiretroviral medications, and who it is buying them from.

The Center for Global Development, an international development think tank, stated in a summary of one of its research reports, "While the U.S. government collects extensive information about how PEPFAR funding is used, only a small share of this data is publicly disclosed. Even PEPFAR staff are not able to access some of the collected data."[108] The annoyances involved in tracking PEPFAR spending were noted by one of the group's researchers, who wrote, "U.S. taxpayers have a right to access information on PEPFAR's funding flows in a machine-readable and open format, without resorting to the Freedom of Information Act (FOIA) for each datum of information (or resorting to hiring full-time research assistance)."[109]

It's not totally clear why PEPFAR's contracts with its "prime partners" are so difficult to filter through. It could just be that each layer of bureaucracy has added a transaction cost and information availability gets lost in

transition. Or it may be because as little as 8 percent of
PEPFAR money gets directly allocated to developing
country governments. The vast majority of the AIDS
relief money that the U.S. "donates" goes back to American
companies and organizations.[110]

Tied Aid

To persuade Americans to support spending money on
foreign aid, the State Department and USAID will funnel
much of their foreign funds through U.S. companies. "Buy
American" language is placed into appropriations bills, which
stipulate that goods must be bought in the donor country.
This practice is called "tied aid."[111]

For years, USAID refused to buy things such as
condoms from companies in developing countries, where
they would cost about two cents apiece, in favor of buying
them from American producers, who charged five cents
apiece. By 2009, Pisani estimated that Americans had spent
an additional $270 million to purchase their foreign-aid
condoms this way. Then, using taxpayer money, USAID
pays to ship those American-produced condoms around
the world. This transportation cost isn't included in the
$270 million bill. Neither is the enormous carbon footprint
left behind.[112]

The "Buy American" philosophy becomes particularly
costly with HIV medications. Instead of purchasing generic
brands that cost about $350 a year per patient, for years the
U.S. purchased HIV drugs from pharma companies such as

Pfizer, Merck, and Bristol-Myers Squibb, which ran up to $15,000 a year per person.[113]* In 1996, about 70 percent of U.S. aid was tied. As it became clear that tied aid increased the costs of development projects by 15–30 percent and the practice became unfavorable in the international community, the U.S. ceased reporting its tied-aid status until 2005. That was the year that the U.S. and many large Western aid donors committed to the Paris Declaration on Aid Effectiveness, an international agreement intended to reduce tied aid.[114] Subsequently, the amount of reported American aid that was tied fell from 68 percent in 2005 to 37 percent in 2014.[115] As the U.S. began spending more of its foreign aid money in other countries to honor the Paris Declaration on Aid Effectiveness and to save cash, companies such as Alabama-based Alatech Healthcare, which used to be the United States' sole supplier for international condom distribution, lost their government contracts to overseas competition.[116]

But just because the U.S. reduced its tied aid doesn't mean most of its foreign funding doesn't still get spent in-house. Tied aid *requires* that money be spent on U.S. products and services. If money is "untied," it can be spent

---

*   Many of the major drug companies eventually relented and began selling their drugs at significantly reduced costs to African countries and AIDS groups. But it took several years for this to happen, and the changes only came after great resistance. Drug companies today advertise their charity, but Bristol-Myers Squibb, GlaxoSmithKline, Roche, and Bayer sure as hell don't ever mention that they sued Nelson Mandela and South Africa in the late 1990s just a few years after apartheid ended, because Big Pharma was outraged that Mandela had the nerve to reduce drug prices for disease-stricken AIDS victims.

anywhere. Usually, it still stays in the United States. A 2011 report suggests as much as 90 percent of U.S. foreign aid was spent through U.S. companies and organizations.[117] In 2008, the top twenty-five recipients of PEPFAR funding received roughly $2.3 billion collectively. Twenty-two of these twenty-five recipients were American-based, twenty-one of which were on the East Coast.[118]

Several of the largest recipients are research universities or nonprofit groups with locations in multiple countries. It's not as if all the aid money that gets spent on American recipients gets directly turned into profitable commodities. However, much of this money goes to groups that directly and indirectly promote condoms as a reliable first measure of defense against HIV, which, as we have seen, is not necessarily the best strategy in some regions of the world.

Condom Sense

One of the reasons condoms continue to be upheld as an attractive option to fight HIV is because people are told that, as long as they use rubbers, they otherwise don't have to change their sexual habits to avoid disease. Condoms are advertised to provide the delights of sexual indulgence *and* the safety to avoid disease. Even in the face of deadly sexual disease, marketers proclaim the carnal joys condoms can facilitate.

At the World AIDS Conference in 1998, attendees were told by pharma companies and condom distributors where they could find "hardcore" bars and "backroom sex." Green states that he has seen pamphlets at AIDS conferences from drug companies that tell men where to go for anonymous gay sex. [119] At an AIDS prevention seminar in Botswana, Halperin saw a "teenage bikini beauty contest" featuring girls who appeared to be in middle school strut across the stage clothed in "strings and tiny patches of fabric" while drunk men in the crowd belted out rap lyrics such as "I want to fuck you, ho!" Halperin noted that the event's emcee told the crowd to "always use a Lovers Plus rubber!"—which is a condom brand USAID contractors sponsor. [120] It is difficult for African leaders to not follow along and promote the products that Western organizations push at them, because the money flowing from these Western donor initiatives can in some cases rival the hosting African country's GDP.

One of the world's biggest social-marketing organizations, PSI, is alleged to receive about $100 million a year, much of it from the U.S. government, to promote condoms in Africa. [121] In past years, they've put up billboards in places such as Botswana, which displayed a boxing glove and a condom next to the slogan "IT CAN TAKE THE FIERCEST PUNCHES." [122] Another ad PSI ran in Botswana in 2007 featured a smiling fourteen-year old girl with the caption, "I am going out with an older man who adds flavor to my life and one thing I do is have protected sex using Lovers Plus condoms everytime [sic]." [123] The ad glossed over the facts that intergenerational sex transfers viruses from generation to generation, that old men in Botswana are *much* more likely to have HIV than young men, that having sex with a girl under sixteen is a criminal offense in Botswana, *and* that when the ad ran Botswana had one of the highest HIV rates the world has ever seen.

Another infamous PSI campaign came about because the organization discovered that one reason Zambians weren't using condoms was because they trusted their partners. PSI developed a campaign to get people to mistrust their partners, pushing the idea that no one could know what their partners were really doing, so less trust and more condom use was the healthy route to go. The campaign was called the "Trusted Partner Campaign." By dismissing messages of partner reduction and faithfulness as tools to fight AIDS, this campaign narrowed the focus on HIV prevention to the product they got paid to promote—condoms—and potentially put Zambians at risk by implying that casual sex was safe as long as a condom was used.[124]

While condoms can be relatively cheap, reliance upon AIDS drugs for treatment of the disease is not. Biomedical companies have incentive to keep the ideology running that condoms slash HIV rates, even though research indicates condoms contribute to a phenomenon known as risk compensation, in which perceived safety leads people to indulge in riskier behavior.[125] A classic example of risk compensation is seat belts leading motorists to feel more comfortable and drive faster, resulting in more accidents and fatalities despite the increased safety measures.[126] Another example is the number of flooding deaths in the U.S., which haven't changed much the past century despite the fact that levees are built much stronger today than they were 100 years ago. Stronger levees attract more people to the floodplains by appearing to minimize the risk of living in those areas, as do subsidized flood insurance and federal disaster relief, which prompt people to accept more risk.[127] Noting that society is full of examples of people adjusting their habits in response to perceived diminished risk, Gabriel Rotello writes, "The more we experiment with technological fixes the more we discover that the very interconnectedness of things often defeats such narrow approaches."[128]*

Both businesses and politicians have institutional incentives to encourage people to rely on pharma products rather than trying to get them to reconsider the risky sexual behaviors prevalent in their culture. After all, *preventing* HIV makes drug companies less money and provides partisan groups less political capital than *treating* it does. Helping people stay disease free is mostly imperceptible to voters, and it's potentially damaging to shareholders if it results in revenue drops. However, providing medicine to suffering people can boost corporate profits while delivering photo-ops that businesses can put in their brochures and politicians can plaster on their campaign posters.[129] Green states that a World Bank study

---

* Rotello argues that the birth control pill led to risk compensation. "The pill was once expected to limit the number of unwanted pregnancies, but instead the number of unwanted pregnancies has soared, to the extent that it is currently estimated that half of all pregnancies in the United States are unplanned. The reasons are complex, but foremost among them is the fact that the pill, like antibiotics, helped usher in a sexual revolution that lowered the age at which people have sex, increased the incidence of premarital relations, and increased the total number of sexual encounters many people have. Then, since not everybody uses the pill and since not everybody correctly and consistently uses any particular form of contraception, the total number of unwanted pregnancies rose dramatically."

found that money spent on Third World textbooks
yields a payoff fourteen times greater than that on
schoolhouses. Yet buildings are more visible than
books, so they get the money. Agencies can take
before-and-after photos—vacant land + funds =
school—and donors can read glossy brochures that
show happy children trooping in for class and teach-
ers with pointers at blackboards. In this way we waste
money and kids go uneducated. Substitute condoms
for schoolhouses and fidelity for textbooks, and you
have African AIDS.[130]

As the "AIDS Industrial Complex"[131] grew, the bureaucracy stuck to initiatives that provided evidence for the necessity of its existence, which some researchers worried crowded
out cheap homegrown African solutions.[132] According to
Epstein, campaigns such as "Zero Grazing," which focused
on promoting faithfulness and reducing sexual partners, are
unlikely to resurface for several reasons:

For one thing, there is no multimillion-dollar bureaucracy to support it. For condoms, there are the large
contractors like PSI with headquarters in Washington
and thousands of employees in plush offices all over
the world. Abstinence-only education is supported by
a similarly well-endowed network of faith-based and
abstinence-only education organizations, mainly in
the US. Zero Grazing was devised by Ugandans in the
1980s, when they were facing a terrible problem, and

had to deal with it largely on their own. Now that AIDS is a multibillion-dollar enterprise, donors with vast budgets and highly articulate consultants offer health departments in impoverished developing countries a set menu of HIV prevention programs, which consists mainly of abstinence and condoms. Beleaguered health officials have no time, money, or will to devise programs that might better suit their cultures.[133]

AIDS epidemics present drug companies several other opportunities aside from direct sales of drugs. These companies can also use the threat of impending epidemics to pressure the FDA into quicker approval for AIDS drugs. Fast-tracking new drug development reduces research costs, which means more profit.[134] More treatment through drugs, as opposed to focusing on prevention through behavior change, also means there are more people with HIV in the population potentially taking sexual risks as they feel better and live longer.[135] That's not to say that antiretroviral therapy (ART) or condoms should be prohibited. When used correctly, ART can make a person less likely to transmit HIV by reducing the amount of virus in a person's body. ART also makes HIV much less deadly by extending the lives of its victims, and by improving their quality of life.[136] However, it's at least worth acknowledging that increasing pharmaceutical treatments can facilitate risky sex and HIV transmission.[137] In an op-ed to the *Washington Post*, the cochair of Uganda's National AIDS Prevention Committee, Rev. Sam Ruteikara, summed up the issue:

Treatment is good. But for every African who gains access to HIV treatment, six become newly infected. To treat one AIDS patient with life-prolonging anti-retroviral drugs costs more than $1,000 a year. Our successful ABC campaign cost just 29 cents per person each year.

International suppliers make broad, oversimplified statements such as "You can't change Africans' sexual behavior." While it's true that you can't change everybody, you don't have to. If the share of men having three or more sexual partners in a year drops from 15 percent to 3 percent, as happened in Uganda between 1989 and 1995, HIV infection rates will plunge... So hear my plea, HIV-AIDS profiteers. Let my people go. We understand that casual sex is dear to you, but staying alive is dear to us. Listen to African wisdom, and we will show you how to prevent AIDS.[138]

Though the number of new HIV infections has continued to decline in many African countries since Ruteikara made this statement, the number of people living with the virus in sub-Saharan Africa remains staggering. About 70 percent of people living with HIV worldwide, which equates to more than 25 million people, live in sub-Saharan Africa, according to WHO.[139] And there are regions, particularly in southern Africa, where people still have a high chance of getting infected.[140] UNAIDS believes that, with enough donor funds, the epidemic could be ended by 2030.[141]* That's quite an ambitious goal, especially considering that billions of dollars have already been spent on campaigns that have mostly fallen short of expectations, and that expansive organizations have to cut through political red tape, which could delay sincere and concerted relief efforts.

THERE'S NO SUCH THING AS A FREE HUMP

When the potential consequences of sex decline, people feel safer taking sexual risks. This phenomenon was witnessed decades before AIDS became known to the public. In one of the greatest accidental discoveries ever, Scottish scientist Alexander Fleming noticed some fungus growing on a petri dish in his lab in 1928. What Fleming found to be peculiar was that the fungus killed the bacteria in his culture. The fungus makes up what we

---

*   UNAIDS' advocacy for biomedical solutions has been so successful that the media now does UNAIDS job for it. From *Vice* specials to *New York Times* editorials, several media outlets still often solely credit worldwide HIV declines to American donors and their medical spending. These outlets make claims such as "The World Could End AIDS if It Tried" and by "tried," they actually mean "donated more money." But these outlets merely repeat UNAIDS press releases while failing to cite specific independent epidemiological studies that show an actual basis for the praise. Instead of noting that the biggest HIV declines in Africa came in countries that received little U.S. funding or bringing awareness to effective low-cost strategies like circumcision or Zero Grazing, many U.S. media publications have found comfort in patting Western AIDS organizations on the back while recycling unquestioned sociological assumptions.

know today as penicillin, and because of Fleming's dirty dishes, sex would never be the same.[142]

About fifteen years after its discovery, penicillin became a widely used treatment for syphilis, which ran rampant in the early twentieth century. From 1947 to 1957, syphilis deaths declined 75 percent and the rate of new infections of the disease dropped 95 percent. In response to the safer sexual climate, those plain-Jane folks from the bland 1950s started taking more risks when they got it on. According to the study *The Wages of Sin: How the Discovery of Penicillin Reshaped Modern Sexuality*, gonorrhea rates began rising in 1957 and increased about 300 percent by 1975. In that same time frame, the ratio of children born illegitimately increased by about 250 percent, and the ratio of births to teenagers increased by about 50 percent.[143]

The 1950s are a decade commonly associated with the kind of conservative values espoused in *Leave It to Beaver*, not radical sexuality. But after syphilis-related deaths fell off, people started having riskier sex, which resulted in increases in children born out of wedlock, STD transmission, and teens getting knocked up. The efficacy of penicillin in treating the most dangerous sexually transmitted disease of the time began a trend of people increasingly relying on chemical solutions to solve one problem, while ignoring how changes in behavior could contribute to other problems. Unwanted outcomes such as increased rates of gonorrhea, teen pregnancies, and illegitimate births were just a sign of things to come, as the consequences of perceived risk-free intercourse would later contribute to HIV epidemics.[144]

The American AIDS epidemic resembled syphilis's grip on the nation early in the twentieth century. Syphilis deaths in the U.S. peaked in 1939 and AIDS deaths peaked in 1995. During those respective years, syphilis accounted for 1.4 percent of all deaths, and AIDS accounted for 1.9 percent of all deaths.[145] Another similarity that these two STDs share is that the drugs used to treat each disease have led to increases in risky sexual behavior. Like penicillin, the availability of AIDS treatment drugs has led people to be less fearful and cautious about contracting AIDS, driving them to engage in more risky sex whereby HIV could be transmitted.[146]

Confronting Ideologies

Though biomedical companies and AIDS groups have incentives to mislead the public to keep cash flowing, the deception mostly happens subconsciously, because these organizations are full of intelligent, sympathetic, honest individuals who are looking to improve the lives of AIDS victims and halt the spread of viruses. AIDS bureaucrats often have genuine intentions, and drugs they've pumped into African nations have helped improve the quality of life for many AIDS victims.[147]* However, as Halperin and Timberg write, "The

---

*   Antiretroviral medications can also help reduce infection by reducing the likelihood of HIV transmission during childbirth.

creation of such an extensive industry creates its own political and financial imperatives."[148]

In a laboratory setting, it's easy to show that condoms will almost always prevent a virus from spreading and that treatment drugs will extend people's lives while lowering their viral load, making them less susceptible to transmit the virus. It makes intuitive sense that condoms would be a good defense against AIDS, and that approach has worked in places such as Thailand and Cambodia.[149] However, in those countries HIV was mostly spread through *commercial* sex, so it was possible to enforce mandatory and consistent condom use in brothels. In Africa, where condoms are often seen as a Western imposition, many couples refuse to use them with their regular partners and only use condoms irregularly, and sometimes incorrectly, during casual sex.[150] In these cases, some use has been worse than no use, because the availability of condoms promotes risk compensation while failing to adequately protect users.

A randomized controlled clinical trial can't accurately capture how culture will impact these kinds of behavioral reactions. That's why observing cultures and examining "natural experiments" is so crucial, and why lessons from Uganda and Zimbabwe are so important. The real-world anthropological evidence indicates that cheap grassroots campaigns *controlled by Africans* have been more effective in reducing HIV transmission in Africa than have the expensive biomedical interventions run by Western donors. Western biomedical products were successful in squashing other diseases, such as polio and smallpox. But unlike polio or smallpox, stopping HIV involves confronting sexual and cultural nuances that make people uncomfortable and that Western money alone can't overcome.[151]

Even if a bureaucrat, donor, or researcher begins advocating for changes in prevention strategy, they will encounter immense political inertia. Any attempt to improve AIDS-prevention strategies will face major roadblocks to becoming reality because sexual politics are log-jammed with zealous orthodoxy from both right and left. The right doesn't want to acknowledge the benefits of condoms in preventing infections in concentrated epidemics, as that could imply they endorse making nonmarital sex safer. The left is concerned with protecting people's rights and freedoms, which in extreme cases leads to the imposition of faux-intellectual, politically correct condemnation on anyone who acknowledges racial differences or sociological taboos, or who dares to suggest sexual activity should ever be curtailed. People who subscribe to these opposing philosophies often find themselves in abstinence-versus-condoms debates, which entirely miss the point that partner reduction (which is unrelated to condoms or abstinence) has likely played the largest role in cutting HIV transmission in Africa.[152]* These debates become so toxic that sometimes organizations oppose certain strategies *just because* their political adversaries promote them.

Malcolm Potts was the first medical director of the International Planned Parenthood Federation and the former CEO of Family Health International, a group that for decades ran condom campaigns in Africa. Potts admitted to Epstein

---

*   Researchers in the *British Medical Journal* write, "Partner reduction has been the neglected middle child of the ABC approach."

that he resisted partner reduction and fidelity programs for ideological reasons:

> AIDS produces so much emotion. It's hard to look at the evidence. We've never really been on an even keel with respect to strategy. There was a sense that promoting fidelity must be totally wrong if it was a message favored by the Christian Right. We've made an emotion-based set of decisions, and people have suffered terribly because of that. And they will go on suffering. Everything we learn about the epidemic goes in slowly and is resisted on the way.[153]

Partisanship isn't the only political nuance that turns AIDS dialogues toxic. Political correctness retards AIDS discussions and misinforms the public. James Chin writes that AIDS programs "have been politically correct and morally motivated but epidemiologically incorrect."[154] The effect of political correctness has been witnessed all around the world ever since the AIDS virus came into public view.

According to Randy Shilts, when AIDS first struck the U.S., people thought they could get HIV through saliva, because the public was repeatedly told that HIV transfers through "bodily fluids," a vague euphemism used by public officials and the media because using precise terms such as "blood" and "semen" made people uncomfortable. Those who thought HIV could be so easily transmitted had yet another reason to avoid contact with AIDS victims, which contributed to the disease's stigma.[155]

In an attempt to get people to care more about AIDS, to

get more funding, and to avoid further stigmatization of gay people, in the 1990s and early 2000s many health officials warned that AIDS would spread to heterosexual populations around the world, even though it was already apparent by then that for most countries a "heterosexual AIDS explosion" was unlikely.[156]* International AIDS prevention programs became vague about target populations, and some programs ignored the fact that HIV spreads much faster among men who have sex with men than it does among men who have sex with women. In India and Tanzania, prevention programs focused so much on heterosexual transmission that some men reported they avoided sex with women and instead had sex with men. They thought gay sex would protect them from HIV because they thought HIV could only transmit through vaginal sex.[157]

Regarding how PC culture halts the progress of AIDS prevention, Pisani writes:

> We don't tell the truth for fear of seeming racist, for fear of losing our jobs or our chance for a promotion to a director's position, for fear of seeing our institution's budget evaporate. We don't tell the truth for fear of upsetting people who are already infected with HIV, or stigmatizing people who belong to groups in which HIV rates are high. We don't tell the truth for fear

---

* Regarding an alarmist report UNAIDS issued in 2002, Piot writes that "our own epidemiologists were unhappy with the prediction that China would have as many as ten million cases of HIV in the not too distant future—that estimate was not based on serious evidence."

of losing clients, access to health care, our marriage.
We don't tell the truth because our religions and our
cultures want us to be prudish about sex and drugs,
whereas, in truth, most of us think they are fun.[157]

Shilts noted similar thought and speech patterns in the
1980s, which he dubbed "AIDSpeak, a new language forged
by public health officials, anxious gay politicians, and the
burgeoning ranks of 'AIDS activists.' The linguistic roots of
AIDSpeak sprouted not so much from the truth as from
what was politically facile and psychologically reassuring.
Semantics was the major denominator of AIDSpeak jargon,
because the language went to great lengths never to offend."[159]
Green writes that terms like "'sex positive'…narcotize serious
thinking," adding, "But that's how ideology blinds people."[160]
Which is a shame, because sexual environments affect
well-being much more than many of the trivial activities that
gridlock Washington. But AIDS has become so politicized
that many of the organizations controlling the money write
about AIDS as if it were divorced from sexuality, omitting
frank sexual talk in favor of discussing "resources," "poverty,"
and "education." By *not* directly talking about sex, it's easier
for powerful money-hungry groups with opposing agendas
to mask their underlying doctrines. The abstinence alliance
assumes that large swaths of the population should, and
will, withhold sex until marriage, while the condom coalition
condemns anyone advocating for anything resembling a sexual
restriction. It's tragic that neither group cares to acknowledge
the cheap solution lying in the middle.

= 4 =

soldier sex

HOW THE U.S. MILITARY INADVERTENTLY
HELPED FORM OUR CONCEPT OF GAY IDENTITY

A hidden consequence of war is its power to influence sexual networks. Pulling young people away from their families and placing them into sex-segregated communities full of strangers has created all sorts of sexuality-related headaches for military leaders, from venereal disease epidemics to losses in manpower as soldiers were historically discharged for their sexual orientation. American generals have tried everything from encouraging abstinence to regulating prostitution in hopes of quenching the desires of lonely troops, oftentimes producing unintended results. But what has baffled U.S. military officials most in their regulation of sexual desire is what to do with gay, lesbian, bisexual, and transsexual (LGBT) servicemembers. Despite attempts to ban LGBT servicemembers from serving and to stamp out all evidence of homosexuality from troops stationed across the world, the military's persecution of gays and lesbians didn't keep same-sex desire in the closet. Instead, it actually helped create a gay minority identity in the U.S., as the military unwittingly brought more visibility and connectedness to the LGBT community than any other organization in the country.

Prostitution in the Military

Though many people are familiar with the "Ah, me so horny," imagery of Vietnamese prostitutes in *Full Metal Jacket* as the embodiment of American soldiers' sexual adventures, the link between prostitution and the American military might actually have peaked much earlier, during the Civil War. Because women at that time depended almost exclusively on their husbands' wages for their livelihood, prostitution was unavoidable for many Civil War–era women as a means to support their families when their spouses went off to combat. According to a *Smithsonian* article by Angela Serratore, Nashville saw the number of its "public women" increase from 198 in 1860 to 1,500 in 1862. In 1863, George Spalding, a military police official in Nashville, was ordered to "seize and transport to Louisville all prostitutes found in the city or known to be here." Spalding was able to round up the prostitutes, but his journey still failed. After word of the ship's cargo reached Louisville's law enforcement, the ship full of prostitutes was banned from docking in Kentucky and ordered to move on to Cincinnati. Ohio didn't want more prostitutes, either, and ordered the ship *back* to Kentucky.

Once again, the ship was rejected, and the prostitutes headed back to where they came from—Nashville.[1]

Because Spalding was unable to find a "home" for them, and because after these women were rounded up others took their place and kept the sex industry alive, Spalding figured he might as well focus on making prostitution *safe*. This decision resulted in the Union Army's creating America's first system of legalized prostitution out of the sheer inability to shut down the sex industry.[2]* In fact, it was so common for soldiers to pay for sex during the Civil War, there's debate about whether the term "hooker" came from Union General Joseph Hooker, whose troops visited prostitutes frequently.[3]†

Around the turn of the twentieth century, however, the military's open relationship with prostitution collided with the morals of the Progressive Era, which aimed to ban the sale of alcohol, "Americanize" immigrants, and censor media for violence and sex. According to historian-sexologist Vern Bullough, around the time of WWI, the War Department promoted abstinence to its troops, but distributed prophylactics only as a last resort. The abstinence policies failed, as soldiers continued to contract syphilis and other venereal diseases

---

* According to Serratore, "Today, the handful of U.S. counties that allow prostitution, such as Nevada's Lyon County, rely on a regulatory system remarkably similar to the one implemented in 1863 Nashville."

† Pornography was also common among Civil War troops. The amount of porn floating about infuriated Union officer Captain M. G. Tousley enough that he complained to his commander in chief that they weren't doing enough to "checkmate and suppress" the "obscene prints and photographs" that were "quite commonly kept and exhibited by soldiers and even officers."

(VD). According to Bullough, demonstrated success in combatting VD came from commanders who ignored the official abstinence policy and promoted prevention and treatment instead. Under General John J. Pershing, the military eventually altered its abstinence policy.[4] Pershing realized the difficulty soldiers faced in serving their country while battling sexually transmitted diseases. After all, Pershing himself contracted gonorrhea twice.[5] However, the military as a whole wasn't preemptive in fighting these illnesses, and it took a VD epidemic to get the War Department to alter its prevention strategies.

Going Down in the Trenches

While the War Department was promoting abstinence by issuing soldiers pamphlets with titles such as *Live Straight if You Would Shoot Straight*, which proclaimed that "all loose women are dirty" and said that by abstaining from sex men "honored and protected the sisters, wives, and future mothers of the race we are fighting for," about one in eleven soldiers were getting infected with syphilis, gonorrhea, or chancroid from 1917 to 1919.[6]* According to Dr. Granville MacGowan,

---

*   According to medical historian Allan Brandt, the high number of soldiers coming down with VD led the military to change its discharge policies. Before WWI, VD was reason enough to reject someone from the military. But because there was a "critical need" for soldiers during the war, and there were so many service-members with sexually related infections, the military began treating infected soldiers rather than expelling them. Another reason for the change in policy was that some military officials at the time feared soldiers would intentionally contract VD to avoid service.

an executive officer of a medical advisory board, "If you were to attempt to get an army without having men who had gonorrhea, you would not have an army."[7] In *Devices and Desires: A History of Contraceptives in America*, historian Andrea Tone estimates that venereal disease cost the military seven million days of lost active duty during WWI. "Only the great influenza epidemic of 1918 ranked higher as a cause of 'lost time,'" she writes.[8]

Pershing was tired of the tolls unchecked sexuality was taking on the military's productivity. "A soldier who contracts a venereal disease not only suffers permanent injury, but renders himself inefficient as a soldier and becomes an encumbrance to the Army," he said.[9] But many military orders at the time focused on combatting VD with abstinence, morality, and entertainment rather than focusing on prevention and treatment. As seen in this passage from General Order No. 34, issued on September 9, 1917:

> It shall be the constant endeavor of all Commanding Officers to develop among the members of this command those better qualities which are characteristic of high moral standards of living. [...] In connection with the instructions laid down in General Orders of the War Department, now in force, there will be provided amusements, reading rooms, entertainments, opportunity for athletic sports, etc., whenever it is at all practicable. While the chief responsibility for supplying opportunities for social recreation, physical and mental occupation, and the giving of

advice directed against intemperance and licentious living rests with company officers, frequent lectures will also be given by medical officers on sexual hygiene and venereal disease, in which continence shall be advised and illicit intercourse with women discouraged.[10]

Under Pershing, the military eventually altered the tone of its sexual policy by focusing the orders on prophylactics and early treatment for sexually transmitted diseases rather than abstinence, morality, and entertainment, as seen in General Order No. 77, issued on December 18, 1917:

All Commanding Officers are directed to give personal attention to matters pertaining to the prevention of venereal disease. They will at all times support the medical officers charged with the management of prophylactic stations and assist in every way possible the prevention and eradication of venereal affections. [...] Men discovered as having venereal disease will be given intensive treatment and if complications exist will be sent to a hospital. [...] Particular attention must be given to these [prophy-lactic] stations which should contain a waiting place protected against the weather, a clean sanitary treat-ment room with privacy, proper equipment, and technique to inspire confidence in the men, who should have impressed upon them the importance of early prophylactic treatment.[11]

Between 1910 and 1915, VD rates generally hovered between 90 and 100 infections per 1,000 soldiers.[12] By 1917, when General Order No. 77 was issued, VD rates fell to about 70 per 1,000. After the order, which reflected a new official emphasis on prophylaxis treatment and education, VD rates fluctuated briefly but then consistently declined until they were cut in half, to about 34 per 1,000 in the mid-1930s.[13] But there was more running alongside the drop in VD than just prophylactic treatment and an official order from Pershing. Soldiers were also allowed to have sex, even with regulated prostitutes, as long as they didn't rape, marry, or take concubines. According to *Families of a New World: Gender, Politics, and State Development in a Global Context*, wherever American troops were stationed, prostitutes were segregated and inspected for venereal disease. Upon seizing Veracruz in the Pancho Villa Expedition of 1916, nurses from the military and Red Cross were "assigned to assist in rounding up all prostitutes and in making the examinations." A surgeon during the Pershing regime described the situation: "The prostitutes were surrounded by a barbed-wire fence, every woman was examined, and only those found uninfected were retained for duty." Brothels were even segregated, with black, white, and Mexican women occupying different neighborhoods so soldiers could go where they preferred. To defend prostitution, one military officer argued, "If prostitution were not provided, these men would disobey orders, go to Mexican villages and get mixed up with the women and thereby possibly bring on war."[14]

Ignoring education and treatment in favor of absti-nence sparked VD outbreaks, as soldiers continued to engage in risky sex but had few options for healing themselves in a culture that likely would scorn open acknowledgement of their behavior. Emphasizing disease eradication and regulating the women that soldiers had sex with helped reduce VD, even as prostitution was encouraged. The *American Journal of Public Health* notes, "The campaign was conducted amid an environment offering in many instances extraordinary opportunities for exposure. General Pershing's determination to return the boys to the United States as clean as when they left their home shores was more than accomplished."[15] But finding the right balance of methods to lower transmission rates of VD often proved elusive. And as baffling as policing straight sex was for generals, trying to limit gay sex in the military proved even more difficult, which in turn brought on significant unanticipated consequences.

Entrapped in the Closet

Although straight sex created struggles for the military, policies on prostitution, abstinence, and VD treatment were at least up for debate throughout American history. What wasn't up for debate until very, very recently was the fact that gay sex would officially get a soldier punished.[16]* So what initially drove the

---

*   Nathaniel Frank argues the military's discharge of homosexuals is as old as the country itself. "Ever since the Revolutionary War, men have been drummed out of

military to adopt such a hard-line stance against homosexuality? And why did they stick to it for so long?

Historian Nathaniel Frank writes, "A crucial part of military culture has also been its self-definition as a realm of strong men. Resistance to allowing women in combat, reluctance to discipline sexual harassment,[17†] refusal to accept homosexuals into service—it often seems that command leaders would rather not acknowledge the presence of anyone but straight males in their midst."[18] Official military policies, which long excluded LGBT people, often have alluded to stereotypes of homosexuality equating with weakness. Policies have also slowly ebbed and flowed with the cultural zeitgeist.

For example, "Don't ask, don't tell" (DADT), which theoretically allowed gay people to serve if they hid their sexuality, was passed in the 1990s, when public acceptance of LGBT people was growing. President Barack Obama's eventual repeal of DADT in 2011 came after several states had approved gay marriage and it became politically viable in some states for politicians to pass nondiscrimination ordinances to protect LGBT people. Of course, these changes in societal perception that ultimately influenced

---

the U.S. military for homosexual acts," Frank writes. "The first recorded incident of a discharge for homosexuality was that of Lieutenant Gotthold Frederick Enslin in 1778."

†   After interviewing LGBT veterans, historian Steve Estes noted there can be an interplay between sexual harassment and sexual-orientation discrimination. In his research, he found that some women in the military who were suspected of being lesbians were coerced to have sex with their superiors to "prove" they were straight.

military policy were led by the gay rights movement. And the gay rights movement relied on a growing gay identity, which, in circular fashion, had been created in part by the military's persecution of gay servicemembers.[19]

Although gay servicemembers have historically been discriminated against, the ways in which they were punished have fluctuated. It wasn't until around the time of WWI that the idea of *excluding* soldiers for *being gay*, instead of just punishing those who engaged in homosexual acts, began to circulate.[20] This change in practice (of the military punishing people for their gay *identity* as opposed to punishing people for same-sex *conduct*) was led by developments in psychiatry at the time, which cast homosexuality as a mental illness.[21]* In response to a police raid at a gay club that found soldiers among the crowd, psychiatrist Dr. Albert Abrams wrote in September 1918:

> Recruiting the elements which make up our invincible army, we cannot ignore what is obvious and which will militate against the combative prowess of our forces in this war... From a military viewpoint, the homosexualist is not only dangerous, but an

---

*   Philosopher Michel Foucault writes that although psychiatry contributed to a stigmatization of same-sex desires, psychiatry "also made possible the formation of a 'reverse' discourse: homosexuality began to speak in its own behalf, to demand that its legitimacy or 'naturality' be acknowledged, often in the same vocabulary, using the same categories by which it was medically disqualified." Foucault also writes, "The sodomite had been a temporary aberration; the homosexual was now a species."

ineffective fighter... It is imperative that homosexual-
ists be recognized by the military authorities.[22†]

During this time, the military began its most infamous
purge of homosexuals in an event that has become known
as the Newport sex scandal. At the naval base in Newport,
Rhode Island, Navy officials in 1919 persuaded enlisted men
to entrap and seduce suspected gay sailors. The plan was
hatched when Chief Machinist's Mate Ervin Arnold discovered a gay subculture at the Newport naval base. Arnold took
this information to his superiors, which eventually culmi-
nated in the assistant secretary of the navy, future president,
Franklin D. Roosevelt, ordering a "most searching and rigid
investigation" into Newport's gay subculture, with the intent
of prosecuting gay servicemembers.[23] Although he's often
viewed as a liberal crusader, as assistant secretary of the navy,
FDR approved gay purges.

Arnold's superiors, Roosevelt included, felt they would
need evidence that would stand up in court if they were to
discharge the uncovered gay soldiers. To get this evidence, they
enlisted volunteer Navy officers to go undercover at popular gay
hangout spots, such as the YMCA.[24†] The undercover soldiers

---

†   To detect homosexuals in order to disqualify them from military service, Abrams
    invented a device that "recorded" the levels of radiation emanating from people's
    genitals. His theory was that the testicles of gay men would emit less radia-
    tion than the testicles of straight men. And that gay men would have "ovarian
    reactions," meaning their testicles would produce the same amount of radiation
    as a woman's ovaries.

‡   The Village People were created by gay music producer Jacques Morali to appeal

were told to keep personal journals and take note of everything that happened. Some of the volunteers staked out the homes of suspected gay soldiers and noted who came and went from the residence. Arnold told his men to "obtain information and evidence pertaining to cocksuckers and rectum receivers and the ring leaders [sic] of this gang arranging from time to time meetings whereas to catch them in the act."[25] He ordered his volunteers to note the full names, home addresses, and military stations of those they suspected to be having gay sex.

To penetrate the gay subculture, Arnold recruited a very specific type of soldier. "Handling this class of work, with reference to perverts, a good looking man from the average [age] of 19 to 24 will be the best people," he said. "Once a man passed 30 and lost his looks, they [homosexuals] usually will not solicit or bother them." Arnold suggested his investigation volunteers try to convince gay soldiers they were "what is termed in the Navy as a 'boy humper,'" so that gay soldiers could be seduced and entrapped, because Arnold's superiors noted that perpetrators would likely have to be caught having gay sex in order to maintain a conviction.[26]

While the volunteers denied being gay themselves, they pursued these commands with zeal, having anal sex and

---

to the gay subculture, and YMCAs were a notorious hookup spot within that subculture. It doesn't take a musicologist to conclude the song has a homosexual feel and inspiration to it. The next time you see old granny doing the letter dance at a wedding, keep in mind she's actually celebrating the expression and sensation of hot, hot, 1970s man-on-man action.

sharing orgasms with the soldiers they set up.* Sailors who were caught having gay sex (which in the Newport case involved entrapment) were court-martialed for sodomy and generally given five-to-six-year prison sentences.[27] Even in the roaring '20s, newspaper writers were perplexed as to why servicemembers were dispatched to trick their own colleagues into criminal acts rather than focusing on defending their country.[28] The Newport scandal alludes to an institutional obsession with homosexuality, and this infatuation crept into later policies that remained on the books for decades.

Military Mind-Sets

The Newport sex scandal was just one isolated example of how the military persecuted homosexuals. Looking at larger, more comprehensive policies, one of the most cited military reports regarding homosexuality is the Navy's 1957 Crittenden Report. The report found "no factual data" to back up the idea that gays "cannot acceptably serve in the military" or posed security risks, but it still recommended discharging gay soldiers.[29†] Why?

---

*   In a contemporary sense, it would appear the volunteers were closet cases in denial. However, it may not be quite so simple. As discussed in this chapter, the modern gay *identity* in America is a relatively recent phenomenon. In the past, men who had sex with men didn't necessarily view themselves as "gay," especially if they adopted the active role (i.e., top/pitcher) during sex.

†   The military has continually altered its reasoning for banning gay service-members. Initially, sodomy was criminalized. Then, with the rise of psychiatry, homosexuality was branded as a mental illness. As it became untenable for the

"The service should not move ahead of civilian society nor attempt to set substantially different standards in attitude or action with respect to homosexual offenders," the report stated.[30]* Reflecting the "standards in attitude" of the time the report was issued, naval officers in the 1950s were instructed, "Homosexuality is an offense to all decent and law-abiding people, and it is not to be condoned on grounds of 'mental illness' any more than other crimes such as theft, homicide, or criminal assault."[31] And if that wasn't clear enough, the report goes on: "Homosexuality is wrong, it is evil, and it is to be branded as such."[32]

Although the condemnatory language was dialed back, official military attitudes about homosexuality didn't change much in the following decades. A 1981 policy stated, "The presence in the military environment of persons who engage in homosexual conduct or who, by their statements demonstrate a propensity to engage in homosexual conduct, seriously impairs the accomplishment of the military mission."[33] In 1989, a Department of Defense research group suggested the military treat gays "as a minority group" rather than view

---

military to link sexual orientation to mental disorders, the military then claimed that gay servicemembers posed security risks. After the security risk hypothesis was disproved, gay servicemembers were accused of undermining unit cohesion. Now that unit cohesion worries are being dismantled, it's unclear what gay servicemembers might possibly be accused of next.

*   According to Bérubé, the report was kept secret and the military said they couldn't locate their own studies on homosexuality. Army officials stated they had "no evidence of special studies pertaining to homosexuals." The report was finally released in 1977 under orders from a federal judge.

homosexuality as "sin, crime (or) sickness." The group's report stated gay people were no more of a security risk or vulnerable to blackmail than were heterosexuals. The Pentagon rejected the report.[34]

In 1993, the United States changed its policy on the treatment of gay people in the military when Bill Clinton passed DADT, a policy that was supposed to reduce discrimination against LGBT personnel. So long as gay troops weren't open about their sexuality, they could serve. But if gay troops were out and open, they were still barred from service.[35] While the policy was intended to allow LGBT people to serve as long as they concealed their sexual orientation, people still continued to be discharged for their sexual orientation until the repeal of DADT under President Obama in 2011.[36†] And even though gay soldiers are now allowed to serve in the military, the long history of discharging gay and lesbian soldiers has had remarkable effects on gay life in America that continue to be felt today.[37‡]

Discharge Difficulties

Before the mid-1900s, soldiers caught committing sodomy (defined as anal and sometimes oral sex between men) were

---

†   According to an entry in the *Oxford Encyclopedia of American Military and Diplomatic History*, "More than fourteen thousand service members had lost their jobs under 'don't ask, don't tell.'"

‡   Frank writes, "The role of lesbians [in the military] is particularly vital. [...] According to statistical analyses of the U.S. census and other data, the proportion of female service members who are lesbian is 5.2 percent, nearly twice the estimated proportion of lesbians in the general population."

often court-martialed, discharged, and sent to military prison. But with the mass mobilization of troops during World War II, courts-martial for each sodomy accusation would have been an unsustainable economic drain on the military. To speed up the process of discharging homosexuals, the U.S. began issuing "blue discharges," which were named for the color of paper that homosexual dismissals were printed on. And to prevent gays from entering the military in the first place, draft boards put processes in place to identify and reject suspected homosexuals.[38]

To "identify" which men were gay, doctors inserted tongue depressors into patients' throats to trigger their gag reflexes, assuming that men who performed fellatio on other men wouldn't gag.[39] Doctors also analyzed responses of suspected homosexuals on how they felt when engaged in the "application of the mouth to the sexual organ" of another guy, theorizing "true homosexuals" gave so many blow jobs they felt pleasure in their mouth while their penises remained flaccid during fellatio.[40] Urinary hormone tests were also introduced, under the theory that gay men would have more estrogen and less androgen than straight men, but the practice was abandoned after the war because correlating hormone levels with sexual orientation was "too uncertain and too expensive to try on every inductee," according to a 1947 *Newsweek* article.[41] Regardless of the efficacy of these identification procedures, with 36 million men eligible to be drafted,[42] and with LGBT people making up about 3.8 percent of the population according to the best research we now have,[43] hundreds of thousands of prospective soldiers faced *potential* exclusion from service because of their orientation.[44]*

By barring gay people from serving their country, the military ensured that only heterosexual men and gay men who hid their orientation from society would die in war.[45] In wars with many casualties, such as WWII and Vietnam, antigay procedures held the potential to save the lives of thousands of gay individuals. Draftees soon caught on, and during the Vietnam War, pretending to be gay became a common tactic draft dodgers used to avoid service. At protests, activist groups chanted phrases such as "Suck cock, beat the draft."[46] The *Realist* stated that being a "hoaxosexual" was the best way to avoid service. In 1967, between thirty and forty men claimed "homosexual tendencies" every day at the L.A. Examination and Entrance Station.[47] One draft counselor quipped, "All of my clients who faked [homosexuality] got their exemption—but they drafted the one fellow who really was gay."[48]† There was even a pamphlet advising dodgers:

> Dress very conservatively. Act like a man under tight control. Deny you're a fag, deny it again very quickly, then stop, as if you're buttoning your lip. But find an

---

*   John D'Emilio argues that gay men were disproportionately represented in the U.S. military during WWII because the military preferred single men with no children.

†   Penile plethysmography, which is used by psychologists to identify deviant sexual desires by tracking changes in blood flow to the penis, was originally developed by Czech psychologist Kurt Freund during the 1950s as a way to determine if men who claimed to be gay in order to avoid military service were, in fact, aroused by other men.

excuse to bring it back into a conversation again and again, and each time deny it and quickly change the subject. And maybe twice, no more than three times over a half-hour interview, just the slightest little flick of the wrist.[49]

While people protested Vietnam and thousands of young men were drafted, the military excluded able candidates solely based on their sexuality, which accidentally provided dissidents another tool to escape service. By placing so much focus on homosexuality, the military brought visibility to LGBT communities, exposing these topics to mainstream America. Through carrying out a rigid regulation of homosexuality, the military continued to unintentionally bolster a gay identity in America.

Breeding Awareness

Ironically, by targeting and excluding homosexuals, the military encouraged gay veterans and those blue-discharged to take on a stronger gay identity, historian Allan Bérubé argues.[50]* Having

---

*   Frank notes, "The majority of these losses [gay discharges] were men, as the majority of uniformed personnel were male. But discharges of women were far out of proportion to their numbers, a fact that highlights the incidence of lesbian-baiting—threatening to tar as lesbian any woman who resisted or reported sexual harassment. It's one of many examples of how fear of homosexuality works to bolster the power of heterosexual men.

"During the late 1980s, women represented a quarter of gay discharges even though they were only a tenth of the military population; in the Marines, they accounted for nearly a third of gay discharges while representing only 3 percent of the force."

to always strategize and conceal their sexuality, gay soldiers realized that being gay was integral to their overall sense of self. The rhetoric and discrimination surrounding blue discharges (where soldiers were often dishonorably expelled, stigmatized, and denied benefits) produced a perceived aura of political legitimacy, where struggling soldiers felt emboldened by antigay stances. The war allowed LGBT soldiers to meet other gay people while also witnessing their heterosexual peers practice situational homosexuality, which led them to conclude their sexual behavior wasn't all that unusual. After fighting discrimination, and finding others who shared their sexual orientation, gay and lesbian soldiers came back to the States with a more concrete sense of their identity and new expectations for their civilian lives.[51†] This new sense of identity inspired some to publicly express their persecution as a discriminated-against minority group in hopes that it would lead to reformed military policies and social changes in the broader American society, Bérubé writes.[52] According to a gay soldier Bérubé interviewed:

> You lived a lifetime of experiences in four years that you would never have lived ordinarily in your own

---

†   Bérubé writes, "The massive mobilization for World War II propelled gay men and lesbians into the mainstream of American life. Ironically the screening and discharge policies, together with the drafting of millions of men, weakened the barriers that had kept gay people trapped and hidden at the margins of society."

    Bérubé added, "Officers who aggressively rooted out homosexuals and exposed them to their draft boards, company mates, and families further destroyed their ability to hide in the closet, forcing them to lead new lives as known homosexuals."

hometown. And to get some awareness of yourself and also, being a homosexual, to learn to be crafty, to be careful, to have fun when you can, be careful when you can't. So that I think I was much more prepared to be an upfront homosexual once I settled here in San Francisco.[53]

Although the military officially excluded gay people, as we saw earlier, the methods used for "identification" were quite crude. The military was also desperate for manpower. So despite draft boards examining millions of people, only 4,000 to 5,000 soldiers were rejected from the draft for being gay during WWII.[54] But during the peacetime years following WWII, the rate for gay discharges more than tripled the wartime rate, indicating that the military placed a higher priority on discharging gay servicemembers when it wasn't as in need of active troops. This point is further illustrated by the fact that the gay discharge rate once again dropped during the Korean War, according to Bérubé.[55]

They may have had to conceal their sexuality to get into the military, but after successfully enlisting, many gay servicemembers had their first homosexual experiences while serving during WWII.[56] Because of strict criteria that didn't allow for married or pregnant women to enlist, a disproportionate number of lesbians served in the military during WWII.[57] In interviews with gay and lesbian servicemembers, journalist Randy Shilts found the prevalence of lesbians in the military became a self-fulfilling prophecy, as some lesbians joined the military primarily *because* they expected to find other lesbians there.[58] Shilts also claims that it was while serving in the military that many troops first heard of the concept of gay identity:

> For the first time in their lives, they heard a new word—a word that not only defined the difference that had lurked secretly within, but also indicated that others like themselves existed. If the word didn't come from fellow G.I.s, the soldiers learned it from gay cruisers who frequented the parks, depots, and YMCAs used as makeshift sleep sites for servicemen. Many a California gay had his salad days in San Francisco then, since the city was the major point of debarkation for the Pacific theater.[59]

Vern Bullough backs up Shilts's "salad days" claim by tossing around the findings of sexologist George Henry. The military consulted Henry about its problem with gay soldiers. According to Bullough, Henry told military officials, "Far more homosexuals served with the armed services than were eliminated before or after induction. In fact, the army had in a sense encouraged homosexuality by making men aware of their sexual orientation. As a result, many men had their first overt homosexual experience while in the army."[60] As sociologist Donald Webster Cory puts it, "It was not until after Pearl Harbor that it [the word 'gay'] became a magic by-word in practically every corner of the United States where homosexuals might gather."[61]

For these reasons, several military personnel Bérubé

spoke with said they felt "more homosexual" after joining the military than they had previously. Some of them then banded together and began speaking out about their shared persecution as a minority group.[62]* Bullough notes that gay organizations grew after WWII because the war gave gay people a chance to meet other gay people and realize they weren't alone, which led to the formation of communities and groups.[63] One of these organizations was the Veterans Benevolent Association, which existed from 1945 to 1954 and is cited by some scholars as one of America's first gay membership organizations.[64]

Although the military discharged only a few thousand gay men each year, those numbers eventually accumulated to about 100,000 disenfranchised veterans by the 1980s.[65] Among them included several LGBT advocates who brought visibility to the gay political movement, including Leonard Matlovich, who won the Bronze Star and the Purple Heart for his service in the Vietnam War. As a decorated service-member, Matlovich's battle with the military became a cause célèbre after he was discharged for publicly acknowledging his homosexuality.[66] The controversy surrounding Matlovich's dismissal led him to grace the cover of *Time* and become the focus of a 1978 TV movie, *Sergeant Matlovich*

---

*   One of the most zealous cases in the military's campaign against homosexuality came in 1958 when the military brought sodomy charges against Admiral Selden Hooper about a decade *after* he retired from the military. Even though the sexual acts in question occurred after Hooper left the military, he was forced to forfeit all his retirement pay and benefits.

vs. the U.S. Air Force. Matlovich died of AIDS in 1988. The statement "When I was in the military they gave me a medal for killing two men and a discharge for loving one" is written on his tombstone.[67]

According to the *New York Times*, Miriam Ben-Shalom was "one of the first two women to serve as drill sergeants in the Eighty-Fourth Division of the United States Army Reserve."[68] Because it was rare for women to hold these types of positions in the 1970s, Ben-Shalom attracted the attention of local press. On the day she graduated from drill sergeant school, Ben-Shalom was interviewed by a TV reporter. During this televised interview, she outed herself as a lesbian. This earned her a discharge.[69†] After her discharge she told the *Milwaukee Journal*, "I joined the Army to prove that gay people can serve along with straight people."[70] Ben-Shalom took her discharge to court and won in 1980 when a U.S. District judge ruled in her favor, but the army wouldn't let her reenlist—triggering years of court battles. In 1987 she won the right to reenter the service, but in 1988 the military once again challenged the decision. Finally, in 1990, Ben-Shalom appealed her case to the U.S. Supreme Court, but it declined to hear the case, effectively ending her military career.[71] After her time in the military, Ben-Shalom cofounded the organization that now

---

† As to why Ben-Shalom admitted to being a lesbian, she told the *Times*, "After the graduation [from drill sergeant school], a reporter asked me how it felt to be a gay person in the military. And I couldn't see any reason to lie. What kind of leader would I be if I lied?"

calls itself the American Veterans for Equal Rights, Inc. and became a vocal opponent of policies such as DADT.[72]

Perry Watkins was an openly gay army sergeant who performed in drag when stationed abroad. Like Ben-Shalom, Watkins won a court battle to stay in the military after getting discharged for his sexual orientation. A federal appeals court ordered Watkins's reinstatement in 1989, which was, according to the *New York Times*, "the first ruling by a full appellate panel that struck at the military's ban on gay and lesbian service members."[73] In 1993, Ben-Shalom and Watkins were co-grand marshals of the New York City gay pride parade. Watkins's story was chronicled in the documentary *Sis: The Perry Watkins Story*.[74]

But the visibility and personal-rights issues these LGBT advocates helped promote was far from being the largest unforeseen outcome of issuing blue discharges. Blue discharges outed people in an era where gay tolerance was nonexistent in most areas of the U.S. For many of these soldiers, living publicly as a homosexual equated to becoming a social outcast. Instead of returning home and answering to fearful, angry, and worried family members, many stayed in the locations where they had been discharged, hoping for a fresh start. And many of these discharges happened to be processed in San Francisco.

According to Shilts, "By the end of World War II, the military establishment had given San Francisco a disproportionately large number of identified gays." It's possible that without the military's insistence on outing and discharging gay soldiers, the largest and one of the oldest gay neighborhoods in America, San Francisco's Castro district, wouldn't have become an "international gay Mecca."[75]*

============ **THE GAY BOMB** ============

Around the time DADT was enacted, the military began developing a theoretical non-lethal weapon at the Wright-Patterson Air Force Base in southwest Ohio. The development plans for this weapon were exposed by a Freedom of Information Act (FOIA) request by the watchdog group the Sunshine Project.[76] According to Sunshine Project Director Edward Hammond, the weapon worked by identifying chemicals already present in the human body in small quantities, "[a]nd by virtue of either breathing or having their skin exposed to this chemical, the notion was that soldiers would become gay."[77] Essentially, the military planned to drop pheromones onto enemy troops, with the intent of making them sexually attracted to each other. One of the researchers involved in the project told journalist Mary Roach, "The idea was to ruin [enemy troops'] morale because they're worried their buddy is going to come in their foxhole and make fond advances."[78]

In the end, the weapon was never developed, and

---

*   San Francisco was not the only port city to develop a visible gay community because of these military discharges. Other port cities such as New York City and Los Angeles also developed visible gay communities through similar circumstances.

the researchers' $7.5 million request to develop this "love bomb" was rejected.[79] The weapon, now dubbed the "gay bomb," gained notoriety by winning a 2007 Ig Nobel Prize, which is a parody of the Nobel Prize and is given to scientists for pursuing unusual or downright useless research.[80]

Out of the Closet

Dealing with issues related to sex confounded generals prior to Pershing and on past Patton, and the sexuality-related issue that has most baffled the military is how to confront homosexuality. Until very recently, this was accomplished by entrapping, excluding, discharging, and denying benefits to gay military personnel. However, as more Americans have become accepting of diverse sexual orientations and LGBT people have gained more legal rights, there has also been a great deal of change in military policy in just the past six years.

DADT lasted until September 20, 2011, when it was repealed under President Obama's administration.[81] Since the repeal, gays, lesbians, and bisexuals have been allowed to openly serve in the military. In 2013, the Pentagon announced it would lift a ban on women serving in ground-combat units,[82] and in 2015 Defense Secretary Ashton Carter ruled that all combat jobs would be open to women.[83] In June 2015, sexual orientation was added to the Military Equal Opportunity policy, which meant that LGBT servicemen and women would be protected from discrimination that prevents them from rising up to higher military levels.[84] In June 2016, the Pentagon ended its ban on transgender servicemembers.[85] In August 2017, President Trump signed a directive reinstating a ban on transgender servicemembers. As of this writing, Trump's ban is being challenged by multiple federal lawsuits.[86]

You can see that, despite the difficulty the world's most powerful military has historically had in dealing with issues surrounding the sexuality of its troops, it has recently become more open and accepting about who can serve.[87]* There's indication the newfound openness can impact the top of the organizational chain, because in May 2016 Army Secretary Eric Fanning became the first openly gay leader of a U.S. military branch.[88]

From regulating prostitution to promoting abstinence, the armed forces have tackled a number of controversial topics and made decisions that affect the way our country's residents perceive sexual issues. But it's in dealing with homosexuality that the armed forces' sexual strategies have created the most surprising effects. "For many gay Americans," historian John D'Emilio wrote, "World War II created something of a nationwide coming-out experience."[89]

While openly gay people weren't allowed to serve, the military unintentionally helped create a gay Mecca, made

---

*   After the military ended its ban on transgender troops, an article in LGBT-interest magazine the *Advocate* stated that the military had "stepped out ahead of most governmental organizations, schools, and companies with this policy to become a leader in social change… This makes it one of the most socially progressive institutions in America. Think about that one for a bit."

scores of gay people aware of their orientation, gave many individuals their first gay experience, brought together gay people who formed advocacy groups, helped create a gay minority identity in America, saved the lives of gay individuals in high-death-rate wars, and gave straight people another route to dodge the draft. What's remained hidden to many people regarding this legacy of intended marginalization is how the prohibitive policies inadvertently brought together gay people who went on to influence their world.

PART II

ECONOMICS

there goes the gayborhood

AN INVESTIGATION INTO THE ECONOMIC PROWESS OF LGBT DISTRICTS

Wₕₑₙ speaking at a forum about Detroit's future two months before the city filed the largest municipal bankruptcy in U.S. history, George Jackson, former CEO and president of the Detroit Economic Growth Corporation, told the audience, "When I look at this city's tax base, I say bring on more gentrification." Jackson continued, "I'm sorry, but, I mean, bring it on. We can't just be a poor city and prosper."[1] That's an undeniable economic fact, but given the city's declining population and tax base, not to mention its high crime rate, what practical steps can the city take to revive itself? And why does research suggest

starting a gay neighborhood could kick-start the gentrification Jackson sought?

For decades, LGBT people have been pioneers in
redeveloping decaying urban areas. That's why for economic,
and not moral reasons, cities should put forth their best
efforts in trying to hook up with gays and lesbians. While
isolated gay districts—city neighborhoods where large
numbers of LGBT residents live often for cultural, social,
or safety purposes—may not be as necessary as they once
were, some queer folk still desire the accompanying social
benefits and visibility. Also, the visible presence of a gay
community signals to artists and other creative types that an
area is accepting. According to research from demographer
Gary Gates and urban theorist Richard Florida, cities with
high numbers of gay people can expect their economies to
grow more than cities with few gay people.[2] This is because
cities that show tolerance (which can be exhibited through
a visible gay community) are able to attract more workplace
talent, which stimulates industry growth.

But unlike many major cities that have seen gay people
redevelop city cores, Detroit lost out on this opportunity
(because of high crime, unwelcoming leadership, and other
municipalities luring LGBT residents away with better amenities), further worsening its chances at recovery. However,
there are specific things Detroit and other cities can do to
make themselves more gay friendly and spur neighborhood
revival—and they range from simple things such as political
acknowledgment of minority groups to more extreme ideas
like building new neighborhoods from scratch.

Gentrifigaytion

After Detroit filed for bankruptcy in July 2013, some people suggested the city should sell off assets, such as the Detroit Institute of Arts' collection or Belle Isle, an island park on the Detroit River the city has owned since 1879, to help meet its $18 billion debt. Just about every method of boosting local business and reviving blighted neighborhoods has been examined, except one: scant attention has been paid to the LGBT community's role in Detroit's economic comeback. Unlike other major American cities, Detroit has few LGBT liaisons or political groups aimed at increasing networking between LGBT people, and public officials have rarely acknowledged the community. When public officials have drawn attention to the LGBT community, their comments have often been homophobic. It's surprising that a city desperate for a resurgence would so blatantly ignore gays and lesbians, given that they've been major drivers of gentrification for decades.

Gentrification typically refers to the restoration and rebuilding of deteriorating areas. Although that definition sounds positive, the term can have negative connotations, because redevelopment can drive up prices and displace long-term residents. But gentrification in Detroit, a city that has lost most of its population, is much different from gentrification in places like San Francisco, where there's a lack of space and a growing population pushes people out of the city.[3]*

---

* A study from the Federal Reserve Bank of Philadelphia found that low-income residents in Philadelphia were no more likely to move out of gentrifying areas than they were to move out of non-gentrifying areas. The study also found that

Considering Detroit has about 80,000 abandoned buildings, it isn't surprising Jackson made the somewhat controversial comment to "bring on more gentrification."[4] After all, Jackson was a prominent official who was expected to assist in urban development and bring the city back to life. His comments came from someone who dealt with Detroit's dire economic climate on a daily basis. He was merely being realistic that the city needs to bring in people to revive itself. But what does that have to do with gay people?

Broadly speaking, there are a few groups of people that often drive gentrification. The theory is that artists and gay individuals are frequently among the first to move to and redevelop blighted areas, because they tend to be more tolerant of risk and are attracted to culturally vibrant and diverse places. But Detroit already has a strong artistic scene. What it doesn't have is a centralized gay district, something Detroit could use, since LGBT people often have incentive to be less sensitive to risk than straight people, and risk is a major stigma the bankrupt, high-crime city of Detroit faces with investors and potential residents.

Why would LGBT people have less reason to be risk sensitive than straight and cisgender (people whose gender

---

the people most likely to move out of a gentrifying area were not people with low incomes, but were people with high credit scores and high incomes who leave the gentrifying area for wealthier neighborhoods. But, as Villanova University economics professor David Fiorenza told CNN, gentrification's benefits depend on context. "Gentrification in Philadelphia is a good thing," he said. "For some other cities, it may not work."

identity matches the sex they were given at birth) folk? The reason generally relates to having children. People with children are incentivized to be more sensitive to things such as crime rates and school districts. Parents become less tolerant of risk than childless people because their decisions affect other human beings, who probably aren't old enough to make their own life decisions yet. Because of their responsibility to provide their offspring with a stable upbringing, people with children have more incentive to flee to safer, albeit more boring, suburbs.

For obvious biological reasons, gay people have kids less often than straight people. Even taking adoption into account, straight couples are about twice as likely as same-sex couples to be raising a child.[5] Because fewer gay couples raise children, they are less likely to be swayed by school districts and crime rates when choosing where to live. It's not that LGBT individuals ignore educational issues or don't care about their well-being. Rather, because they are less likely to have children, they have less reason to attend school board meetings or start neighborhood watches.

Because LGBT people are less likely to have children, LGBT couples are less likely to have one person staying home to watch a child. This allows LGBT people to have greater labor-force participation than straight couples. One study shows people in same-sex couples are either working or looking for work at a rate 13 percentage points higher than those in straight relationships.[6] Because LGBT people are working more and having fewer children (which take up a considerable amount of time and income), it's possible they have greater net disposable income to spend than straight people do.[7]* Historically, LGBT people have spent their time and income in urban areas, and in the process they've helped redevelop several neighborhoods throughout major American cities.

THE DOWNSIDE OF GENTRIFICATION

Gentrification is a buzzword that can imply "revitalization" to urban developers and "human-rights violation" to gentrification opponents. Critics point out that redeveloping economically depressed areas drives up home prices and taxes, which displaces long-term residents. Debates between those wanting to fix up blighted urban neighborhoods and the people who have lived there for decades can become extremely intense. The Peabody Award–winning documentary *Flag Wars* covers this issue as it relates to Columbus, Ohio. In *Flag Wars*, the rhetoric gets very heated as a long-term resident tells the local news that gentrification in his neighborhood is similar to ethnic cleansing in Bosnia. (This comment is quickly juxtaposed with a new

---

*   LGBT people have often been portrayed as wealthy and educated, but the reality is much more complicated. Research on the incomes of LGBT people is mixed. Some researchers say that LGBT people have more disposable income because having fewer children equates to less income being saved. However, other research shows that there is a sexual-orientation wage gap, because some studies show that LGBT people make less than their straight counterparts. Meanwhile, other studies show lesbians on average make more money than straight women.

gay homeowner telling a realtor, "Isn't it wonderful what fags in the urban area can do?")

Like Columbus, Detroit has also seen tensions arise between longtime residents and newcomers. The *Detroit News* reported in 2013 that buildings in gentrifying areas such as Midtown and Corktown were spray-painted with slogans like "Stop Gentrification in Detroit," "Respect Our Roots," and the word "Hipster" circled in red with a slash going through it.[8]

To be fair, many opponents of gentrification have legitimate frustrations. With new residents coming in, zoning boards and homeowner associations sometimes begin enforcing codes that have been ignored or nonexistent for decades. Realtors see a hot piece of asset and begin issuing edicts as they worry that things such as ethnic signs and broken-down cars might limit rising home prices, curtailing their profits. These attitudes can make the people who have lived in the area for years feel like they're being driven out of their own neighborhood. And as prices rise, some long-term residents can't keep up and are forced to give up their homes.

Being driven out by price increases isn't limited to long-term residents. Oftentimes, the very people who helped rebuild the area can no longer afford to live there. The author of a *Boston Magazine* article, who identifies as bohemian, complains about new people moving in who casually pay $11 for cocktails and walk around with little dogs in sweaters, which makes the neighborhood unhip and unaffordable.

Many patrons arrive in their luxury SUVs, dine, and drive away again. They don't look like the kind of crowd that first drew transplants like my wife and me to the South End. One summer evening, as we strolled past the patio scrum at Stella [a restaurant], she said aloud what I was thinking: "Who the hell are these people, and what are they doing in our neighborhood?"[9]

As a new wave of gentrification comes in, fear brews among the locals over yuppies making the place uncool and generic. Look at the reaction in London's Brixton district after the area underwent another round of gentrification:

Locals gathered in the street, catcalling as the first of the residents were bundled through the doors. Bins were set alight, windows broken, walls spray-painted. "YUPPIES OUT," they spelled out, one letter at a time. Then "BURN THE BAILIFFS."[10]

Because rising prices continually force people out, multiple gayborhoods often develop within individual cities as previously attainable neighborhoods become too expensive for the majority of residents.[11] Aside from Dupont Circle in Washington, DC, a well-known LGBT-friendly neighborhood, there is also Shaw and Logan Circle. In Chicago, Boystown is the most notable gay-oriented neighborhood, but LGBT people have also helped redevelop Andersonville and parts of Hyde Park and South Shore. But given the Brixton and Boston commentaries, it seems gentrifiers are as dismayed as long-term residents when "their" neighborhoods start changing.

Solutions to limiting the impact of gentrification on long-term residents would likely involve rezoning, establishing community land trusts, creating cheap public housing, or using rent controls for long-term residents. Also, getting homeowner associations and zone board members to quit acting like middle school hallway monitors who diligently enforce previously ignored rules could help prevent long-term residents from feeling they're being driven out of their own neighborhoods. While controls can be put in place to reduce the negative effects of gentrification, it's illogical to assume that gentrification can be stopped altogether or that it only hurts the poor and favors the rich.[12]

Displacing long-term residents sounds horrifying. But having a city riddled with blight doesn't sound grand either. In reality, there is a give and a take. If an area becomes safer and more developed, prices will rise. If no one redevelops impoverished areas, then prices will remain stagnant, as will tax revenue, because no one new will come to the area, which is problematic when cities have outstanding pension obligations. And without redevelopment, crime will be less likely to fall. As Kelefa Sanneh writes in the New Yorker, "The opposite of gentrification is not a quirky and charming enclave that stays affordable forever; the opposite of gentrification is a decline in prices that reflects the transformation of a once desirable neighborhood into one that is looking more like a ghetto every day."[13]

There are valid criticisms against how gentrification can play itself out. But to *always* oppose the process altogether (regardless of specific contexts) is to vote against urban revival and progressive change and to favor keeping everything as it currently is. As the *Detroit News* points out, "Non-gentrification, on the other hand, hasn't worked all that well in a city that hundreds of thousands of people have sprinted to escape."[14]

Municipal Makeovers

If Detroit is successful in attracting and mobilizing gays and lesbians to help redevelop the city, it certainly won't be the first to do so. Here are a few brief examples of city areas that have been gentrified in large part by LGBT populations.

During the mid-twentieth century, the South End of Boston was described as a diverse "working-class slum" home to blacks and immigrants from the Middle East and Eastern Europe.[15] By the late 1970s, the area became "Boston's gay ghetto," as real estate values gradually rose and the South End went from an impoverished area to some of the city's most expensive real estate.[16] As a wealthier crowd moved in, first led by LGBT people, they filled the area with shops, restaurants, and excellent public amenities thanks to increases in tax revenue.[17] Now preserved historic homes in the area sell for more than $3 million.[18]

Parts of Washington, DC, have also been gentrified by gay individuals. After race riots erupted in the city following the assassination of Martin Luther King Jr., Washington's Dupont Circle began to fall apart, just like many other American neighborhoods that were stricken by riots in the late '60s.[19] Then in the '70s, gays and bohemians moved in and began fixing up the area. The revived area attracted more residents and investment throughout the next few decades.[20] Now Dupont Circle features some of Washington's most sought-after property.[21]

And don't think gay makeovers happen only to coastal cities. The gay community in Chicago has redeveloped several neighborhoods, none more prominent than a former working-class section in Chicago's Lakeview district. In the 1970s, gay men began residing near and starting businesses down Halsted Street, gentrifying the area. So many gay-owned businesses sprang up that the area eventually became known as Boystown. This area helped make Chicago the Midwest's gay hub.

The Midwest's Gay Mecca

Tom Tunney is Chicago's first openly gay alderman, and he represents the city's Forty-Fourth Ward, which happens to include Boystown. Tunney has been an involved member of Chicago's gay community for decades. Prior to becoming a politician, Tunney was an entrepreneur who owned restaurants (including ones near Chicago LGBT districts Boystown and Andersonville) and worked as an AIDS activist.[22]

Tunney says Chicago's political establishment first became openly accepting of the LGBT community when Jane Byrne was elected mayor in 1979.[23] But while Byrne and other mayors like Harold Washington were seen as gay friendly, no one went out of their way as often to acknowledge the gay community as Richard M. Daley, who served as Chicago mayor from 1989 to 2011.

However, Daley's relationship with Chicago's gay community wasn't always smooth. After Daley announced his retirement in late 2010, Chicago's oldest operating LGBT newspaper, the *Windy City Times*, chronicled Daley's relationship with the gay community during his career. The story noted that during his first term in office, AIDS activists confronted Daley and let him know that they thought he was showing poor leadership on AIDS issues. The *Windy City Times* reported, "At a meeting of the gay Chicago Professional Networking Association (CPNA), held in early 1992 at the Vic Theatre, critics also lambasted Daley. And in a spontaneous verbal attack on Daley, more than two months later about 40 AIDS activists screamed insults at him."[24]

A few months after this meeting, Daley boosted AIDS funding by $2.5 million, more than doubling the city's efforts in fighting the epidemic. Daley also appointed official LGBT liaisons, started a committee for gay and lesbian issues, and began openly recruiting LGBT police officers in an effort to reduce homophobia and hate crimes.[25]

Daley became extraordinarily welcoming toward gay residents and was the first Chicago mayor to participate in the city's pride parade.[26] He went so far as to say, "Every quality-of-life issue, the gay community has stepped forward as great leaders."[27] The city's openness to all types of sexual orientation didn't go unnoticed, as Chicago was chosen to host the Gay Games in 2006. The Gay Games are sporting and cultural events organized every four years by and for LGBT people. According to the *Daily Beast*, the games tend to attract about 100,000 visitors and bring $50 million to $80 million to the hosting city.[28]*

After getting the Gay Games to come to Chicago, Daley wasn't shy about letting visiting LGBT people know how much he valued diversity, newcomers, and, of course, places in Chicago where they could spend money. Below is an abbreviated version of Daley's remarks at the opening ceremony for the Gay Games. It's almost as if he is directly recruiting gay people to move to Chicago:

> On behalf of all the people of Chicago, I'm delighted to welcome you to the seventh Gay Games. [...] Our entertainment, shopping and cultural attractions are world-class—so there will be plenty to keep you

---

* Any study proclaiming an "economic impact" from an event is suspect because these studies are usually commissioned by someone with an agenda to sell the event's importance. These studies, common in sports, often fail to account for substitution effects, meaning money being spent at a certain event doesn't mean that money wouldn't already be spent elsewhere in the local economy. However, Cleveland pledged $700,000 to give itself an edge over other candidates like Boston and Washington, DC, as the games' organizers were nearing a decision in 2009, so there might be value in hosting these games. Cities get advertising out of the events, which allows them to show off their welcoming attitude, diversity, and openness.

occupied when you're not at the games… We have distinctive neighborhoods, a multitude of religions and a variety of lifestyles. And we're fortunate to have a very large and active gay and lesbian community… I'm proud that Chicago has been in the forefront when it comes to meeting the needs and aspirations of the members of the gay and lesbian community. We provide domestic partnership benefits to city employees and we outlaw discrimination on the basis of sexual orientation or gender identity… Members of the lesbian, gay, bisexual, and transgender community have contributed to Chicago in every imaginable way—in business, education, the arts, and neighborhood development. They deserve to have the city of Chicago standing on their side, and it will continue to do so, as long as I am mayor.[29]

Chicago's image as a diverse, tolerant city attracted LGBT people to the region, but Chicago is also attractive to LGBT people because of accepting leaders like Daley, says Tunney.[30] "He was politically astute and grew on the job," Tunney says. "He realized the importance of the LGBT community and that they were a political and economic force to be reckoned with." Tunney, who served on Daley's economic development committee, adds that Daley was effective at mobilizing the area's gay community: "He was a blue-collar mayor from Chicago. Not New York or San Francisco, where people expect such open acceptance of the gay community. When he said 'What's the problem with gays?' that opened the eyes to Middle America that it's OK to be gay... When he speaks, Middle America listens."[31]

Chicago's gay community is so prominent now, "It's hard to quantify all the parts of neighborhoods they helped revitalize," says Tracy Baim, cofounder of the *Windy City Times*.[32] Chicago's political leaders, who continue to publicly show support for their LGBT residents, further bolster the community's visibility. In 1991, Chicago opened the first municipal Gay and Lesbian Hall of Fame in the U.S.[33] It also built a $20 million gay community center on Halsted Street in 2007.[34] And in 2014, the city opened an affordable senior housing complex for LGBT people.[35] Since becoming the Midwest's LGBT hub, Chicago's gay scene has also become a tourist destination. LGBT-focused events such as International Mr. Leather, Miss Continental, Northalsted Market Days, and the Chicago pride parade bring hundreds of thousands of people to the city annually.

Since gay neighborhoods have become economic boons for several major cities such as Midwestern Chicago, why doesn't financially troubled Detroit have a recognizable gayborhood?

Detroit's Lack of an LGBT District

As mentioned earlier, gay communities have helped develop areas of Chicago, Washington, DC, Boston, and many others. But unlike all of these cities, Detroit doesn't have a centralized gay district. At least, not anymore.

Until the mid-1980s, Detroit had a gay enclave in its Palmer Park neighborhood. Gay businesses, gay bars, historic houses, and art deco apartments lined the area. But like many other things in Detroit, the gay neighborhood in Palmer Park disintegrated for some of the same reasons Detroit ended up bankrupt.

In trying to pinpoint why Detroit's gayborhood split up, sources cite everything from lack of mass transit to white flight. But a few themes repeated throughout.

One: High crime rates in the 1980s drove people into the suburbs. While there had already been an exodus out of the city post-1950s, rapidly rising crime accelerated it. Crack cocaine and the drug trade around it became popular to the point where people in places like Palmer Park were getting murdered and beaten regularly.

Two: Unwelcoming leadership. It's no secret that Detroit has had some of America's most corrupt politicians over the past few decades. Former mayor Kwame Kilpatrick, who served from 2002 to 2008, was sentenced in 2013 to twenty-eight years behind bars for racketeering, bribery, extortion, and tax crimes.[36] Kilpatrick also repeatedly disparaged the gay community. He once said he didn't want his children to see "that kind of lifestyle."[37]* Comments like this didn't exactly bring LGBT people into the city or convince gay people already living in the city to stay.

Three: Ferndale (a Detroit suburb) and other nearby cities (such as Chicago) capitalized on Detroit's loss. Detroit

---

*   Kilpatrick defended himself by saying, "There are things that my impressionable children don't need to see at this age—a man kissing a man, a woman kissing a woman. That's not hatred. It's just that I want to raise strong, proud men that love women."

lost residents to other cities, particularly Chicago, because they were safer, had more visible gay communities, and were in better shape financially, which allowed them to provide better public services and amenities. As for Ferndale, a 2007 article for the *Detroit Metro Times* titled "Affirming Ferndale: How a Once-Faltering Suburb Became a Hub for Gay Community" lays out the history of Metro Detroit's gay community and how an enclave blossomed in Ferndale, which helped redevelop the suburb.[38] Ferndale directly borders Detroit and starts on the north side of 8 Mile Road, the infamous dividing line between city-proper Detroit and the burbs. As high crime in the 1980s drove gays out of Detroit, many moved to Ferndale because it was close and cheap. At the time, Ferndale hadn't been developed as fully as it is today. Low rents, open space, and a more welcoming political environment brought in working-class gays and lesbians who immediately got to work improving their neighborhoods.

Just as LGBT people redeveloped areas of major cities, they helped turn Ferndale into one of Detroit's busiest suburbs. Before gays and lesbians began migrating to Ferndale throughout the 1980s and '90s, Ferndale "was littered with empty retail shells," according to the *Detroit News*.[39] Nowadays, few buildings are vacant in Ferndale, as bars, retail stores, and restaurants line the main drag. But the flight of LGBT residents from Detroit to more accepting locations is just one issue the Motor City's gay community has. Another is that the community lacks visibility.

CLUELESSNESS AND LGBT PREVALENCE

Many people believe roughly 10 percent of the U.S. population is gay. However, no recent credible researcher or poll has ever found the number that identify as LGBT to be even 5 percent. In a 2015 Gallup poll looking at America's top 50 metro areas, San Francisco, the gayest city in America, had the highest percentage of LGBT people at 6.2 percent, which was still well short of the 10 percent statistic people throw out.[40] The most cited academic studies regarding LGBT statistics come from demographer Gary Gates and the Williams Institute at UCLA, which estimate 3.8 percent of America identifies as LGBT.[41]

Americans are so grossly unaware of the actual size of our national gay population that many people drastically *overestimate* the 10 percent myth. Gallup polls in 2011 and 2015 found that more than half of Americans believe one in five people are gay.[42] And more than a third of Americans believed that at least *25 percent* of the population is gay (which would make America statistically as gay as the Freddie Mercury–led band Queen).

The *Atlantic* put out a policy-based think piece in response to Gallup's 2011 poll titled "Americans Have No Idea How Few Gay People There Are." The article argues that Americans' overestimation of the prevalence of LGBT people can actually contribute to homophobic fears. Here's why:

Such a misunderstanding of the basic demographics of sexual behavior and identity in America has potentially profound implications for the acceptance of the gay-rights agenda. On the one hand, people who overestimate the percent of gay Americans by a factor of 12 seem likely to also wildly overestimate the cultural impact of same-sex marriage. On the other hand, the extraordinary confusion over the percentage of gay people may reflect a triumph of the gay and lesbian movement's decades-long fight against invisibility and the closet.[13]

Given the overestimates of LGBT people, it's clear that gay people are no longer invisible to mainstream society as they were prior to New York's Stonewall riots, which sparked the gay liberation movement in 1969. However, while overestimating implies increased visibility, the overestimates also illustrate a radical misperception that's at least partially inflamed by fear and ignorance.

The Importance of Visibility

Detroit is a huge city, taking up 142.9 square miles, an area large enough to fit Manhattan, Boston, and San Francisco *ALL* within its limits.[44] So while a great many Detroiters are accepting enough that gay people generally feel comfortable living all over the city, the large size and lack of visibility means finding other gay people in Detroit isn't always easy. "The gay community is not integrated in Detroit, it is invisible," says Joe Posch, a gay entrepreneur who lives in Detroit. "And that is a huge difference. Without visibility, where can you reliably go to meet new people, for friends or dating? Or if you are new to the city, how do meet other gay people or get involved with the community if it isn't easy to locate?"[45]

A gay district would benefit the area's LGBTs for social and business reasons, Posch says. He would like to see a district with gay bars, restaurants, coffee shops, and businesses. "Having businesses with gay appeal within close proximity would help promote business for everybody," he says. "It would be good for networking, which would help promote business growth."[46]

Posch also thinks a gay district in Detroit could add value to the gay community by offering services that cater to the unique needs of LGBTs. Having gay doctors, places that share information on HIV prevention, education, and testing, and community centers where gay people can congregate are some social services a gay district could offer, he says. But it all comes back to visibility. "Detroit's gay community needs a voice, and that only comes from banding together," Posch writes.[47]

Urban studies researcher Richard Florida believes so strongly that large populations of LGBT people can indicate economic growth that he developed a Bohemian-Gay Index, which Stephen Colbert quipped "may sound like another name for the San Francisco phone book." The index, which is measured by concentrations of LGBT people and artist types, correlates with rising home values, according to Florida.[48] Although it wasn't Florida's intention to do so, he claims his indices helped real estate agents identify hot real estate.[49] This echoes what real-estate agents told Erik Bottcher, a former New York City LGBT community liaison: "If you want to find a new area to invest in, follow the gay community."[50] It's also why Colbert jokes, "The same-sex chickens have come home to gentrify their roost."

Given the fact that many gays have left Detroit, it's not surprising the area's concentration of LGBT people ranks in the bottom half of the nation's fifty largest metro areas.[51] While Metro Detroit's rank of thirtieth might not seem too terribly low, it's relevant to recall that unlike most metro areas, many LGBT people in the Detroit area are concentrated in the suburbs rather than the city. With that in mind, the rank of thirtieth is actually very generous as far as Detroit *city* is concerned. Policy makers aren't unaware of this. In 2003, the Michigan Department of Labor and Economic Growth sponsored an event called the Creating Cool Conference: Linking Culture, Community, and the Economy, where Florida was the keynote speaker. More than 1,400 city planners, community organizers, arts organization reps, politicians, and developers attended the conference, according to *PrideSource*, Michigan's main LGBT newspaper.[52] At the conference, Florida told the crowd that Michigan needs to be more accepting of LGBT people. "It's like 'Queer eye for a straight city,'" said Florida. He added, "It is not just important that a city have gay people—there must be visible, open gay couples and people who are known to be gay."[53]

Although gay enclaves have historically developed organically, a group of Detroit community leaders are betting that a gayborhood can be built and refurbished like the very homes gays often fix up when gentrifying areas.*

If You Build It, They Will Come

Curtis Lipscomb is a gay man in Detroit who runs a black gay pride parade and is the founder and executive director of LGBT Detroit, a center for LGBT individuals in Detroit. For several years, he's been meeting with a group of people from the banking, nonprofit, and community development sectors of the city who want to build a gay district in Detroit.

The district, which could include retail locations, housing, cultural institutions, places of worship, and gay

---

* Several sources I talked to hinted that LGBT people, particularly gay men, are more sensitive to design, fashion, and architecture. Because of that, gay men love fixing up historic homes, they said. Which would be another reason why they're more attracted to old city districts than the general population. *Flag Wars* has a great anecdote about this concept where two gay aspiring homeowners talk about gay gentrification and restoring homes. For simplicity's sake, I will call them "Adam" and "Steve."

 Adam: I've seen this in other cities too. It's the gay community that actually goes in…

 Steve: It happens all over. I saw it happen in Boston.

 Adam: Yeah, where no one else will go into these neighborhoods.

 Steve: I think a lot of us just have that ability. We can look at a building that other people would say, "Oh, what a dump." And I would look at it and say, "Oh. That's a beautiful building." You know. And I would, like, almost feel compassion for the building and want to save it.

bars, would likely be developed in northwest Detroit. Regardless of which neighborhood in Detroit this group decides to start a gayborhood in, they're going to have to convince people to get over all the bad press about Detroit if people are to move there. But Lipscomb is convinced Detroit has positive qualities its suburbs don't, such as better night-life, more gay bars and art venues, and cheaper rent. And he's not the only gay person who sees more value in living in Detroit than in its suburbs.

In a 2006 *PrideSource* article, a gay Metro Detroiter talks about wanting to move out of Metro Detroit because of the city's lack of a major gay district.[54] And what the gay-friendly suburb Ferndale offers isn't inclusive enough to sway this man, who told reporters, "It [Ferndale] doesn't have a solid chunk of gay businesses all within walking distance of each other. It doesn't compare to Lakeview in Chicago or the North End in Columbus, Ohio... The complaints I've heard from a lot of young gay people who want to move [are] the lack of a gay neighborhood, the sprawl—how you have to drive everywhere to get anything and the [poor] quality of gay nightclubs."[55][†] To address

---

† Many popular news outlets have run stories about how young professionals dislike urban sprawl and prefer dense, walkable cities over the suburbs. However, as Harvard economist Edward Glaeser notes, there are many "creative" people (who Richard Florida claims are central to growing economies) who like living in the suburbs, relying on automobiles, and residing in good school districts with low taxes. "After all, there is plenty of evidence linking low taxes, sprawl, and safety with growth," Glaeser writes. While the metro Detroiter quoted by *PrideSource* has a point that Detroit is sprawling while many gayborhoods (e.g.,

these complaints, the group behind the gayborhood development *can* contribute to bringing a centralized gay district
together and improving the quality of gay nightclubs. But
Detroit's physical sprawl is out of their hands, as are many
other issues (such as high crime, urban blight, and under-
funded city services) affecting LGBT people, and people in
general, in the area.

Other ways cities can make themselves more gay friendly
are by having LGBT liaisons in multiple sectors of city
government, training police to be sensitive to hate crimes, and
establishing LGBT committees in chambers of commerce.[56]
Detroit briefly had a LGBT representative in the mayor's
office. It also implemented a liaison in its police department.
But with the city's high debt, realistically it probably cannot
afford to add liaisons or fund more police training. A more
realistic route for debt-ridden cities like Detroit to become
more gay friendly is to focus on increasing LGBT visibility
and perceived acceptance.

Lipscomb says people in city government—city council
members, police chiefs, and those in the mayor's office—
have expressed support for the project.[57] He hopes these
public officials, as well as business and community leaders,
can help him and his colleagues identify more resources,
partners, and companies by supporting the campaign and
helping to advertise it.

---

the Castro, Boystown) are in dense areas accessible by mass transit, there are also
other prominent gayborhoods (e.g., West Hollywood, San Diego's Hillcrest) that
are spread out and only accessible by automobile.

THE ALLEGED DEMISE ═══
OF LGBT DISTRICTS

Most of the gay-driven economic developments in the U.S. happened decades ago in neighborhoods like New York's Greenwich Village, Boston's South End, San Francisco's Castro, Washington's Dupont Circle, and Los Angeles County's West Hollywood. Today, as LGBT people gain more acceptance, there is less incentive for gay people to congregate together, because a major reason many gays and lesbians originally moved into centralized areas was for safety purposes. Because increased gay acceptance now allows LGBT people to safely live anywhere among the masses and blend in, gay districts are now irrelevant, some people say. Although the necessity of gayborhoods has declined for some gay people, Amin Ghaziani, sociologist and author of the book *There Goes the Gayborhood?*, whose title inspired the name of this chapter, disagrees that gay neighborhoods are no longer necessary or that gay people feel safe living anywhere in America.

Although overall acceptance of gays has increased, LGBT people still face discrimination. Ghaziani points out that a 2011 study found that gay couples are 25 percent more likely to be rejected by landlords looking for tenants than straight couples are.[58] However, when gay couples apply for housing in gay neighborhoods, their rates of rejection plunge. Gay marriage may now be legal, but it could take years for Americans' acceptance of LGBT people to catch up to the law. As of

2011, 20.4 percent of Americans still preferred to avoid having gay neighbors.[59] And Florida says that about 45 percent of his survey respondents said their communities were "bad" or "very bad" places for LGBT people to live.[60] "If our society is truly and totally post-gay, then in theory these [LGBT] households would be randomly dispersed," Ghaziani writes. "But such is not the case."[61] Rather than being evenly dispersed throughout the U.S., LGBT people are currently concentrated in California, south Florida, and throughout the Northeast, which are areas tolerant of diversity.[62]

There are scores of think pieces lamenting an eventual extinction of gayborhoods, but the real test as to whether gayborhoods will survive depends on whether LGBT people think gayborhoods are still necessary and worth supporting. In a 2013 Pew survey of LGBT Americans, only a minority (19 percent) said "there is a lot of social acceptance for the LGBT population today." The majority (59 percent) acknowledged "some" acceptance, while 21 percent said there is "little to no acceptance today."[63] Given the low levels of perceived acceptance, it makes sense that a majority (56 percent) of the LGBT people polled by Pew agreed that "it is important to maintain places like LGBT neighborhoods and bars." Although gayborhoods are certainly changing, it's a bit premature to project their extinction.

Selling a Bankrupt City

Detroit's monumental downfall has been well documented. In about a hundred years, it went from "the Motor City" to "Motown" to "Rock City" to "bankrupt city." But there still are things about Detroit that make the city attractive to LGBT and progressive people. And in turn, LGBT and creative individuals can help bring Detroit back to prominence.

With annual deficits, massive debt, and an aging and declining population, Detroit's problems reflect those of many American cities. Except of course, Detroit's are much more pronounced. The bankruptcy may have helped get things rolling by restructuring financial woes. But it cannot correct long-term demographic problems. Detroit needs people. And Detroit needs cash. And if the city continues to raise taxes on those who live there, then even more people might defect and take their business elsewhere.[64]* Which means instead of raising taxes, more people are needed *to tax.*

But with high crime and abysmal public schools, people with children aren't likely going to be moving in soon. However, Detroit's strong music and art scene, deep history, and cheap housing make it attractive to artists, young professionals, and childless folks. Many of these people prefer authenticity over comfort. They don't like strip malls and Chili's restaurants cluttering up their downtown. And one thing Detroit has in abundance is its own flavor.

Most stores and restaurants in Detroit are locally owned, not franchised. In neighborhoods like Indian Village and

---

*   Detroit already taxes its residents more than any other city in Michigan.

Woodbridge, there are beautiful, weathered houses being sold for chump change. Detroit is also the birthplace of the American automobile, iconic pop music, and Prohibition smuggler routes and speakeasies. While ruin porn and dilapidated factories like the Packard Plant get much attention, some abandoned buildings such as Michigan Central Station have a haunting elegance that isn't found in your run-of-the-mill American city. On top of that, Detroit has a gorgeous riverwalk down Hart Plaza where people can stroll across marble squares as they look southward to Canada over the clear-watered Detroit River.* And just a breezy three-hour drive north of the city lies Northern Michigan, where the Great Lakes, rolling hills, and changing leaves create some of the most picturesque scenery in America. There's so much hidden potential in Detroit that for a second you forget about the murders, crumbling factories, corrupt politics, and crippling population loss. But that hidden potential is useless to LGBT and creative people if there isn't an atmosphere of tolerance. And that perception is for better or worse largely determined by public figures.

That's why, when Mayor Mike Duggan was campaigning prior to the 2013 primary election, Posch told Duggan he needed to make a statement saying gay people were welcome in the city. Considering it was 2013, Duggan thought LGBT people felt accepted in the city, he told Posch. Duggan didn't think he needed to release a statement on the issue, figuring that it was somewhat common sense in today's age that

---

*   Not a typo. Windsor, Ontario, is south of Detroit.

everyone should feel accepted. But being a gay man in Detroit, Posch thought differently. "Given the ignorant comments of Kwame Kilpatrick and the avoidance of the topic by other officials, the perception of many gay people was that Detroit was hostile toward them," Posch says.[65]

On November 5, 2013, Mike Duggan was elected mayor of Detroit. In his acceptance speech, he made what Posch claims was the first positive mention of gay people by a Detroit mayor in recent history, or perhaps ever. "The way we are going to rebuild this city is to value every single person in our community," Duggan said. "It will no longer matter if you are black, brown, or white. It will no longer matter if you are Christian, Jewish, or Muslim. It will not matter if you are gay or straight. We want all of your talents. You're all going to be equally valued and welcomed, because only in that way will we rebuild the kind of Detroit everyone in this city deserves."[66]

To many people, Duggan's single sentence mentioning sexual orientation might not be a big deal. But to Posch, an active member in Metro Detroit's gay community, the statement meant enough to inspire him to write an editorial for the state's largest newspaper, the Detroit Free Press.

So, if Detroit's development leaders are serious about attracting people to the city to combat its dwindling tax base, it would be in their best interest to continue to engage the area's LGBT residents in a very public fashion. Though it may be too late for a gay-driven economic force to develop organically in Detroit, it's not too late for the city to try to connect to and benefit from its LGBT residents.

Lipscomb and his group will face many obstacles in

building an LGBT district from scratch, which means it may take a lot of time and money to pull off. And even *if* they are able to bring it all together, a gayborhood won't "save" Detroit, because no single group, policy, or business plan alone can correct the city's deep-rooted structural dysfunction. But perhaps Detroit can take another affordable step toward recovery by recognizing the economic power of its LGBT people.

= 6 =

the power of porn

A LOOK AT HOW EROTICA SHAPES OUR TECHNOLOGY AND EVERYDAY LIVES

Because of its taboo reputation, porn analysis is controversial in a country where many people oppose even basic sexual education in public schools. This polarization runs all the way to the Oval Office, where strategic leaders use emotion provoked by pornography debates as political capital. Held over the head of constituents by politicians, porn's dividing power is further fueled by agenda-driven groups and ignorant and overworked media members, which contributes to an obliteration of the public's understanding of statistical reality. Americans simply have no idea how the frequency of sexually related behaviors—such as rape, divorce, or contraceptive use—has changed over time. And that increased porn access, which many assume is associated with sexual violence, actually correlates with *fewer* rapes. Data about sex-related behaviors get lost in shouting matches as people twist research findings to promote disguised personal moral imperatives.

Despite all the conversations that porn provokes, its true power remains hidden to most people. Porn isn't just a sexual commodity that elicits shame or orgasm. It's an incredibly influential economic force that shapes everyday habits by subtly dictating behaviors such as how people view movies and purchase consumer products.

Presidential Porn Commissions

Porn and politics go together like matches and gasoline— when they mix, the result is often explosive and dangerous. The human aversion to rationally examining the social and societal effects of porn and to avoid emotional moralizing can even be seen in America's most powerful political positions. In the 1970s and '80s, two presidential commissions set out to examine the effects of porn on society. The conclusions from both commissions ended up supporting the party platform of the president in charge during each respective commission's inception.

President Lyndon Johnson set up a "Commission on Obscenity and Pornography" to study things such as the effect of porn on "crime and other antisocial conduct."[1] Published in 1970, the report found "no evidence to date that exposure to explicit sexual materials plays a significant role in the causation of delinquent or criminal behavior among youths or adults."[2] The report concluded that porn wasn't a big social problem, that there was no evidence that it was harmful, and that Americans should focus more on improving sex education than on legislating obscenity.[3] By the time the report was released, Richard Nixon had taken over the White House. Nixon, a Republican, was not pleased with the report's conclusions:

> I have evaluated that report and categorically reject its morally bankrupt conclusions and major recommendations. So long as I am in the White House, there will be no relaxation of the national effort to control and eliminate smut from our national life... Smut should not be simply contained at its present level; it should be outlawed in every State in the Union.[4]

Given Nixon's visceral reaction to the idea that porn might not be overtly harmful, and his pledge to head a "citizens' crusade against the obscene,"[5] it shouldn't be terribly surprising that when fellow Republican Ronald Reagan set up his own porn commission years later, it found results more in line with the GOP's values. In 1986 Reagan's commission released the Meese Report (named after then U.S. Attorney General Edwin Meese), which concluded that pornography was harmful to society by causing rape, facilitating prostitution, and being linked to organized crime.[6*]

---

* An ironic thing about the porn-condemning Meese Report is that the nature of the report itself was quite pornographic. Kauffman noted, "The taxonomic skills of the commissioners would inspire envy in Sade: they alphabetized the porn,

As gender-studies scholar Linda Kauffman notes, although both commissions could be viewed as political spectacles, the Meese Report under Reagan was "flagrantly ideological."[7] (Two members of the Meese Commission who rejected the report were Judith Becker, a Columbia University clinical psychologist who treated victims of sexual crimes, and Ellen Levine, then editor of *Woman's Day* magazine. Because the Meese Report was quickly thrown together within a year and had a mere $500,000 budget, they claimed a "full airing of the differences" between its members was impossible, adding, "No self-respecting investigator would accept conclusions based on such a study.")[8]

Adjusted for inflation, the commission under Johnson had sixteen times the resources as the commission under Reagan.[9] Johnson's team spent two years going over results, funded more than eighty studies examining porn's effects, and included a mix of liberals and conservatives (which included clergy members, former congressmen, sociologists,

---

detailing in *Dragnet*-style prose the acts, positions, and perversions involved." After the commission's *Final Report* came out, ACLU lawyer Barry Lynn stated, "I fully defend my government's right to publish filth." Feminist activist Susie Bright quipped, "I masturbated to the Meese Commission Report, until I nearly passed out—it's the filthiest thing around! And they know it." The *New York Times* reported that religious bookstores, who typically agreed with the commission's call for an anti-porn campaign, were "refusing to stock or display the book for fear that the vulgar language in it and its graphic descriptions of sexual acts will offend their customers." A manager of a Christian bookstore told the *Times*, "We got two copies in but I don't want to put them out on the shelves. I agree with the commission's findings, but there are many things objectionable in the book."

criminologists, and lawyers) to research and discuss the social effects of porn. It commissioned original research, invited more than a hundred organizations to express their views, and used a quarter of its report as a proposal for sex education. Reagan's team funded no original studies.[10]

The Meese Report recommended that states change obscenity verdicts from misdemeanors to felonies and that anyone found guilty serve a minimum one-year jail sentence.[11] These recommendations aren't surprising, considering the chairman of the report, Henry Hudson, was known for suing video stores for renting pornos, and the report's executive director, Alan Sears, sent letters to drugstores and convenience stores warning them that if they sold *Playboy* they would be identified in the commission's report as pornography distributors. Another commissioner, Rev. Bruce Ritter, suggested the government condemn pornography as well as homosexuality—before it came to light that he used funds from a charity he founded to have sex with young male prostitutes.[12]

From collegiate town-hall debates to presidential commissions, loud political rhetoric gets people's attention. But as common as it may be, it's a poor lens for examining porn's actual effects on society. To get at what's actually going on, it's best to ignore politicians and focus on social science and data.

Porn Up, Rape Down

For many years, people have accused porn of being associated with the worst kinds of human behavior. "Pornography is the theory, rape is the practice," feminist Robin Morgan wrote in 1977.[13] The authors of *The Porn Trap: The Essential Guide to Overcoming Problems Caused by Pornography* imply that porn contributes to divorce and irresponsible sex. Feminist author Andrea Dworkin insisted porn leads to sexual abuse of women.[14] According to former U.S. Senator Rick Santorum, "Pornography is toxic to marriages and relationships. It contributes to misogyny and violence against women."[15] And a whole host of experimental studies show correlations between porn consumption and sexual aggression. So why hasn't the internet's massive proliferation of porn led to a *Mad Max*–like dystopia full of rape, debauchery, and abandoned women? And why is it that instances of rape have actually declined as porn use has risen?

Northwestern University law professor Anthony D'Amato found that reports of rape declined 85 percent per capita in the U.S. from 1980 to 2004, while porn availability significantly increased during this time because of the internet. To show the importance of internet access (which is associated with porn access) in reducing rape, D'Amato compared rape occurrences in states with the highest internet access and states with the lowest internet access. The four states with the highest internet access saw a combined 27 percent decrease in rape reports, while the states with the lowest internet access saw a combined 53 percent increase.[16]

Taking D'Amato's findings further, economist Todd Kendall found that, from 1998 to 2003, U.S. rape rates fell most for the groups of people who put in a lot of time and risk to access porn prior to the internet.[17] In other words, the rape incidence by teenagers who lived with their parents fell more than rape incidence by older adults. The main reason: pornography was more restricted for teenagers prior to the internet. Kendall found that for every ten-percentage-point increase in internet access, reported rape declined 7.3 percent. Not only did states that quickly adopted the internet see rape rates decline faster, but the effect was largest in states with high male-to-female ratios. This implied that in environments with few potential mates, males were more likely to substitute porn viewing (which was easier to access, thanks to the internet, and was typically coupled with masturbation) for sexually assaulting women. He did not find similar correlations between internet access and declines in other crimes. These findings led Kendall to argue for internet access as a *substitute*, not a motivation, for rape.

In a meta-analysis of experimental studies and real-world violent crime data, criminal-justice researchers Christopher Ferguson and Richard Hartley conclude, "Evidence for a causal relationship between exposure to pornography and sexual assault is slim and may, at certain times, have been exaggerated by politicians, pressure groups, and some social scientists… It is time to discard the hypothesis that pornography contributes to increased sexual assault behavior."[18] Looking beyond American statistics, sex researcher Milton Diamond examined pornography's effects in Canada, Japan, Czech Republic, Croatia, Denmark, West Germany, Finland, China, and Sweden, and concluded, "It has been found everywhere scientifically investigated that as pornography has increased in availability, sex crimes have either decreased or not increased."[19]*

These studies point toward porn being a *potential* substitute to rape for *some* men, because of its ability to release sexual tension. But these large-scale, real-world statistics have many confounding variables. The causation behind the correlation remains uncertain. D'Amato theorizes that porn may have demystified sex and made it less appealing for some people to seek no matter the consequence. He also mentions declining crack usage, women being taught to avoid dangerous situations, increased incarceration rates, and sex education. But without taking into account increased porn access, none of those factors could explain the significant drop in rape, he writes.[20]

Although these researchers have shown that increased porn usage is not associated with increases in sexual assault, there are still many people who insist that porn causes sexual violence.

---

*   It is important to note that increases in porn availability signal many things aside from mere tech advances. In some cases, they indicate a country is becoming more progressive. Some of the countries mentioned above legalized porn after ridding themselves of communism. In these instances, increased porn availability accompanied many political, economic, societal, and psychological changes. Also, declines in porn can mimic declines in violent crime in general. Anytime different cultures and countries are compared over different time periods, there are going to be too many variables to draw a direct *cause* between them. Nevertheless, Diamond and other researchers have found an interesting, seemingly universal trend: that as porn access increases, sexual crime rates tend to decrease or stay put.

Pornographic Lab Studies

Critics of D'Amato, Kendall, and Diamond point out that decades of lab research shows that watching porn increases aggressive attitudes in men, thus leading men to resort to sexual violence against women. It's this "wealth of research" that people such as Santorum refer to when they want to use porn as a tool to sway votes. The problem with citing "research," without providing any actual citations or further context, is that the studies concluding that porn turns men into inconsiderate sex fiends and the studies correlating declines in rape with increased porn accessibility measure entirely different things.

If you look through the academic literature on porn and aggression, you'll typically come across studies like this: A group of male college students take a questionnaire regarding their attitudes toward women. The students then watch some porn, and take a similar questionnaire immediately after that. After watching porn, young men report feeling more aggres-sive. Therefore, porn is said to cause sexual aggression in men.

But measuring attitudes in a lab setting while artificially limiting people's regular responses (in this case, the natural response would be to masturbate to the porn) has little generalizability to the *real world*. As the economist Steven Landsburg wrote, "The experience of viewing porn on the internet, in the privacy of one's own room, typically culmi-nates in a slightly messier but far more satisfying experi-ence—an experience that could plausibly tamp down some of the same aggressions that the *pornus interruptus* of the labora-tory tends to stir up."[21] However, most institutional review boards (committees who review and authorize research projects while axing proposals that could get their institution into ethical or legal trouble) will not approve of research that involves college kids jerking off, so academics are handcuffed in obtaining any actual telling data here.

Though there's evidence that an increase in porn availability coincides with a decrease in rape, there could be other hidden factors driving this relationship. And even if porn is an alternative outlet for some potential rapists, there may be other individual sexual deviants who become more likely to victimize others after watching porn.[22]* There's certainly too much uncertainty to declare unequivocally that *porn prevents rape*. But because so many people believe that porn *causes* sexual violence, it's important to know *real-world* statistics show that, if anything, the inverse appears more likely to be true and that, in some cases, porn may act as a substitute for rape.[23]† Given the common misperceptions large chunks of

---

*   To assume rape is *only* influenced by sexual factors would be wrongheaded, as rapists also can have a lust for power and can exert all sorts of abnormal psychology. However, rape isn't about power *or* sex, which is a false dichotomy along the lines of virgin *or* whore, evolution *or* God. In many cases, rape is about power *and* sex, and the mix between the two varies per perpetrator. As anthropologist Donald Symons writes, "Sex and power are not antithetic; human motives are complex, intertwined, and often conflicting, and perhaps no human act results from a single, pure impulse. Surely no completed rape has ever occurred in which the rapist did not experience some sexual feeling, and very likely no rape has ever occurred in which this was the only feeling the rapist experienced."

†   Even real-world stats are not infallible. Rape is underreported for many reasons ranging from social stigma to distress brought on by the legal system. However, underreported rape doesn't negate the research discussed in this chapter, because it's

the population have regarding porn and its alleged association with sexual violence, it makes sense that porn's true influence slips by undetected, even as it guides our everyday lives.

=== STATISTICAL SLIPPAGE ===

There is a big demand for messages purporting that
porn is associated with all sorts of negative sexual issues
such as disease, abuse, and divorce. But despite what
many believe, as porn access increased, there have been
improvements in many of these areas.

Divorce rates are one statistic that is grossly misun-
derstood by the public. When giving the dish on the last
celebrity breakup, TV news reporters like to generalize
Hollywood's romantic struggles by informing viewers
that divorce rates are "50 percent and climbing." But
contrary to popular belief, divorce rates aren't rising.

---

hard to rationally argue that there's much less reporting of sexual crimes today than
in the past. If anything, given the increased emphasis on education, prosecution, and
victim rights, it seems likely that victims would report crimes *more often* today than
in past decades. On the flip side of unreported rape and rapists escaping prosecution,
there are other things muddying stats like the *occasional* false-rape accusation, as
seen in high-profile cases at Duke and the University of Virginia. These select cases
are dangerous to the wrongly accused as well as to the many sexual-assault victims
who seek justice. As Harvard Law professor and former U.S. federal judge Nancy
Gertner writes: "If there is a widespread perception that the balance has tilted from
no rights for victims to no due process for the accused, we risk a backlash. Benighted
attitudes about rape and skepticism about women victims die hard. It takes only a
few celebrated false accusations of rape to turn the clock back."

Divorce has considerably declined since the 1970s and 1980s, when no-fault laws first became common. And many of those divorces in the early 1980s were initiated by people, primarily women, escaping bad marriages that would have been more difficult to end previously.[24]

Out of marriages that began in the 1990s, about 70 percent reached their fifteenth anniversary, up from 65 percent of 1970s and 1980s marriages.[25] Marriages in the 2000s are dissolving less often yet, and if the trend continues, economist Justin Wolfers predicts that among people who are currently getting married, about two-thirds of today's marriages *won't* end in divorce.[26] According to the authors of *Sacred Cows: The Truth about Divorce and Marriage*, the "50 percent" factoid is a myth generated by the media's reliance on statistics that come from family-focused special-interest groups. Young couples today are actually expected to have fewer divorces than their parents' generation.[27]

Another common claim among "pro-family organizations" is that porn helps facilitate a hypersexualized culture where our youth will go wild. But according to the Centers for Disease Control and Prevention, in the past quarter-century, rates of several STDs,[28] abortion,[29] and teenage births have declined.[30] Today's youth also use contraception more often,[31] have less sex,[32] and use drugs and alcohol less often[33] than previous generations. The point here isn't that increased porn access has led to these changes, but that people are able to lobby for political position by linking porn to sexual assault, divorce, and just about anything involving sex, for that matter, because the public has no clue as to how frequently these behaviors actually occur in our society or how they've changed over time.

It's Been around the Block

If prostitution is the world's oldest profession, then porn is the world's oldest art form. And it's an art form that has always been at the heart of innovation. According to Patchen Barss in *The Erotic Engine: How Pornography Has Powered Mass Communication from Gutenberg to Google*, "From the earliest known examples of human beings using a medium to express themselves—painting, carving, drawing—sexual representation has been at the heart of advances in communication. It has never stopped."[34] While there's evidence that erotica helped popularize early technological advances such as printing presses, the research on ancient technologies is thin on data and relies on inferences and projections. So we'll stick to modern technologies, because the evidence is clearer in showing how porn drives many products we use in everyday life.

Pornographers don't usually invent the technologies (such as the VCR and e-commerce services) they help make popular. Rather, their influence comes from being early adopters. Because pornography is somewhat taboo and many people are ashamed to admit usage, pornographers risk lots of money to adopt uncertain technologies that make porn access easier and more private. Here are a few of them.

The VCR

While major movie studios now rely heavily on home-video releases to boost revenue, they initially opposed releasing their films for use in private homes. "I say to you that the VCR is to the American film producer and the American public as the Boston Strangler is to the woman home alone," the president of the Motion Picture Association told Congress in 1982.[35] It took a Supreme Court decision in 1984—*Sony Corp. of America v. Universal City Studios Inc.*—to determine that viewers recording shows at home didn't violate copyright law. With a 5–4 decision in favor of Sony's Betamax, the Court ruled that home recordings and storage of copyrighted material were legal and "fair use" of a product, and that any product "capable of substantial non-infringing use" could be legally sold, even if the product was often used to infringe copyrights.[36] The ruling of this case paved the way for websites like YouTube, Netflix, and iTunes to upload and distribute copyrighted works. Had one more justice decided to dissent, the videocassette player wouldn't have gotten the opportunity to hook up with porn peddlers, and movie-studio business models would probably look much different today, as would much of the internet.[37]

After the film companies' narrow victory, pornographers partnered with VCR manufacturers. According to Frederick Wasser in *Veni, Vidi, Video: The Hollywood Empire and the VCR*, it was pornographers, not major movie studios, who built up the necessary infrastructure for trading prerecorded tapes.[38] Adult video stores started exchanging recorded tapes years before Hollywood studios cooperated with video rental shops. The adult stores created club memberships to obtain credit information from customers, which gave the stores leverage against customers who chose to hold onto tapes past their due date.[39] Mainstream video retailers such as Blockbuster and Hollywood Video would eventually adopt this business model. Another way pornography helped build video-store infrastructure is that in the early days of the VCR, sex tapes constituted a sizable part of rental stores' inventory. Through the mid-1970s, about 90 percent of videotapes purchased in America were pornographic. While that percentage would significantly drop, in the mid-1980s X-rated titles still accounted for about half of all videotape sales.[40]*

The popular story regarding porn and VCRs generally goes like this: Betamax and VHS were battling for market share. Although Beta had better video quality and debuted before VHS, VHS overcame Beta by distributing porn before Beta. By the time Beta began to sell porn, it was too late. Beta's market share had been decimated, and VHS triumphed—so much so that many people born after 1980 have never even heard of Betamax.

It's not an outlandish story, given the way porn can sway consumer habits, but it's not exactly true. And it actually sells porn's influence short.

---

* As one technology is embraced, oftentimes another is discarded. The VCR transformed the adult entertainment industry by bringing pornography out of theaters and into living rooms and bedrooms. "It is estimated that there were 1,500 theaters devoted to adult movies in 1980. By 1985 there were an estimated 700 such theaters, down to 250 in 1989," Wasser writes.

Both VHS and Beta offered porn early on. Even though Betamax had higher video resolution, VHS beat Beta because VHS had superior marketing, offered cheaper machines and tapes, and allowed longer recording times.[41] Porn alone didn't lead VHS to victory over Beta. Rather, after VHS started dominating the consumer market, "porn companies simply followed the money," said Frederick Lane, author of *Obscene Profits: The Entrepreneurs of Pornography in the Cyber Age.*[42] Porn's influence was actually greater than leading one company over another. Because the entire VCR market—both VHS *and* Beta—would have likely folded early on without porn availability.[43]

Less than 1 percent of households owned a VCR in 1979, yet home videos survived because early adopters kept the market alive.[44] Many of these early adopters were pornography viewers who paid top dollar for both the machine and accompanying tapes, forking over as much as $300 for a single pornographic video in 1979, according to Barss.[45] That's about a thousand bucks in 2018 dollars. It's hard to imagine people ever paying those sums given all the free porn that's now easily accessible, but early technology adopters always pay big premiums to be on the cutting edge. Although initial VCR sales were low, enough revenue came from the loads of cash blown by porn consumers to encourage investors. Porn kept the VCR market afloat with its high prices even when 99 percent of Americans didn't own a VCR. "Pornography played a major role in the initial years of VCRs by providing customers with a product, and, at the same time, justification for acquiring costly equipment," writes technology historian

Jonathan Coopersmith.[46] Porn also played a major role in popularizing several online technologies.

Internet Influence

The internet's history can be traced all the way back to *Sputnik*'s 1957 launch by the Soviet Union.[47] After the Soviets launched Earth's first artificial satellite, President Dwight Eisenhower promptly created an agency, the Advanced Research Projects Agency (ARPA), in 1958 to develop emerging technologies for the military.[48] Because computers in the late 1950s and early 1960s were primitive, and different networks often had no way to communicate with one another, in the late 1960s the military hired tech company Bolt, Beranek, and Newman to develop a reliable communication network between the military's computers.[49] This network, ARPANET, significantly sped up information transfer between computers and laid the foundation for what eventually became the internet. In the internet's infancy, access was mostly limited to military and university experts.[50] Though the internet's doors were open to commercialization before porn entered the picture, it wasn't until people began sharing smut online that the internet really began transforming from an arcane puzzle that only highly computer-literate individuals could operate to a household fixture that ten-year-olds now find intuitive.[51] As Anthony Lane writes in a *New Yorker* film review, "To make a documentary about the internet that scarcely mentions sex… is like writing a history of gardening and turning your nose up at the roses. (And the manure.)"[52]

Think of the military as the inventor and porn as the entrepreneur who brings the inventor's new technology to the masses. Commercialization of the internet largely stemmed from pornography. During the early to mid-1990s, porn sites were among the only web ventures that "consistently made money," according to Lane. In 2001, Lane wrote, "There is no doubt that adult Web sites have succeeded in turning the internet into a viable place for commerce. It's not simply that profits are being earned by online pornography sites, it's that *a lot* of money is being earned."[53] Without demand for porn, the concept of e-commerce might have died out. Here are some major ways porn influenced online technologies, and in turn, many of contemporary society's everyday habits.

Enter E-Commerce

Porn companies are essentially media companies. And media companies—and many businesses in general, for that matter—usually need a steady flow of advertisers to become profitable. To get advertisers online, porn companies needed to obtain information on customer habits. Most web ventures in the mid-1990s were unable do this, and lost money.[54]

In the internet's infancy, most companies didn't invest in e-commerce services, because they didn't have much incentive to do so. Most people weren't yet comfortable with shopping online, and the revenue-generating potential of e-commerce was very unclear. For most consumer products, there was little upside to gain by taking the risk to purchase a product through an uncertain platform. But porn users were more willing to venture out into the unknown and take risks by purchasing their smut online, because unlike books, CDs, and most other consumer products, purchasing porn in public carried a stigma.[55] The internet gave porn users a route to privatize their taboo purchases and consumer habits, which is why porn users were more willing to put up with the risks and annoyances associated with the early days of online shopping. And, in turn, porn companies were among the first businesses to aggressively pursue customers online.

Porn companies like Cybererotica and Danni's Hard Drive began developing and popularizing tools like web cookies, which stored little pieces of data on customer's browsers so porn companies could see whether customers were new or habitual and what else they liked to browse for online.[56] Using this information, pornographers engaged in affiliate marketing, which is a referral tactic where a business pays another business for bringing traffic to its site. Because pornographic websites drew so much traffic, non-porn companies started placing ads all over porn sites, hoping to lure customers in. This strategy would become a major component of e-commerce as non-porn websites such as Amazon and eBay made it an instrumental part of their business models.[57]*

---

*   "Non-porn" companies were also some of the biggest pornographic profiteers in the 1980s and '90s. In a 1997 article, Eric Schlosser found that as porn use shifted from public theaters and bookstores to being consumed at home via videocassettes, television, and phone hotlines, big profits were being made off porn by businesses outside the sex industry. Local video stores, phone carriers like AT&T, cable companies like Time Warner, and hotel chains like Holiday Inn earned millions by supplying adult content.

Another major aspect of e-commerce pornography has influenced is online credit card transactions.[58]* Porn was about the only thing people were willing to pay for online in the early to mid-1990s.[59] But porn companies faced huge chargeback issues in setting up their own transaction software. Chargeback fraud occurs when a customer purchases a product, but then denies having purchased the product and complains to their credit-card company, demanding a refund. Banks and credit-card issuers absorb the financial losses, and in turn raise fees on their members to recoup the lost funds. Chris Mallick, a former executive of financial intermediary company Paycom Billing Services and whose life story loosely formed the basis of the 2009 movie *Middle Men*, told the *New York Times* in 2002 that porn-related chargebacks often

---

The *New York Times* noted in 2000 that, through subsidiaries like DirecTV, General Motors sold more porn films than *Hustler*. And EchoStar Communications Corp., which relied heavily on Rupert Murdoch's money, made more money on porn than *Playboy*. "We're in the small leagues compared to some of those companies like General Motors or AT&T," *Hustler* publisher Larry Flynt told the *Times*. None of the major "non-porn" companies would go on record for the article. When pressed why, an AT&T official said, "It's the crazy aunt in the attic. Everyone knows she's there, but you can't say anything about it."

* According to a 2001 *Forbes* article by Seth Lubove, Congress inadvertently incentivized people to use credit cards when purchasing porn. When Congress attempted to regulate online porn with the Communications Decency Act of 1996, they "endorsed the use of credit cards for age verification purposes, presumably because kids can't get credit cards," Lubove writes. And even though the Supreme Court struck down the Decency Act, Lubove notes that "porn operators are still shielded from accusations of peddling obscene material to minors so long as they require a credit card."

occur because husbands get buyer's remorse after their wives find out about their porn bills.[60] Paycom Billing Services was just one of many businesses that sprang up to deal as middlemen between porn websites and credit card companies.[61] By operating as "legitimate" and allegedly impartial companies working in the background, the middlemen could represent porn companies' best interests in negotiating fraudulent charges with banks and credit card issuers. Years later, after pornography showed that e-commerce wasn't just a fad but a potentially lucrative business, web giants such as Yahoo! began using third-party payment systems to allow consumers to safely purchase products online with credit cards.[62†]

Accelerating Bandwidth Growth

As important as pornography's influence was to marketing and e-commerce, its biggest online influence comes from increasing bandwidth.[63] Bandwidth is a conduit that allows people to share files online. It's like a pipe that connects computers and networks. Having more bandwidth (widening the pipe) allows people to share bigger files and move them more quickly. Without increasing the demand for bandwidth, porn's online influence would be limited, because file sharing and the internet itself would be significantly restricted without bandwidth advances.[64]

During the early 1990s, when the internet was quite

---

†   Porn is also associated with several other undesirable behaviors such as spam, copyright infringement, fraud, and piracy.

primitive, porn got people sharing more pics and videos online, which created a demand for more bandwidth so consumers could share higher quality and higher quantities of porn. It's no accident many of the first popular interactive chat rooms were porn-centric, or that porn sites pioneered video streaming technologies.[65]

As bandwidth increased, the internet's non-pornographic potential became more evident. "Only when the bandwidth and users were already in place was the internet ready for non-porn services such as YouTube, CNN.com, and Flickr, all of which depended on sending images, text and videos through the very pipelines that were created through the buying, selling, stealing and trading of pornography," Barss writes.[66] Porn got people to demand more bandwidth, which spurred investors to expand the Web's infrastructure. Tech giants like Google and Facebook continue to benefit from the groundwork laid by pornographers. There's no question of whether porn has driven technology. The real question is: What future technologies will pornography influence?

LIBRARIES, PHONE LINES, AND PORN

The last few sections of this chapter show how porn has influenced popular technologies and business strategies. But porn's influence didn't stop at home video recording and the internet—it affected many other technologies that are less visible, but no less interesting, in today's society.

Without dedicated voyeurs wanting to hide nude pictures, society's archiving abilities would possibly be worse off. Microfiche, which libraries use to archive materials, stems from nineteenth-century optical devices called Stanhopes, which allowed people to view microscopic photos without a microscope. Shrinking images to microscopic sizes allowed people to view photographs discreetly. Stanhopes became popular largely because most contained erotic photographs.[67]

Another example of how pornography has influenced technology is how the demand for phone sex affected developing countries' telephone infrastructure. In 1987, Congress introduced the "Telephone Decency Act," which made "obscene" and "indecent" phone calls illegal.[68] "Dial-a-porn" company Sable Communications sued the FCC, which was in charge of screening for lewd phone calls, for violating the First Amendment. Their case, Sable Communications of California v. FCC, reached the Supreme Court in 1989. Justice Byron White delivered the majority opinion and wrote, "Sexual expression which is indecent but not obscene is protected by the First Amendment."[69] Although "indecent" phone calls were now made legal, the Court still upheld the ban on "obscene" phone communication.

Rather than risk crossing the precarious legal zone between "indecent" and "obscene," phone sex providers looked to other countries for business. According to Lane, in 1993 the island of São Tomé brought in $5.2 million worth of sex calls made by Americans being redirected to operators in São Tomé. The island's government made about half a million dollars from its share and used the money to build new telecommunications systems.[70] By trying to stop Americans from having phone sex, Congress inadvertently redistributed income to poorer nations.

There're also plenty of news stories about how adult content popularized CD-ROMs, video game consoles, cameras, and pay-per-view TV. However, the effects of porn on these technologies often get exaggerated as those quoted in the press typically have a vested interest in promoting the power of porn, including the organizer of an international trade show for pornographic CD-ROM products who told the New York Times, "Over all, the adult area of CD-ROM is spearheading quite a bit of growth of general CD-ROM technology."[71] Although it may be true that porn actually pushed CD-ROM technology, it's worth questioning the reliability of the trade show organizer's statement, because porn's proponents exaggerate the economic impact of adult content.

However, while it's easy for adult industry spokespeople to overstate porn's tech influence, it's much harder for anyone to exaggerate porn's ubiquity. Porn is so prevalent in Western society that University of Montreal researchers examining men who never watched pornography had to alter a 2009 study because finding participants was impossible. "We started our research seeking men in their twenties who never consumed pornography," one of the researchers told reporters. "We couldn't find any."[72] With such widespread popularity, porn creeps into lots of economic nooks, many of which we're probably still unaware of.

Where Will We Go from Here?

After experimenting with virtual-reality headsets at the E3 video game tradeshow, a porn executive told *Wired*, "The first thing I think of when I hear of new technology is 'How can I fuck with it?' or 'How can I let people watch me fucking on it?' Usually there's one or the other application if you think hard enough."[73] As porn producers ask themselves similar questions in an era of rapidly expanding technology, what can we expect next from the adult industry?

Most adult content currently focuses on sight and sound. Innovators are trying to expand the senses affected by pornography. In a field called "teledildonics," computer-controlled sex toys guide participants to remote-controlled orgasms. Sometimes the process of adding senses, particularly touch, to the pornographic experience is done through biofeedback. Which is where people gather information about their bodies (e.g., heart rate, skin temperature, etc.) using data-collection tools such as sensors and electrodes so they can alter, manipulate, and improve their experiences.[74] Biofeedback, usually used for health purposes, can also be utilized to control sexual releases.

Relying on bodily data, teledildonics via biofeedback hopes to enhance orgasms through science. This area currently remains more experimental than practical. It also faces opposition from patent trolls, which are lawyers and companies who profit off frivolous lawsuits over vague patents. A 2015 *Gizmodo* article summarizes the practice of patent trolls: "They buy overbroad patents, sue people for infringing, and bet that their victims won't have the money to challenge the patent itself. So the victims just pay the fees, and the trolls get rich."[75] By filing lawsuits based off broad patents, patent trolls can slow down innovation and limit what products come to market.

Current teledildonic products do things such as track people's vital signs during sex and allow users to rate their sexual experience. After enough data gathering, users can compare their vital sign statistics for poor, average, and great experiences, seeing what correlates with being turned on most.[76] Users can monitor these devices while having sex, so they can be cognizant of where their vital signs are relative to their peak sensation levels, which sexual positions most often lead to orgasm, and how many calories they burn during sex.[77] Other products aim to do things like chart muscle activity during sex, so that the data can be sent to a remote partner who can manipulate a sexual device from afar (via a computer or smartphone app) to recreate sexual sensations.[78] These devices could revolutionize "phone sex" by giving people new ways to share sexual sensations with long-distance partners.

Teledildonics has the potential to significantly expand the breadth of haptic technologies.[79] And sometimes the effects of these emerging haptic technologies are realized in odd places—such as expecting parents preparing for childbirth.[80] In 2013, the diaper company Huggies came out with a pregnancy belt that uses touch technology to stimulate the experience of pregnancy.[81] Expectant fathers put on the belt to feel what it would be like to have a baby kicking in the womb.

Another expanding area of technology that people speculate will soon lend itself to pornography is virtual reality (VR). Ever since there's been news about VR headsets that use computer-generated graphics to immerse people in digital worlds that feel "real" to users, there have been accompanying articles exploring VR's pornographic potential. Though most current VR products are crude, there were already porn products tailored to the Oculus Rift, a VR headset acquired by Facebook, even before the headset was made available to the public.[82] Several companies are working to create human-lookalike sex avatars both within VR headsets as well as in real life.[83]

It's been theorized that in the future people will be able to purchase sex "bodysuits" hooked up to haptic interfaces, which allow people to feel the bodily sensations of their partners many miles away. In *Love and Sex with Robots*, artificial intelligence expert David Levy says that in the future, instead of asking "Do you have a condom?" people about to have sex will instead ask their partner, "Is your bodysuit strapped on?" and "Are you connected to the haptic interface?"[84] It's possible that as these products gain traction, sex in virtual worlds, sex through electronic devices, and sex with AI robots could reduce the demand for human prostitution.[85]

Pornographers must continue to innovate if the industry is to maintain profits. New technologies usually have allowed the industry to expand by charging a premium for making porn consumption more privatized, but the internet has been a double-edged sword for the pornography industry.[86]* It increased porn's prevalence and popularity but also facilitated easily accessible free porn and user-created sexual content. As porn producer Colin Rowntree told *Wired* in 2015, "People no longer wanted to pull out their credit cards. But they said: 'Oh, there's this thing called YouPorn. It may be grained and shitty, but at least I can masturbate.'"[87]

Aside from free porn sites such as YouPorn and RedTube, subscription porn sites face competition from people sexting photos and videos, naked pictures on Snapchat, and risqué Instagram accounts. "We have met the future of porn and it is us," Lane says.[88] The rise of free and user-created porn has led to a decline in revenues for the mainstream adult entertainment industry. *The Huffington Post* estimates that since porn's financial peak in the mid-2000s, 80 percent of porn companies have gone defunct or faced significant financial struggles. And a managing editor at adult-entertainment trade publication *XBIZ* says industry revenues were about cut in half from 2004 to 2014.[89]

To combat the ubiquitous free content, porn companies are creating more live and interactive experiences that

---

* Privacy is also a double-edged sword when it comes to porn use and technology. Before VCRs, people had less privacy when consuming porn in that they had to visit a public theater to see movies. But it could be argued that people watching porn on their laptops today actually have less privacy than theatergoers had because websites track endless amounts of information about their visitors, whereas theaters left no paper trail when attendees paid in cash.

require payment. This is done through selling novelty goods from shoots (like the dildo that was used during a specific sex scene), putting on education seminars (to teach couples things such as the dynamics of rope bondage), giving studio tours (live and virtual), opening strip clubs, bars, store-fronts, and restaurants, live web-camming with porn stars, expanding into podcasts and radio, hosting events, crowd-funding content, and creating custom porn packages in which consumers pay premiums to act as pseudo-directors in pornographic films.[90]

The Paradox of Porn

Everyone knows about porn's prevalence, but few realize its true power. According to Coopersmith, "If it were not for the subject matter, pornography would be publicly praised as an industry that has successfully and quickly developed, adopted, and diffused new technologies. But because the subject matter was pornography, silence and embarrassment have been the standard responses."[91]

People have been conditioned to talk about porn in a conspiratorial way. They recite easily remembered mantras such as "pornography causes sexual violence" while conveniently ignoring that fact that rape has declined as porn access significantly increased. But just because real-world data shows increasing porn access *correlates* with rape reduction doesn't mean porn promotes socially desirable behavior or that all anti-porn groups proclaim falsehoods. It just means that instead of relying on the accusation that porn incites violence, anti-porn activists should probably look for a more sound and honest reason to oppose pornography—of which there are many. Most are based on individual morality, which is an entirely different realm from studying social behavior.

The discussion of porn in society is driven by ideology. Although most people have used porn casually, the ones who get quoted in the news belong to two extremes—pro-porn lobbyists and anti-porn zealots hoping to sway voters to their cause. Porn's greatest power isn't in influencing crime rates, one way or the other—it's in influencing many products and services that guide our lives. Until society looks past its steamy content and to its true significance, the actual impact of erotica will remain unheard.

—7—
invisible handjobs

EXAMINING THE HIDDEN RELATIONSHIPS
BETWEEN GOVERNMENTS,
MARKETS, AND BIRTHRATES

n 1968, Donald Duck starred in a short Disney film that implied large Hispanic families cannot support themselves, and will work to exhaustion "if the number of children born is left to chance." The film concluded, "In fact, it [family planning] actually improves the health of mothers and children, because both are better off if children are not born too close together."[1] That same year, *The Population Bomb* made its author Paul Ehrlich a celebrity and a championed guest on Johnny Carson's *Tonight Show* by selling a forecast of overpopulation, mass starvation, and doom that never came true.

Consequences of high birthrates, such as maternal death and resource shortages, remain relevant in the developing world, where high birthrates are needed to replace high child-hood death rates. In those countries, where modern agricul-tural, medical, and technological advancements are often not accessible, leaders want to improve health conditions, slow birthrates, and have fewer people fighting for finite resources. But regarding the world's wealthiest nations, there's a growing body of research warning the exact opposite of what Donald Duck and Ehrlich feared—that if birthrates don't pick up in most Western nations, there could be economic catastrophe because of an aging population with few young workers to support it.

Both countries with unsustainably high birthrates and countries with fertility rates significantly below replace-ment level have incentives, albeit much *different* incentives, to nudge residents into birthing at a particular frequency to benefit their country's economy. Economics often comes off as an arcane and dry subject. But the components of GDP—consumption, investment, government spending, net exports—are affected by how many working-age people live in an economy. And the *number* of working-age people is a function of sexuality and incentives. Examining sex and family formation is critical, because no other unit of capital affects economies like *Homo sapiens*.

Big Brother Birthing

In some areas of Germany, the population has aged so drasti-cally that, about ten years ago, the state instituted a govern-ment program to convert local prostitutes into elder-care nurses to help offset a shortage of workers to care for the large group of retirees. "They have good people skills, aren't easily disgusted, and have zero fear of physical contact. These characteristics set them apart. It was an obvious move," a spokesperson for the welfare program that runs the nursing homes told the *Independent*.[2]

Although the tactic of converting prostitutes into nurses is a pretty exceptional way to address aging concerns, what isn't exceptional is Germany's demographic situation. In many countries, parenthood has become increasingly expensive, which has contributed to aging populations and sagging fertility rates. As policy analyst Phillip Longman writes, "The high cost of parenthood largely results from institutional arrangements designed to better society—equality for women, expanding educational opportunities, income support for the elderly, and heightened concern for child safety and welfare."[3]* The unintended pressure these "arrangements designed to better society" place on fertility rates is problematic, because

---

*   While this chapter examines *political policies* that aim to affect birthrates, it's important to recognize there are *many* other factors influencing fertility rates. Increases in women's education and workforce participation, as well as increased access to contraception and abortion services, tend to be associated with decreases in birthrates. As infant mortality declines and life expectancy climbs, birthrates tend to drop. Countries and states whose residents tend to be religious usually have higher birthrates than similar areas with less religious participation. When areas become more urbanized and fewer people farm for a living, fertility levels drop, as the pool of workers relying on their children for free labor shrinks. People also have fewer children during economic recessions and depressions than when the market is healthy.

as populations start shrinking, there become fewer and fewer workers to support the social welfare, healthcare, and pension benefits of retirees.[4]* With so many countries' fertility rates below replacement level, there's been a recent surge of desperate pro-natalist policies aimed at increasing reproduction, which demographic journalist Jonathan Last catalogues in *What to Expect When No One's Expecting*.[5]†

In 2007, Russia created a family-formation holiday, "Family Contact Day," where workers were given time off and encouraged to get it on. If they had babies nine months later, on "Give Birth to a Patriot on Russia Day," they could win things such as a TV or an SUV, according to Last. Putin then declared 2008 the "Year of the Family." Special benches designed to subtly slide couples closer together were displayed in a Moscow park, billboards were installed that told people to have kids, and July 8 was branded as another new holiday, "Family, Love, and Fidelity Day," to encourage

---

*   While a shortage of young workers is certainly problematic, the "dependency" of elderly people often gets exaggerated by demographers who fear population decline. In many models, the "dependent" population is just those who are at least sixty-five years old. However, as people continue to live longer and healthier lives through advancements in science, they also have become more productive as they age. To correct for the ever-changing nature of "dependency," Winter and Teitelbaum propose that "dependency" should be measured when "remaining life expectancy drops below 15 years rather than the constant of 65 years."

†   Pro-natalist policies are often framed as being in the best interest of working families. However, pro-natalist policies have also been implemented by dictators out of fear that low fertility rates could threaten their countries' political and military power. Hitler, Stalin, Mussolini, and Mao were all aggressively pro-natalist.

people to form families.[6] In 2010, the Korean Ministry of Health, Welfare, and Family Affairs did something similar by turning out the lights in its office buildings at 7:00 p.m. once a month in an attempt to encourage its workers to go home and make babies.[7] According to a *Smithsonian* article, in 2012, Singapore sponsored a "National Night" party where young couples were told to "let their patriotism explode" so their country could achieve the "population spurt it so desperately needs."[8]‡

In Japan, attempts to incentivize babymaking have been even stranger.[9]§ While American parents worry their youth are too obsessed with sex, many Japanese officials fear their country's youth are too apathetic about shagging. According to one survey, more than one-third of Japanese males ages sixteen to nineteen say they have no interest in or are averse to sex.[10] And almost half of women aged sixteen to twenty-four "were not interested in or despised sexual contact."[11] On top of that, about 30 percent of Japanese people under thirty have never even dated.[12] And Japan's National Institute of Population and Social Security Research claims that 90

---

‡   The "National Night" event was sponsored by Mentos—The Freshmaker.

§   Interesting thing about Japan: During its post-WWII occupation, Japanese officials were pressured by American policymakers to legalize abortion. These Americans feared Japan could become hostile if the country became overpopulated and undernourished. So Japan legalized abortion in 1948, well before other industrialized nations followed suit. But it took more than fifty years, until 1999, for the country to legalize birth control pills. Among the major opponents to oral contraception were Japanese abortion doctors who feared that legalizing the Pill would lead to fewer abortions and cut into their income.

percent of young Japanese women believe being single is "preferable to what they imagine marriage to be like."[13]* In a 2013 article in the *Observer*, Abigail Haworth theorized why marriage has become so distasteful in Japan:

> Marriage [in Japan] has become a minefield of unattractive choices. Japanese men have become less career-driven, and less solvent, as lifetime job security has waned. Japanese women have become more independent and ambitious. Yet conservative attitudes in the home and workplace persist. Japan's punishing corporate world makes it almost impossible for women to combine a career and family, while children are unaffordable unless both parents work.[14]†

The sex and dating aversions of Japanese adults have contributed to Japan's low fertility rate of 1.4 births per

---

*   About 60 percent of Japanese women under thirty have never been married. In most Western countries, typically only 30 to 40 percent of women under thirty have never been married. The lack of young Japanese women getting married is a big problem for Japan's fertility rate because births outside of marriage are very rare in Japan. In many Western countries, 30 percent to 50 percent of babies are born outside of marriage, but in Japan, just 2 *percent* of births happen outside of marriage.

†   Low gender equality plus rising female education is a recipe for low fertility all over the world. Teitelbaum says, "Societies in which traditional expectations prevail about women's primary responsibilities for family and childrearing while female education and labor force participation have risen substantially are settings in which work and family are most incompatible and the opportunity costs of childbearing are higher for increasingly well-educated women."

woman, which is well below replacement level and is one of the lowest in the world.[15] The country's population has already peaked, and a Pew report projects Japan's population will age significantly while also losing 15 percent of its people by 2050.[16] The Japanese government predicts the country's population will shrink from 128 million people to 87 million people by 2060, and the government expects that nearly half of those 87 million people will be 65 or older.[17] While demographic projections can be wildly off when predicting so far out in the future, Japan's population has already aged so dramatically that analysts predict adult diapers will outsell baby diapers by 2020,[18] and by 2040, there will likely be a Japanese person more than 100 years old for every Japanese baby born.[19] The country's elderly population has grown so much in recent decades that in 2003 Japan's finance minister, Masajuro Shiokawa, suggested sending retirees to the Philippines. "Japan is aging, and there are so few people to care for them [retirees]," Shiokawa said. "There are so many young people in the Philippines."[20] The director of the Clinic of the Japan Family Planning Association even warned Japan "might eventually perish into extinction" over its sexless ways.[21] So to combat this sex apathy and economic disaster, Japan's government has tried many things to generate a stimulus package between the sheets.

The Japanese government has proposed increasing child allowances, daycare support, and childcare leave in an effort to increase birthrates.[22] While increasing practical benefits such as maternity leave has the potential to influence women in the workplace to have more children (because increased maternity leave theoretically makes it easier for expecting mothers to put work on hold), the potential of these policies to increase fertility rates is lost if the culture in which the policies are implemented isn't supportive of working women in the first place. The practical pro-natalist measures that Japanese officials have proposed will have trouble achieving tangible results, because Japan has been notoriously unsuccessful in achieving gender equality, ranking 111th out of 144 countries, according to the World Economic Forum.[23] There are reports of married women in the workplace being called "devil wives," and about 70 percent of Japanese women leave their jobs after their first child because of inflexible hours and a judgmental corporate culture that makes it difficult for women to combine career and family.[24] Japanese women report that their chances of earning a promotion disappear once they become married because employers assume they'll get pregnant and leave.[25] Former Minister of Health Hakuo Yanagisawa certainly didn't help ease any perceptions of misogyny when he referred to women as "birth-giving machines" in 2007.[26]*

In an attempt to increase fertility rates, Prime Minister Shinzo Abe has advocated for a three-year maternity leave, which would be more likely to work if a three-year absence wouldn't derail the careers of these women, because climbing up the corporate ladder is much more difficult for women in Japan than it is in many Western societies.[27] To promote motherhood, the government considered distributing

---

*   In a follow-up press conference, Yanagisawa told reporters, "My wife scolded me."

notebooks to young women that instructed them on when to have children, warning that it was dangerous to a woman's health to postpone marriage and motherhood. These "Women's Notebooks" also implied that career-oriented and childless women were selfish.[28] By appealing to health fears and cultural shame, the notebooks were supposed to persuade women that they should have children before it's too late. There's no evidence that any of the quirky pro-natalist tactics tried in Singapore, Russia, Korean, or Japan have influenced fertility rates, Last concluded.[29] But not all pro-natalist policies fail. There are a handful of governments that have successfully nudged people into popping out young-lings as part of their civic duty.

Government-Sponsored Babymaking

Some people perceive France to be the world's art center, where modernity is celebrated, and religion and tradition are dismissed. However, the French appear quite committed to parenthood, as France has one of the highest birthrates in Europe, with a 2.0 total fertility rate, which is about 25 percent greater than the European Union average.[30†] "For the economy, Germany is the strong man of Europe, but when it comes to demography, France is our fecund woman," demographer Ron Lesthaeghe told the *Guardian*.[31]

In the 1970s, the French government started giving

---

† France's fertility boost got help from immigration, because immigrant fertility is believed to be higher than that of French natives.

couples stipends for each child they had.[32] That program was later replaced with state-run daycare centers and a family allowance plan that paid families who had two or more children under age sixteen. The family allowances increased with each additional child. In France, both parents are offered paid leave, and mothers can take up to three years off from work (unpaid) and still have their jobs waiting for them when they come back. [33]*

Beginning in the late 1980s, Canada's French-speaking province Quebec began making payments for each child born to parents, eventually topping out at $8,000 (Canadian dollars) for the family's third child.[34]† Researchers claim these payments increased a couple's chance of having a first child by 16.9 percent and a third child by 25 percent.[35] Scandinavian countries, such as Sweden, have also boosted fertility rates by providing child-care services and parental leave from work, and Estonia introduced a fifteen-month paid maternity leave in 2004 that helped boost the country's fertility rate by 20 percent.[36]‡

---

* The majority of the paid leave comes after the baby is born. For example, mothers typically get three to six weeks paid leave *before* the baby is born and ten to thirteen weeks paid leave *after* the baby is born. Fathers receive fewer paid leave days, which range from eleven to eighteen days.

† The $8,000 that parents were paid to have a third child came in twenty quarterly installments of $400. A report from the C. D. Howe Institute, a nonprofit that specializes in policy research, estimates that Quebec's pro-natalist policies were responsible for generating about 93,000 births between 1989 and 1996.

‡ Subsidies are not always this effective. A study of European countries found that a 25 percent increase in benefits increases fertility by 0.6 percent in the short run, and a 4 percent increase in the long run.

Austria is another European country that's been able to increase fertility rates through policy changes. In 1990, Austrian officials got creative with their country's maternity leave policies in an effort to increase birthrates. Their government had already given first-time mothers a year of maternity leave and a stipend since 1961. But in 1990, Austria changed its policy to give mothers a second year of leave if they had a second child within two years of their first.[37]

To prevent people from gaming the system, Austria declared that if your first child was born in June 1990 or earlier, you had to follow the old rules (less maternity leave for the second child). And if your child was born any time after July 1, 1990, you followed the new rules (more maternity leave for the second child). The changes weren't proposed until late 1989, so Austrians didn't have time to plan their first child's birth in reaction to the policy.[38]

What happened in response was that mothers who had their child *after* the June cutoff became 15 percent more likely to have a second child within the next three years than were mothers who had their children *before* the June cutoff.[39] According to a study by economists Josef Zweimuller and Rafael Lalive, Austria's policy increased both short-run fertility (by 4.9 percentage points within three years) and long-run fertility (by 3.9 percentage points within ten years), proving that just a little bit of an economic incentive can alter sexual practices within a population.[40] Giving Austrian mothers extra time off work lessened some of the logistical hurdles that motherhood presents to working women. For some women, more paid leave was just enough to push them toward having a second child.

So why are similar initiatives unlikely to succeed in Japan? Nations such as Austria, Canada, and France rank high in gender equality, while Japan fares poorly.[41]* In France, allowing a mother three years off from work might be enough of a nudge to make her consider having children, because the woman knows she probably won't face discrimination when she re-enters the workforce, and because France has subsidized day care, which makes it more affordable to raise children. In Japan, women might not even bother with such proposals, because they know they'll likely become stigmatized and will give up their chance of climbing the corporate ladder if they have children and take so much time off.

Although Japanese officials have failed to boost fertility rates, their policies have at least avoided spurring significant unintended cultural consequences. The same cannot be said for the world's most populous country.

One-Child Policy

Although many countries are now trying to raise their fertility rates, it's important to keep in mind that "increasing birthrates" are not necessarily economically superior to "decreasing birthrates." Whether a government wants to increase or decrease

---

* Demographer Laurent Toulemon told the *Guardian*, "The ability of society to adapt is crucial. If family traditions cannot be adjusted to suit the new political reality of gender equality, it results in a de facto refusal to bear children." Toulemon pointed out fertility rates in Europe are high where women have equality and feel free to work if they choose and childcare costs are manageable.

its birthrates depends on specific context rather than on universal truths.[42†] While fertility boosts can be economically beneficial in the long run by bringing more workers into the economy to support the entitlement payments of retirees, it's worth noting that fertility declines can also produce benefits and are "associated nearly everywhere with greater rights and opportunities for women," according to *The Global Spread of Fertility Decline* authors Jay Winter and Michael Teitelbaum.[43‡] Having fewer children also frees up more women to join the labor pool, allows adults to put more of their resources into investments, and allows parents to provide better education and health care for each child they do have.[44] And of course, politicians advocate for decreasing birthrates in places where there are food shortages, where maternal death is common, and where people fear overpopulation.

Just as governments can incentivize citizens to have more children, they can also persuade people to stop having

---

†   The effectiveness of any particular policy is also dependent on how prevalent women are in the workforce and whether the father or mother makes the final decision to bear children. For example, if the final decision is made by the father in a traditional society where women rarely work outside the home, then transfer payments and tax cuts that boost income may provide the best incentive to getting people to have children. But if the final decision is being made by women in societies where women make up a huge part of the workforce, then extending maternity leave and making day care more affordable are the best boosts to increasing fertility rates.

‡   Marriage rate declines can also produce benefits for women and society. According to Rebecca Traister, single and late-marrying women have been instrumental in social change movements such as the abolition of slavery, civil rights, and education and labor reforms.

children. The *Wall Street Journal* described a "policy U-turn" in Mexico that began during the mid-1970s that helped keep the country's population in check.[45] Traditionally, population expansion was seen in Mexico as a policy goal and a religious obligation. But after the government set up family-planning clinics, gave out free contraception, set sterilization goals for clinics, and began advertising slogans such as "The small family lives better," Mexico's birthrate fell from 4.7 per woman in 1980 to 2.2 by 2014.[46]

Not all efforts to control population growth are this subtle. China is one example of a nation that has taken a much more direct approach to manipulating its population size. In just thirty years after the Communist Party took control of China in 1949, the country's population exploded from 540 million to 940 million.[47] By the late 1970s, about a quarter of the world's population lived in China even though the country occupied just 7 percent of the world's arable land.[48] And because the large Baby Boomer cohort was entering its reproductive years, Chinese officials had another reason to be concerned that exponential population growth would deplete the country's resources. So in 1979, China introduced a one-child policy to curb birthrates.[49] As Mara Hvistendahl documented in her book *Unnatural Selection: Choosing Boys over Girls, and the Consequences of a World Full of Men*, the country's National Population and Family Planning Commission aggressively promoted abortion as a way for families to adhere to the one-child rule. In the 1980s, village walls displayed pro-abortion slogans to send a message that having multiple children was absolutely not to be tolerated.

Some messages included: "BETTER TO LET BLOOD FLOW LIKE A RIVER THAN TO HAVE ONE MORE THAN ALLOWED" and "YOU CAN BEAT IT OUT! YOU CAN MAKE IT FALL OUT! YOU CAN ABORT IT! BUT YOU CANNOT GIVE BIRTH TO IT."[50]*

In some ways, the policy accomplished its goals. Prior to its introduction, Chinese women had an average of more than four children throughout the 1970s. By 2015, the birthrate had dropped to 1.6.[51] However, it's tough to tell how much of the fertility rate drop stemmed from the one-child policy, because urbanization, rising incomes, and increases in contraception use also contributed to China's massive fertility decline, and China's fertility rate was already dropping before the one-child policy was implemented.[52] China claims about 400 million births were prevented by "one-child," while several demographers claim the actual number is about half that.[53]

While *many* factors drove China's fertility rates down, the tradition of preferring sons over daughters, combined with the one-child policy, led many parents to practice sex-selective abortion so they could have sons.[54] The resulting shortage in women has brought on economic and cultural burdens, which have led Chinese officials to replace their abortion advertisements with messages such as "Boys and girls are both treasures" and "Caring for girls starts with me."[55] In other words, because the country has a shortage of women, the narrative has shifted from getting rid of "surplus" children

---

*   During this time "female factory workers were forced to show their stained menstrual napkins to prove they weren't pregnant," wrote Barbara Demick.

at all costs to promoting the value of women. In recent years, the one-child restrictions have become less restrictive. In 2014, couples were allowed a second child if *either* parent was an only child, and in 2015, the Chinese government stated it would eliminate more restrictions and allow *all* couples to have a second child.[56]* But these changes may be too little, too late, as the one-child ideal has become a part of Chinese culture and values.[57]† After parents who themselves were an only child were allowed a second child in 2014, only about 1 million couples (of an eligible 11 million couples) applied to get government permission to have a second child, which was below forecasts.[58] In the year following the announcement that all couples were allowed to have a second child, 17.9 million children were born in China, which was an

---

*   While headlines implied the policy was ended in 2015 (e.g., the *Wall Street Journal* ran a story titled "China Abandons One-Child Policy"), that's not an entirely accurate way to view the situation. Sure, Chinese couples were allowed another child, but that only became possible very recently, and even then, couples are still restricted to just two children. Also, regardless of what policy China puts in place in the near future, the mind-set behind "one-child" will continue to permeate cultural preferences and produce unintended consequences. For these reasons, and because the effects of "one-child" will remain relevant for decades, we refer to China's childbearing rules as the "one-child policy."

†   Mei Fong, a Pulitzer Prize–winning journalist, writes that part of the reason China took so long to end the one-child policy was because "[b]irth planning had been so baked into the business of ordinary governance, its revenue contributions so necessary, that unwinding all this posed a challenge." China's National Population and Family Planning Commission employed about half a million people. And at the grassroots level, about 85 million people worked part-time in the birth planning industry.

increase of 1.3 million births over the previous year. But the increase fell short of the 20 million births that Chinese officials had hoped for.[59] "Many people have been brainwashed by one-child policy propaganda, including my mom," a Chinese mother told the *Washington Post*. "When I told her I was having a second child, she thought it was unacceptable. She didn't call me or talk to me for a month."[60]

With a strong cultural preference for single-child families, abortion became so ingrained into Chinese culture the procedure became routine for eliminating unwanted pregnancies. In Nie Jing-Bao's *Behind the Silence: Chinese Voices on Abortion*, a Chinese person comments that abortion is "a very natural thing, like eating and drinking."[61] In a questionnaire given to more than 600 Chinese men and women, Nie found 29 percent of respondents believed if pregnancy affects the mother's appearance, then abortion should be permitted. Thirty-four percent believed morning sickness was grounds for abortion. And 75 percent agreed, "Under some situations, it is necessary to force a woman to have an abortion."[62]

With many families restricted to having just one child, the pressure to pass on the family name and lineage through a male child increased. This desire for sons over daughters drove a gender imbalance that in 2004 reached 121.2 boys born for every 100 girls born.[63] Rural areas reported ratios as high as 140 boys for every 100 girls.[64] Though the ratio of boys to girls born in China has dropped from its historic high, it still hovers around 115 boys for every 100 girls, which is still a major imbalance.[65] By 2020, demographers predict there will be a surplus of 30 million young men in China.[66]

That means within half a decade, China could have more excess single young men without an available mate than there are people in the state of Texas. Other estimates place the amount of extra males even higher, with some anticipating 55 million surplus Chinese men by 2020.[67]

These son-preference tendencies are so instilled in some cultures that they don't disappear even when people move to a country without son preference. A husband-and-wife team of economists, Lena Edlund and Douglas Almond, at Columbia University found that Asian immigrants in the U.S. have normal sex ratios for the birth of their first child. But if their first child is a girl, the chance their second child will be a boy jumps about 17 percent. And if the first two children are both girls, then the chance that the third child will be a boy becomes so great that the gender ratio in these instances is 151 males to every 100 females.[68]

Of course, the sex of a child is not determined by the gender of that child's older sibling, and the ratio of 151 boys for every 100 girls could only be possible through human intervention, which likely involves screening and aborting female fetuses until couples conceive a son. Across a large population, the preference for sons eventually creates a drastic gender imbalance within the society—and the consequences for those imbalances can be far-reaching and unpredictable.

Race to the Bottom

The preference for sons isn't unique to China, and can be seen in several Asian countries. A slight change in sex ratios can be enough to affect relationship quality, length, and the occurrence and frequency of sex in any country.[69] But in Asian countries, where women are in severe shortage and countries look abroad to find mates for their men, unbalanced sex ratios can have a more insidious effect.

The governments of some Asian countries encourage the importation of brides to balance gender ratios, and to increase low fertility rates, according to Hvistendahl. A South Korean province sponsored trips to Vietnam for its men to search for women. The South Korean government even sets aside $23 million for adaptation programs of foreign brides, which are meant to assimilate them to Korean culture. And Korean roadways have sported ads such as: "FAST AND SUCCESSFUL MARRIAGE WITH FILIPINO, CAMBODIAN, AND VIETNAMESE WOMEN."[70]

South Korean and Taiwanese men visit Vietnam on one-week "marriage tours," where they pay their newly chosen spouse's family in exchange for their daughter. The money the family receives raises their social status and wealth, making the practice lucrative, as the business of imported wives, who are euphemistically referred to as "marriage migrants," is now an established industry.[71]* Men from Singapore use companies such as J & N Viet-Bride Match-Making Agencies, First Overseas International Matchmaker, and Ideal Marriage Centre to find brides, while South Koreans

---

* It was estimated that in 2003 about one-third of all marriages in Taiwan were between a local and foreigner. The majority of these marriages were between local men and imported foreign women.

prefer Interwedding, and Taiwanese men frequent Lotus 200. It's estimated that there are a few thousand international marriage agencies in South Korea.[72] The brides are purchased from many countries, including Vietnam, Thailand, the Philippines, Uzbekistan, Russia, Malaysia, and North Korea.

A shortage of females can also lead to increases in sex work and trafficking. The director of the Durihana Association, which provides aid to North Korean refugees, estimates that about 80 percent of North Koreans living in China are female.[73] They arrive without money or jobs and often end up as sex workers or bought as brides and traded. There are anecdotal reports of refugee women in China being sold for ten times the amount of money that they were being sold for about twenty-five years ago. [74]

Brides in places such as Vietnam become a money transfer. According to Hvistendahl, the husband gets the mate he desired, the marriage broker is paid off, and the bride's family takes home cash—usually between $1,000 to $2,000—in exchange for their daughter. The money flow doesn't stop after marriage. Many women continue to send money home, and on visits back home, brides sometimes brings back as much as $10,000, which is about five times the per capita income in Vietnam.[75] Doo-Sub Kim, a human migration scholar who specializes in Asia's marriage trade, told Hvistendahl that the trading of poor women in South Korea, Taiwan, and Singapore could set off a frenzy: "In the next twenty-five years, if the situation we have here [in Korea] continues in China, there's going to be a huge migration from Southeast Asian countries to the mainland. It's going to be total chaos."[76]

The global marriage trade could set off a race to the
bottom as men search for women in the poorest areas on
earth. In 2008, John McGeoghan, a project coordinator for
the International Organization for Migration, told reporters that the international marriage trade has "become a
big business. We now see that these marriage brokers are
popping up in Cambodia. This is a new market for them,
and there's a lot of money to be made."[77] With the increased
demand for girls, some parents in these areas see having
daughters as economic opportunities.

"Daughters nowadays are more preferable than sons
because daughters can marry abroad and help families
economically," a Vietnamese villager told Tran Giang Linh, a
researcher examining the international marriage trade.[78] But
many of these daughters fall into sex work because a lack of
women drives an increase in demand for prostitution.[79]* In
Sex Slaves: The Trafficking of Women in Asia, author Louise
Brown writes that among some castes in Nepal:

The traditional South Asian lament at the birth

---

* In 2010, prostitutes in the Chinese city of Wuhan protested government
crackdowns on prostitution. "This kind of suppression will never last," wrote a
protester. "With the gender ratio out of proportion, sexual constraints on single
[men] have created enormous social demand." Hvistendahl notes that throughout
history, prostitution has boomed in societies where men significantly outnumber
women. Nineteenth-century France saw an increase in sex workers after indus-
trialization, which brought on urban migration, making cities disproportionately
male. The same thing happened around Shanghai in the 1930s, and as a result
one out of every thirteen women in the city was a prostitute.

of a daughter and the celebration at the birth of a son is reversed. A pretty daughter is no longer a liability—by selling sex she has become an asset... Increased poverty, higher material expectations, and greater knowledge of economic opportunities mean that whole impoverished communities in less-developed Asia see their girls as a way to survive and sometimes simply as a way to comfortable living.[80]

The demand for sex workers isn't just driven internationally. Women are actually predominantly traded *within* countries, according to Brown.[81] East China and Northwest India are two areas Hvistendahl points to that demonstrate how women get shifted around within a country. Both areas have poor gender ratios at birth, meaning there are more men being born than women in these areas. However, over time the gender ratio of the cohort shifts, and eventually, twenty to thirty years later, there are nearly as many women as men in the group.[82] Why is that?

Many baby boys born in East China and Northwest India eventually become men who, because of a shortage of women in their area, import their brides from a poorer region in their country. By 2030, scholars predict China's poorest provinces will have 50 percent more bachelors over age thirty than will the richest provinces.[83] This disparity is made possible through the trade and trafficking of women.

With the high demand for women, perhaps parents from these countries will sense the economic opportunity daughters present them and will use the same technologies Chinese

and Indian families use for the opposite purpose—to screen
their fetuses with the goal of producing female offspring to
sell to wealthier families. *If* parents from Asian countries
begin screening their fetuses in order to have more daughters, this practice could *potentially* balance out gender ratios
and could *possibly* even reverse current trends so that eventually these societies will have more women than men. But
even if parents begin screening for female fetuses and gender
ratios become balanced as a result, women would still bear
the brunt of the consequences of sex selection. If people
begin having daughters just because "sex work has given
them a market value," a female underclass would develop,
where women would disproportionately be born poor and
sold to rich families.[84]* The sexually related side effects of the
one-child policy are pervasive and affect the lives of millions
of people. But the influence of one-child restrictions isn't
limited to sexual side effects.

---

* While the international marriage trade has its costs, it has also challenged status
quos and homogenous states that have strong national loyalty, which is associated
with race. Biracial children in Korea used to be scorned. The children belonging to
American military men serving in the Korea War and local Korean women were
ostracized. But international marriages are now increasing in South Korea, and
they produce more children than the average South Korean marriage, which has
been welcomed because South Korea had low fertility rates. And in India, some
believe international marriage is slowly eroding the country's oppressive caste
system. Indian archaeologist Sharada Srinivasan told Hvistendahl, "Now because
of [female] scarcity you see marrying outside of caste. Some of these barriers that
go back a long time are beginning to weaken, and in some cases women are being
married without dowries. So there might be some good coming out of this."

═ HONG KONG'S MAN SHORTAGE ═

While mainland China has a shortage of women, Hong Kong actually has a female surplus, with roughly 855 men for every 1,000 women.[85] The gap is predicted to widen to 763 men for every 1,000 women by 2036. According to a 2013 article in the *Atlantic* titled "Hong Kong's Troubling Shortage of Men," this disparity is driven by cultural norms and immigration. Many of the surplus women in Hong Kong are female migrants from the Philippines and Indonesia. Also, there is a cultural norm where men are expected to marry women with lower socioeconomic status and women are expected to marry men with higher socioeconomic status. But many of Hong Kong's women are educated and independent. So even though the raw numbers tip in men's favor, many Hong Kong men have trouble finding a wife with lower earning power than their own.[86]

According to Yong Cai, a University of North Carolina demographer studying China's sex ratios, "Men at the bottom of society get left out of the marriage market, and that same pattern is coming to emerge for women at the top of society."[87] As a result, men from Hong Kong import more traditional and less educated women from mainland China to marry. These types of marriages account for more than 30 percent of all registered marriages in the city.[88]

Instead of rejoicing about living in an area where the odds of finding a mate are highly in their favor, Hong Kong men import women from the mainland, further reducing the number of women in an area already short on females. The surplus women in Hong Kong are left searching for men with higher socioeconomic status, who are in short supply. The popularity of plastic surgery and liposuction has increased on the island, and reality TV shows follow lonely women in their thirties seeking advice from "love coaches," which are trends that can be traced to the intense competition for wealthy, successful men.[89] With too few women in mainland China and too many in Hong Kong, there's a market inefficiency for single people in China's dating scene to exploit—if they can move past cultural norms.

Bad Boys

Under China's one-child policy, crime rates have nearly doubled in the last twenty years.[90] A paper published by the Institute for the Study of Labor found a 1 percent increase in sex ratios (in other words, more men being born than women) in people aged sixteen to twenty-five led to a five-to-six-point crime increase in China. "The increasing maleness of the young adult population may account for as much as a third of the overall rise in crime," the study's authors concluded.[91] According to the *New Republic*, areas with the most surplus men "have more gambling, alcohol and drug abuse, prostitution, rape, bride abduction, and human trafficking."[92] Researchers have called for a "gender rebalancing" to bring about reductions in crime.[93]

Contemporary China isn't the first country to have

abnormal gender ratios that led to increases in crime. Anthropological research shows that societies with many mateless men tend to be high in crime. A study published in a journal run by the Royal Society stated, "Faced with high levels of intra-sexual competition and little chance of obtaining even one long-term mate, unmarried, low-status men will heavily discount the future and more readily engage in risky status-elevating and sex-seeking behaviors. This will result in higher rates of murder, theft, rape, social disruption, kidnapping (especially of females), sexual slavery, and prostitution. As a by-product, these men will probably engage in more substance abuse."[94] This effect is evident in India, where out-of-whack sex ratios can predict which areas will have high murder rates better than poverty levels.[95]

One of the takeaways from the book *Bare Branches: The Security Implications of Asia's Surplus Male Population*, by political scientists Valerie Hudson and Andrea Den Boer, is that high male-to-female ratios can lead to autocratic government structures as political leaders attempt to reduce rising crime. The *New Republic* points out that male youth "bulges" have led to "European imperial expansion after 1500, Japanese imperial expansion after 1914, and cold war–era revolutions in Algeria, El Salvador, and Lebanon."[96] Some researchers even theorize that excessive amounts of unmarried men could eventually bring domestic uprisings or military expansion to China.[97] And, apart from these effects, having too many men in a society can also create economic consequences.

Saving for Sons

A 2015 *Newsweek* cover story noted, "China's household savings rate affects everything from international capital flows to its massive trade imbalance, to U.S. exports and therefore employment. Put simply, if Chinese consumers spent more and saved less, Beijing's trading partners, the U.S. included, would sell more goods and services to them."[98] It's clear that China's savings rate holds economic importance, but what's less clear to many people is how China's one-child policy affects the country's savings rate.

A shortage of women brought on by the one-child policy has ramped up competition among men searching for a wife. There are reports that bride price has significantly increased in China, and that families with daughters now demand that male suitors be financially well off.[99] When bride price increases, wealthy men gain another dating advantage, because poor men get priced out of the mating market. But to prevent their sons from being excluded from the mating market, many Chinese families are saving their income with the intent that their son will use their saved-up money to attract a wife.

China's savings rate has almost doubled in the last twenty years and is among the highest in the world. Parents saving money to secure their sons mates may account for *half* of the increase in household savings China experienced in the past twenty years, according to a study coauthored by Asian Development Bank chief economist Shang-Jin Wei.[100] "We found that not only did households with sons save more than households with daughters on average, but that households with sons tend to raise their savings rate if they also happen to live in a region with a more skewed gender ratio," Wei writes.[101] By influencing savings rates, the one-child policy holds international economic significance, because the high Chinese savings rate affects international trade imbalances, as the *Newsweek* story noted.[102]

Given that China is the world's most populous country, it isn't shocking to find that a sexual and demographic experiment as prominent as the one-child policy reaches into so many areas of domestic life. Other effects surely remain underexplored and are waiting for clever social scientists to tease them out as the first generation born under the one-child policy continues further into adulthood.

Procreation Possibilities

The one-child policy and other fertility rate experiments show that governments try to influence how frequently their residents have children.[103]* They show that many births are a response to environmental, cultural, economic, and political circumstances, and data suggest birthrates aren't random. In societies with readily available contraception, most kids don't

---

*   Whether or not governments *should* attempt to influence birthrates is another topic altogether. There's a major concern among environmentalists that there are already too many people on the planet, and increasing birthrates would contribute to more climate change. There are merits to the concerns environmentalists have regarding overpopulation. However, the intent of this chapter is to focus on economics and unintended cultural consequences, not humanitarian ethics.

just come about as an unexpected passionate shot in the dark. They're more likely to be a product of careful planning.

Governments can indeed influence birthrates, but if governments exert too much control and the economic nudges morph into sexual manipulation, birthrate policies can create unintentional effects that extend outside sexuality, which is what happened in China when its one-child policy led to increases in crime and savings rates. "The great tragedy of population control, the fatal misconception, was to think that one could know other people's interests better than they knew it themselves," writes Columbia University historian Matthew Connelly.[104] Rather than resorting to coercion, governments that want to reduce birthrates can instead make contraception freely available, raise the minimum age of marriage, and increase women's education, which Connelly says is the biggest factor in lowering fertility rates.[105]

While China has put a lot of effort into reducing their birthrates, many countries in the West have an opposite intention and want to increase the number of babies born in their country. But as journalist Mei Fong noted in her book about China's one-child policy, "Countries that switched from anti-natalist to pro-natalist policies have so far found that turning *on* the baby tap is far more difficult than turning it off."[106] Many pro-natalist policies simply fail. If a policy is to succeed in increasing birthrates, the country must show a long-term commitment to increasing fertility, according to Last.[107] Austria, Quebec, Sweden, and France were able to increase their birthrates because they made parenthood more practical by extending maternity leave and making daycare affordable. Japan's and Singapore's pro-natalist policies failed because they relied on gimmicks such as "women's notebooks" and insincere holidays that did nothing to ease parental burdens. "The government *cannot* get people to have children *they do not want*," Last writes. "However, it *can* help people have the children *they* do *want*."[108]

The act of having children is often viewed as divine or coincidental. While that may be true at times, there's more to the story, because the decision to have kids or not is also often driven by economics. If governments realize that and act accordingly, perhaps they can save their stimulus packages and fiscal-cliff cuts, and instead focus on fixing the economy by incentivizing people to indulge in or refrain from having children (depending on the economic context of the country). Regarding childbearing decisions, many people side with God in the book of Genesis when He said, "Be fruitful and multiply." But what many business and political leaders ignore is that people multiply much quicker when it's fruitful for them to do so.

PART III

RELIGION AND CULTURE

sex, drugs, and corn flakes

THE INFLUENCE OF ACCIDENTAL INVENTIONS ON SEX AND COMMERCE

S ex is tied to innovation, both directly and indirectly. From ancient cave paintings to modern beer commercials, it's visually apparent that sex has influenced people's thoughts, behavior, and aspirations for thousands of years. But by examining indirect sexual inventions, we can go beyond predetermined rhetoric and belief systems and incrementally examine a force that guides lives in many mysterious and hidden ways.

The following case studies illustrate the power of religious zeal and the potential of sexual sublimation, as well as how marketers and medical companies harness and guide sexuality when even the smallest of opportunities presents itself. These case studies also show that sexuality pops up in surprising ways, as the origins of Viagra, vibrators, graham crackers, and corn flakes are opposite of what one might expect. Viagra, vibrators, graham crackers, and corn flakes all share a common trait—they thrived and flourished for unexpected reasons. However, unlike graham crackers and corn flakes, vibrators and Viagra weren't intended for sex.

One Crazy Cracker

As a clergyman-physician in the early 1800s, Sylvester Graham mixed medicine and spirituality. A popular lecturer and dietary reformer, Graham believed that most health problems derived from sinning, and that most sins stemmed from lust.[1] Graham's lecturing drew huge crowds who listened to him rant about how certain substances (such as alcohol, coffee, and tea) and sexual activity debilitated the body.[2] His followers became so numerous they got their own name—Grahamites.[3] According to Graham, sex should always be avoided, even within marriage. In *A Lecture to Young Men on Chastity*, Graham lays out many horrors that stem from too much *husband-and-wife* action:

> Languor, lassitude, muscular relaxation, general debility and heaviness, depression of spirits, loss of appetite, indigestion, faintness, and sinking at the pit of the stomach, increased susceptibilities of the skin and lungs to all the atmospheric changes, feebleness of circulation, chilliness, headache, melancholy,

hypochondria, hysterics, feebleness of all the senses, impaired vision, loss of sight, weakness of the lungs, nervous cough, pulmonary consumption, disorders of the liver and kidneys, urinary difficulties, disorders of the genital organs, weakness of the brain, loss of memory, epilepsy, insanity, apoplexy,—and extreme feebleness and early death of offspring,—are among the too common evils which are caused by sexual excesses between husband and wife.[4]

Graham believed that the best way to avoid the sexual urges that caused these ills was through proper diet. Graham taught that meat caused carnal desire because it made people carnivorous, salt caused salaciousness, and spices excited sexual urges the same way they excited the taste buds.[5] According to sexologist John Money in *The Destroying Angel: Sex, Fitness, and Food in the Legacy of Degeneracy Theory, Graham Crackers, Kellogg's Corn Flakes, & American Health History*:

Graham didn't invent his dietary prohibitions. He borrowed them from books he read. Some of them were hundreds of years old—for example, the prohibition against eating the flesh of three unclean animals, the hare, the hyena, and the weasel. Here are the ancient theories regarding the consequences of eating the meat of these unclean animals.

If you eat the meat of the hare (or rabbit), you will become an adult lover of the underaged and you will be unclean, having anal intercourse with an adolescent boy, because these animals grow a new anal opening each year, one for every year they have lived.

If you eat the meat of the hyena, you will become unclean and will practice seduction and adultery with both men and women, because this animal changes its sex every year; one year it copulates with males and the next with females.

If you eat the meat of the weasel, you will commit unclean sexual acts with your mouth, or have unclean sexual acts performed on you by mouth, because this animal conceives through its mouth.[6]

These theories gave Graham the foundation to build his dietary recommendations. Desperate people hoping to avoid disease flocked to see Graham because he guaranteed that his methods of sexual abstinence and dieting could ward off cholera.[7]* As cholera became an epidemic in the 1830s, people tried anything—even avoiding spicy foods or sex—if it had a chance at preventing the illness.[8]

Graham's theory that bland foods had the power to reduce evil sexual urges came during the height of degeneracy theory,

---

* But not everyone loved Graham's talks. Puritan types wanted Graham to tone down speeches because he openly spoke about masturbation in front of female audiences. Butchers loathed Graham because his preaching against meat hurt business. Bakers also wanted Graham's head because he preached their white bread should be avoided because it grew on "debauched and exhausted soil, artificially stimulated with animal manure," Money wrote.

which was based on many pseudoscientific theories, including the idea that sex led to ailments, insanity, and eventually, early death.[9†] Some theorists believed masturbation was degeneracy's main cause.[10] To fight sexual desires, Graham suggested a bland vegetarian diet, which led him to invent Graham bread.[11] Made of only wheat grain, Graham bread was high in fiber, free of additives, and seemingly, free of taste. Eventually Graham bread evolved into sugary graham crackers. [12]

In trying to prevent sexual urges, Graham unintentionally created a popular food item. As time passes, the link between sexual impurity and bland food increasingly fades. Graham's influence waned too, but not before his ideas influenced another food industry titan.

They're Gr-r-reat (at Reducing Masturbation)!

John Harvey Kellogg lived a colorful life. Before his days as a breakfast cereal icon, he became a popular American health reformer and abdominal surgeon while holding prominent positions in the Seventh-Day Adventist Church.[13] He predicted the harmful effects of smoking decades before the

---

†   It's not just "sex-negative" theorists who view sex through partisan lenses and come up with irrational theories and justifications. According to Jack Cashill, "Alfred Kinsey encouraged the sexual torture of small boys. Masters and Johnson created an imaginary heterosexual AIDS crisis. Planned Parenthood buried Margaret Sanger's plan to sterilize the radically and genetically 'impure.'" As Andrew Greeley put it, "The hedonist's injunction, 'Enjoy, enjoy,' is as absolutely moralistic as the puritan's 'Deny, deny.'"

rest of the medical community.[14] And, like Graham, Kellogg lectured on the relationship between dieting and sexuality. Also like Graham, he isn't remembered much for health theories, but rather for a food bearing his name—Kellogg's cereal. Though cereal is now removed from its sexual origins, understanding Kellogg's philosophies helps explain why we now wake up to a bowl of Wheaties.

Like Graham's teachings, Kellogg's dietary recommendations were influenced by degeneracy theory. Kellogg believed sex was always bad. Period. In his book *Plain Facts for Young and Old*, he wrote, "The reproductive act is the most exhausting of all vital acts. Its effect upon the undeveloped person is to retard growth, weaken the constitution, and dwarf the intellect."[15]

Kellogg practiced what he preached. Rather than have sex on his honeymoon, he wrote a book. His marriage was never consummated.[16]* Kellogg sought to prove sex wasn't necessary for a healthy life. This is probably why he never spoke of love or human affection, despite writing extensively about sexuality.[17]

Because Kellogg subscribed to degeneracy theory, and like Graham he believed bland diets could reduce masturbation,[18]†

---

*   That is not to say that Kellogg was never aroused. Some research suggests he was a klismaphile, which is someone who is aroused by enemas.

†   Kellogg believed that, to curb masturbation, young boys should be circumcised and young girls should have carbolic acid poured on the "sensitive parts of the sexual organs." He also writes, "In younger children, with whom moral consideration will have no particular weight, other devices may be used. Bandaging the parts has been practiced with success. Tying the hands is also successful in some

he set out to produce a health food. In 1895, he introduced a food called Granose at a conference held by Seventh-Day Adventists at the Battle Creek Sanitarium, which was a health center in Michigan that Kellogg was then in charge of.[19] After three years, Granose hit the public market and took the name "Corn Flakes." By 1906, the product we now associate with Kellogg had been perfected.[20]

John Harvey Kellogg was more interested in experimenting with recipes than trying to commercialize his product. However, his brother Will Keith Kellogg was more zealous about turning a profit. So, to avoid business tasks, John Harvey delegated the commercial part of company to Will Keith.[21] But mixing family and money proved disastrous for the Kelloggs. Will Keith broke away and formed his own company, which eventually became the Kellogg Company that dominates the breakfast industry to this day.[22]

Facing pressure from competitors such as C. W. Post,

cases; but this will not always succeed, for they will often contrive to continue the habit in other ways, as by working the limbs, or lying upon the abdomen. Covering the organs with a cage has been practiced with entire success. A remedy which is almost always successful in small boys is circumcision, especially when there is any degree of phimosis. The operation should be performed by a surgeon without administering an anesthetic, as the brief pain attending the operation will have a salutary effect upon the mind, especially if it be connected with the idea of punishment, as it may well be in some cases. The soreness which continues for several weeks interrupts the practice, and if it had not previously become too firmly fixed, it may be forgotten and not resumed. If any attempt is made to watch the child, he should be so carefully surrounded by vigilance that he cannot possibly transgress without detection. If he is only partially watched, he soon learns to elude observation, and thus the effect is only to make him cunning in his vice."

Will Keith reengineered Corn Flakes to make them less
bland and give them a broader commercial appeal. Will
Keith produced Corn Flakes using sugar, in direct opposition to John Harvey's beliefs about dietary restrictions. The
new version of Corn Flakes made Will Keith a multimillion-
aire.[23] Wanting his share of the profits, John Harvey fought
Will Keith twice in court, losing both times.[24] The brothers
never made up before John Harvey's death. And Corn Flakes
forever carried the Kellogg name, even though their creator
despised its final formula. As Money puts it:

> Henceforth, to the doctrinally faithful of the health-
> food cults, corn flakes were so contaminated by
> containing commercially refined sugar that they
> would be held in contempt as junkfood [sic]. Just as
> surely as if their name had been changed from corn
> flakes to porn flakes, they had lost their virtue as the
> diet of chastity, abstinence, and sexual purity.[25]

Corn flakes popularized the concept of breakfast cereal
and revolutionized the food industry, and John Harvey
Kellogg became more associated with Tony the Tiger than
any of his religious, sexual, or dietary theories. While intend-
ing to create an anti-aphrodisiac, Kellogg instead changed
America's eating habits. Corn flakes and graham crackers
show how the inspiration to create a sexually based commodity can lead to the creation of a product that people use for
nonsexual purposes. But the reverse can happen too. Goods
not initially intended for sex can end up influencing sexual

practices. That's how a device invented to save professional men time and effort ended up becoming one of the most popular female sex toys in history.

Good Vibrations

One in four nineteenth-century women were believed to have the same disease.[26] Symptoms ranged from hallucinations and paralysis to insomnia, muscle spasms, irritability, loss of sexual desire and appetite, and a "tendency to cause trouble."[27] Luckily for women, the incidence of this disorder declined remarkably in the twentieth century. What led to the decline of this catchall disease called "hysteria" wasn't improvements in women's health care. Instead, improved diagnostic techniques and a greater understanding of psychological disorders led the American Psychiatric Association to drop hysteria from its list of recognized conditions in 1952.[28] But before this disorder was debunked, it led to the creation of a device used to "treat" hysteria—the vibrator.

Prior to the vibrator's popularization, many Victorian women wouldn't masturbate because of their society's disapproval of masturbation, but they let doctors manually massage their vaginas in hopes of relieving symptoms of hysteria.[29] But massages weren't the only remedies that doctors recommended to women to help them get off and reduce their hysteria-related tension. Basically, anything that created friction around the crotch was fair game for treatment. Aside from "pelvic massages," hysteria patients sought relief through horseback riding,[30]* dancing, and spraying water into their vaginas.[31] Although doctors had various tactics in their arsenal, doctors typically relied on "massages," in which they essentially fingered women's vaginas until climax, relieving hysterical symptoms such as fluid retention, irritability, nervousness, and loss of desire for food and sex.[32]

In 1903, physician Samuel Howard Monnell noted the difficulty doctors had in getting women to climax when he wrote, "Pelvic massage (in gynecology) has its brilliant advocates and they report wonderful results, but when practitioners must supply the skilled technic with their own fingers the method has no value to the majority."[33] Another doctor, Samuel Spencer Wallian, wrote in 1906 that a pelvic massage "consumes a painstaking hour to accomplish much less profound results than are easily effected by the other [the vibrator] in a short five or ten minutes."[34] In *The Technology of Orgasm: "Hysteria," the Vibrator, and Women's Satisfaction*, historian Rachel Maines writes, "At no time did physicians show any real enthusiasm for treating hysteria in their women patients. All the evidence points to their having generally considered it a tedious, difficult, and time-consuming chore and

---

*   According to Rachel Maines, horseback riding has a history as a treatment for sexual issues. "Krafft-Ebing and George Beard both reported that some of their male patients were aroused to orgasm by equitation, and historians John Haller and Robin Haller report that horseback riding was one of the nineteenth-century treatments for impotence."

having made efforts to delegate the task to subordinates or machines even in ancient and medieval times."[35] More concerned with increasing the amount of patients they could see in a day than with pleasing their female clientele, male doctors made efforts to quicken the process and cut massage time down by relying on vibrators to treat hysteria. As Tanya Wexler, the director of *Hysteria*, a 2011 film loosely based on the vibrator's invention, told the *Daily Beast*, "The funny thing is that the vibrator was kind of invented for a guy as a laborsaving device."[36]

Eventually, in 1869, help came from a steam-powered device invented by physician George Taylor called the "Manipulator."[37] Essentially, the Manipulator was a motorized table. In the center of the table was a hole where a vibrating ball sat. Patients were laid across this buzzing sphere to achieve stimulation.[38] Though the Manipulator was an improvement over manual stimulation by physicians and got "treatments" headed in the right direction by relieving doctors of exhausted wrists, its dining-table size prevented it from gaining popularity.

In 1880, Dr. Joseph Mortimer Granville invented the first electromechanical vibrator, which superseded the Manipulator. This vibrator was still quite large because it had to be attached to a 40-pound wet-cell battery to receive power.[39] The vibrator itself looked like a thermostat hooked up to a syringe-like appendage.[40] "The vibrating mechanism is basically just a sloppy electrical motor," Maines told *Big Think*.[41] Though impractical by modern standards, the 40-pound vibrator invented by Granville reduced the duration of vaginal "massages" from an hour to about ten minutes.[42]*

After Granville's device became public, businesses realized there was serious money in marketing vibrators directly to women rather than to doctors. In men's magazines, advertisers recommended vibrators as gifts for women that benefitted men by giving their ladies bright eyes and pink cheeks.[43] Though sales didn't really take off until the 1980s, vibrators increased enough in popularity that many women quit going to doctors for hysteria treatment.[44]† Instead, women bought vibrators in Sears catalogs, saving money by relieving themselves at home.[45] While women finally relieving themselves at home could be viewed as a progressive moment, the vibrator might not have been invented if women had always avoided doctor-aided orgasms and pleased themselves at home instead. Sure, had these women not been conditioned to view sexual self-expression negatively, they might've stayed home, saved the awkwardness, saved money, and relieved themselves. But had that happened, the vibrator as we know it might not have been invented, and women now could have fewer tools in their masturbatory arsenal. Without strict Victorian sexual rules where sexuality was medicalized, today's women *might* have been deprived of a very common and effective tool used to get off.

---

*   Most doctors of the era did not recognize that the vibrator-aided massages were sexual. They tended to view the massages as treatment for an illness, and the subsequent orgasms were seen as evidence of the disease.

†   Hysteria no longer being recognized as an illness also contributed to a decrease in women seeking a physical release from doctors.

The vibrator is an example of an everyday household product that found its current usage by accident. Graham crackers and corn flakes were initially invented with a sexual application in mind, but only ended up convincing school kids to drink more milk. Vibrators were intended to help male doctors, but today the only doctor they help is Doc Johnson.‡ And there's another popular sex product whose origin is even further removed from sexuality than the vibrator's.

One Pill Makes You Larger

Pfizer researchers started testing a blood-pressure medication during the mid-1990s, but were disappointed with its efficacy in treating hypertension and chest pain. But the researchers did notice that patients in the clinical trial kept trying to take this ineffective cardiac medicine home with them after the studies were complete. Patients wanted more of the drug for the damnedest of all reasons—it gave them long-lasting erections.[46] What started out as heart medicine turned into phallus-driven gold. And that's how Viagra was born.

On its journey from birth to billions, Viagra relied on researcher-consultants and creative marketing techniques. But the organization to which Viagra most owes its success is the U.S. Food and Drug Administration (FDA). After the FDA lifted its ban on direct-to-consumer broadcast advertising in 1997, Viagra commercials began appearing on TV, making penile problems more public than ever.[47]

---

‡   Doc Johnson is the name of one of the largest sex toy companies in the world.

Because of Viagra, phalluses became a pressing public issue, even in politics.

Viagra came to America's attention during Bill Clinton's presidency. Rather than piggyback off the middle-aged president's virile sexual appetite, Pfizer chose Clinton's political opponent Bob Dole as its spokesperson to appear in Viagra ads throughout the late 1990s. According to sociologist Meika Loe's *Rise of Viagra: How the Little Blue Pill Changed Sex in America*, Pfizer chose Dole for several public relations reasons. "With his Republican family values, Bob Dole was advocating sexual relations in a sanitized, controlled, normal, and noncontroversial (read: penetrative heterosexual) way. Clinton, on the other hand, seemed to fit perfectly with negative stereotypes of out-of-control male sexuality. Let's just put it this way—in 1998, Pfizer would never have wanted Clinton selling Viagra."[48] When Clinton denied Lewinsky's blow jobs and Dole supported penis pills, they became the biggest political stories of 1998.[49]*

The selection of a sanitized spokesperson was just one of many strategic tactics Pfizer used to boost Viagra's public visibility and acceptance. Pfizer had a popular and nonthreatening salesman, but it still needed medical backing for the public to embrace a sex drug. To obtain medical legitimacy, Pfizer consulted with prominent researchers, who then

---

*   After Clinton raised taxes during his first term, Dole campaigned to cut them in the 1996 election. Two years later, the candidates once again found themselves on opposite ends of an issue. Dole wanted to get his dick up, Clinton couldn't tame his down.

conducted studies that showed sexual dysfunction was prevalent in the U.S. These researchers also appeared in TV shows, magazines, and medical journals, where they recommended Viagra as a treatment for the allegedly common ill of sexual dysfunction. Meanwhile, the public remained unaware that these researchers were getting paid by Viagra's parent company, Pfizer.[50]

Branding a Condition

Fortunately for Pfizer, some researchers weren't scared about showing off products aimed at alleviating sexual disorders. At an American Urology Association (AUA) conference in Las Vegas in 1983, fifty-seven-year-old Giles Brindley brought attention to impotence research by exhibiting that old age wasn't preventing him from getting it up. For his research presentation, he was to demonstrate the effectiveness of injectable drugs in treating impotence.[51†] Naturally, he injected himself with the drug, commanded the stage, threw off his pants, and proudly showed off his erect penis. "I was wondering why this

---

† Brindley's demonstration isn't the only time a doctor self-treated an erectile problem. According to the TV special "Sex, Pills, and Love Potions," endocrinologist Mac Hadley wanted to develop a drug that would cause erections as well as tanned skin. "I decided to take one of these products home to get the project moving by experimenting on myself," Hadley said. "I made a slight miscalculation, and the chemical was much stronger than I planned. I didn't develop a suntan right way, but I did develop an erection very rapidly. I developed an erection that lasted eight hours… I couldn't reduce it with ice cubes. I reached up and said, 'We're going to be very rich!'"

very smart man was giving his talk in a jogging outfit," a conference attendee told *Fortune*. "Then he stepped from behind the
podium. It was a big penis, and he just walked around the stage
showing it off."[52] About fifteen years later, Pfizer found other
shameless researchers to back Viagra.

A major reason doctors began dishing out Viagra to
old men faster than a parent hushing their kid with bags of
Skittles is because a 1994 study by recognized sex experts
Edward Laumann and John Gagnon found that between 30
and 50 percent of American adults complain of sexual dissatisfaction.[53] In 1999, Laumann expanded on this study and
claimed that 43 percent of women and 31 percent of men
were sexually *dysfunctional*.[54*] In response to what prompted
the study that found high sexual dysfunction rates, Laumann
told Loe, "I was invited to the international academy of sex
research by Ray Rosen, who was president at the time, and
I was his speaker. He told me that the information from the
1994 study on sexual problems did not exist in the medical
literature, so let's do something about it."[55]

Around that same time, another researcher made headway
for Viagra. Urologist Irwin Goldstein told the AUA that
impotence was a "new field of medicine about to explode."[56]
Goldstein became a medical celebrity as *Time*, the *New York
Times*, *Playboy*, and *Good Morning America* broadcasted his

---

*   These studies enabled Pfizer to claim that, in the late 1990s, 30 million men
        in America suffered from erectile dysfunction. But just a few years ago, prior
        to Viagra's release, pharma companies pushing injectable impotence products
        claimed that 10 to 20 million American men were impotent.

opinions on impotence without much questioning. Goldstein said, "Impotence should be considered as a major health concern." And that Viagra was "a dream practitioners in this field didn't think possible" and "the start of an exciting revolution."[57] Goldstein and other charismatic researchers legitimized the drug to the public by openly talking about sex with authority and telling them impotence was a serious dysfunction that should be treated with pills. Pfizer used these researchers' credibility as leverage to win public favor in its campaign to relabel impotence as "erectile dysfunction."[58†] This change in language further cemented Viagra's status as a reliable drug to treat a major disease.

What Laumann and Goldstein didn't tell the American public was that they were consultants working for Pfizer to sell Viagra.[59] As the practice of drug companies paying superstar academics to promote their products became common, former National Institute of Mental Health official Loren Mosher told *Mother Jones* in 2002, "They [researcher consultants] are basically paid for going on TV and saying, 'You know, there's this big new problem, and this drug seems to be very helpful.'"[60]

Laumann and Goldstein certainly aren't unique in being renowned researchers who accept drug company money. When a group of researchers met in 2000 to discuss

---

†   Impotence isn't the only natural sexual function now considered a disease. Premature ejaculation is only "premature" in modern partner-pleasing settings. As Jesse Bering argues, cumming quickly had evolutionary advantages, because it allowed men to inseminate multiple females in a short time span. As long as it was in before shots fired, there was nothing premature about it.

how female sexual dysfunction should be classified in the Diagnostic and Statistics Manual (DSM), "95 percent of them had financial relationships with the drug companies hoping to develop drugs for the very same condition," write health industry journalist Ray Moynihan and drug assessment specialist Barbara Mintzes. "The conflicts of interest for this group were clear. As they met to work out what could best be described as normal female sexuality, and what might better be labeled as a dysfunction, many of them had been taking money or receiving other support from companies with an interest in seeing the boundaries of this new condition broadened as widely as possible."[61]

When journalists have asked Goldstein point-blank about his ties to pharma companies, he does not deny his connections or get defensive. He just doesn't see his relationships with drug companies as a conflict of interest. "Serving as a consultant to pharmaceutical companies helps me ensure that the research they're performing or [the] results they're interpreting match what we in the field understand about women's sexual function," he told *Mother Jones*.[62] While researchers like Goldstein can provide valuable experience and information to help drug companies better understand diseases, once experts join the pharma payroll, it becomes much more difficult for them to stay objective. "It's not so much that the industry is there in some Machiavellian way," psychiatrist David Healy told *Mother Jones*. "But if you spend an awful lot of time with pharmaceutical companies, if you talk on their platforms, if you run clinical trials for them, you can't help but be influenced."[63]

According to a *Fortune* article, "In many cases, they [researcher consultants] sign nondisclosure agreements that block them from divulging data that might conflict, say, with a company's carefully crafted statements about new drugs."[64] Some of these researchers even invest in the companies they're consulting for, which creates conflicts of interest that are usually hidden from the public.[65] A 1996 meta-analysis in the *Annals of Internal Medicine* examined a few thousand drug-related studies to see how often researcher consultants shill for the drug companies that pay them. It found that 98 *percent* of studies conducted by drug company–sponsored researchers supported the drug in their study, while researchers without drug company sponsors supported the drug in their study less often, 79 percent of the time.[66] A 1998 *New England Journal of Medicine* article concluded that 96 percent of researchers who published studies that supported a group of cardiac drugs had financial ties to the company of the drug they supported. Of authors who were critical of cardiac drugs, only 37 percent had financial ties to the drug's manufacturer.[67] Research has also shown that doctors who receive money from pharma companies are also more likely to request that the company's drugs be added to their hospital's list of medications.[68]

The dubious nature of the relationship between researcher consultants and drug companies still gets glossed over today. Laumann's studies that estimate high rates of sexual dissatisfaction were used by outlets such as *ABC News* in 2014 to give authority to the necessity of new libido-enhancing products undergoing clinical trials.[69] In

2015, the FDA approved a pink pill called Addyi, made by Sprout Pharmaceuticals, that was nicknamed "female Viagra."[70]* Goldstein, one of the popular urologists who helped Pfizer sell Viagra, was a consultant for Sprout and once again made rounds in the media promoting the virtues of a new sex dysfunction product.[71]† Other sex products and procedures, such as injections aimed at boosting female sexual desire, continue to piggyback off Viagra's success and

---

*   Because of Addyi's severe side effects of inducing low blood pressure and faint-
      ing, the pill comes packaged with a "black box warning," which is the strongest
      warning the FDA labels drugs with. The FDA had previously rejected the drug
      twice because of its lack of effectiveness and serious side effects. In a clinical study,
      Addyi users reported an increase of only about one satisfying sexual encounter
      per month, and because of its side effects Addyi can't be used alongside alcohol
      or by women on the birth control pill, which makes the drug's use impractical for
      many women. But after the second rejection, the FDA was accused of "gender
      bias for ignoring the sexual needs of women," according to the *New York Times*.
      The main group accusing the FDA of sexism was a nonprofit called "Even the
      Score," which was sponsored by Sprout.

†   According to a 2015 Reuters article, "The chief executive of Sprout, Cindy
      Whitehead, cofounded the company with her husband Robert Whitehead
      in 2011 after selling another small drugmaker they had founded called Slate
      Pharmaceuticals, which had received repeated warnings from the FDA about
      its marketing tactics." A day after getting FDA approval for Addyi, Sprout was
      purchased by Valeant Pharmaceuticals International for a billion dollars. In
      2016, the *New York Times* reported that Addyi sales were well below forecasts
      because "a series of missteps after the deal [with Valeant], along with turbulence
      from aggressive accounting practices, unusual business relationships, and big
      egos, derailed one of the most intriguing new pharmaceuticals in a generation."
      According to the *Times*, Valeant is "under federal investigation, as are its drug-
      pricing policies, which have been described by lawmakers as predatory."

rely on the same studies run by drug-company consultants. Pharma companies are able to continue relying on compromised research because few people notice the conflict of interest. Rather than uphold sex products to thorough examination, the popular press has often promoted these products through attention-grabbing two-minute sound bites devoid of critical thinking.[72]

Pfizer has extended its sponsored research internationally. Although overall international sales of Viagra dropped 24 percent in 2014, Viagra sold well in China, with a 47 percent increase over the previous year.[73] Behind the sales boosts are messages like those found in the Pfizer-sponsored "China Ideal Sex Blue Book," which states Chinese men are overworked and suffering from high levels of impotence. The report claims that only about half of its respondents could achieve full erections that were "like a cucumber."[74] Pfizer claims that about 28 percent of Chinese men aged thirty to sixty suffer from erectile dysfunction (ED).[75] That puts the potential urban patient population (those who are most likely to be able to afford drugs) at about 68 million people, according to *Bloomberg*.[76] But when the *New York Times* contacted the doctor behind the "Blue Book" study, he "declined to say exactly how Pfizer supported the survey or why the report recommended the company's products as a first line of treatment."[77]

From the start, Pfizer has been very adept at promoting Viagra, which brought in about half a billion dollars in sales in its first year.[78] By 2000, Pfizer was so confident in Viagra, the company named the drug the "official sponsor of Valentine's

Day."[79] The success of Viagra's marketing campaign is now a case study in what critics call "disease mongering," which refers to the practice of broadening disease categories in an attempt to expand the market for treatment products.[80] An article titled "The Art of Branding a Condition" in *Medical Marketing Media* applauds Pfizer's ability in "condition branding" Viagra.[81] The article gives tips on how to conceptualize and market medical conditions alongside emerging pharma products. In branding the ED condition, Pfizer even sent representatives to the Vatican to see how the Catholic Church would respond to the pill. Luckily for Pfizer, the Vatican approved of Viagra because of its ability to improve marital sexual encounters.[82]* A writer in *Pharmaceutical Executive* summarizes Viagra's "condition branding" prowess:

> How many people knew ten years ago that there would be such a term as "erectile dysfunction"? That's brilliant branding. And it's not just about branding the drug; it's branding the condition, and by inference,

---

* Catholic Church doctrine, which is often based on natural law, forbids sex before marriage, masturbation, and contraception upon this "natural law" basis. According to the celibate men who make these policies, unmarried people engaging in sexual releases such as intercourse or masturbation (regardless of whether it's at the height of childbearing years or when sexual urges are at their strongest) violate "natural law." Senior citizens taking an artificial laboratory construction to fight the aging process and induce an erection they couldn't previously achieve, obey "natural law." Apparently it's more "natural" for a ninety-year-old to sport an eight-inch wood than for a fifteen-year-old to soil a sock when fluctuating hormone levels make him feel frisky.

a branding of the patient. [...] What kind of patient does a blockbuster create? We're creating patient populations just as we're creating medicines, to make sure that products become blockbusters.[83]

By "creating patient populations," Pfizer successfully turned Viagra into a blockbuster drug. Through limiting the effect that aging has on sex and convincing swaths of ordinary people that they're sexually dysfunctional, Viagra altered society's perception of sexuality and became a cultural phenomenon.

Viagra's Cultural Impact

Through relying on clever marketing and researchers who subtly misrepresented themselves to promote a product, Viagra sales surged. Although its marketing was packed with deception, the product benefitted people by improving the sex lives of many couples, particularly the elderly.[84†] No longer would scores of aging men lose the ability to sexually satisfy their partners, and they also wouldn't need to undergo any invasive medical procedures or use dangerous, poorly researched enhancement products to make their penises stay stiff.[85‡] The prevalence of Viagra also brought sex into the

---

† Viagra can also have nonsexual benefits, as doctors have used to the drug to treat various heart and lung conditions.

‡ As recent as the 1980s, impotence treatments included vacuum pumps and penile surgeries. Surgeries often involved cutting the ligament that attached the penis to the pubic bone. Several inches of penis that lay within the body cavity would then

public eye.[86]* Erectile dysfunction entered the lexicon, and
it became commonplace to see erection references on TV
commercials, billboards, and race cars.

Aside from its record-setting sales, Viagra influenced
American culture in myriad ways. The market for treating the
"disease" of ED attracted many similar drugs such as Cialis
and Levitra, which had ads that portrayed old men getting
boners as innocent as a father trying to throw a football
through a tire-swing.† Along with prescription drugs such as
Adderall, OxyContin, and Prozac, Viagra plays to the Band-
Aid quick-fix mind-set of modern American medicine. But
as Mary Roach points out in *Bonk: The Curious Coupling of
Science and Sex*, ED isn't a purely biological phenomenon, as
marketers imply. "In truth, plenty of cases of psychologically
based impotence exist, and it's relatively simple to sort out
which ones they are," Roach writes. "If a man is medically
impotent—because his smooth-muscle tissue is damaged,
say, or there's a problem with his nerves—then he won't get

---

be reeled outside the body. These surgeries were as much about looks as they
were about functioning penises. For men so desperate to go through this painful
and expensive procedure just to achieve better perceived sex, the introduction of
Viagra must have been a huge load off their chests.

* According to Shereen El Feki, in Egypt, Viagra has "become so much a part
of the culture that it serves as an alternative currency in some circles. I know
of one man who carries a pocketful of the real thing, picked up in America,
for baksheesh; the pills are especially useful, he says, for bribing bureaucrats to
finish paperwork on time."

† Those commercials made it confusing as to whether ED drugs helped clients get
an erection or improve aim. Apparently old men missed the hole before Levitra.

erections in his sleep. If the problem is purely psychological, he will."[87]‡ But instead of testing nocturnal erections or examining whether a patient's medical symptoms are related to psychological issues, many doctors write scripts.

Studies have also shown a placebo effect among Viagra takers, meaning that at least part of the drug's effectiveness is due to conditioned psychology and the patient's *belief* that it will work.[88] A meta-analysis found that for about half of the men who took Viagra, the drug led to more "successful" attempts at intercourse, and about one-tenth of the men who took the placebo had more "successful" intercourse attempts.[89] In one study, nearly 40 percent who took the placebo reported enhanced sexual function.[90] Rather than examine the cause of impotence, doctors and drug companies convinced people to pop pills instead—which isn't a hard sell, because drug treatments are *convenient* for everyone involved.

Patients like using drugs as their primary way to combat conditions because drugs aren't time consuming, require little effort, and they allow people to overcome biological symptoms without having to confront psychological issues that can be uncomfortable to acknowledge. Doctors like deferring to drugs because writing a script takes much less time and

---

‡   One way doctors have tested for nocturnal erections is by wrapping a small roll of postage stamps around the patient's penis. If an erection did occur at night, doctors would theoretically be able to tell because the penis would bust through the perforations that connect the stamps. But if the perforations remained intact, that meant either that the man did not get an erection or that he was unable to fuck his way out of a roll of stamps.

effort than trying to get patients to change their behavior, which allows doctors to treat more patients, which brings in more money to their medical offices. Pharma companies like patients using drugs because pushing product increases quarterly profits.

Systematically deferring to drugs as a first measure of defense against illnesses (and other conditions that are being branded as illnesses) reinforces a culture that finds mental illness taboo but physical health conditions excusable, as many people want a quick medical fix instead of exploring their inner self. Marketers capitalize on these preferences by advertising diseases directly to consumers. Labeling a naturally occurring process as a medical disorder creates treatment demand, which results in high profits for drug companies.[91]* This cycle contributes to a pill-popping culture and a McDonaldization of medicine. According to the *New York Times*, some Americans have "supersized" medicine cabinets to keep up with their prescription drug habits.[92] Even though its origin lies in blood pressure rather than boners, Viagra is a great anecdote of how sex topics can illustrate bigger issues within society.

---

*   According to Loe, "In the 1970s and 1980s, profitability of Fortune 500 medicine merchants (measured by return on revenues) was two times greater than the median for *all* industries in the Fortune 500. By 2000, it had jumped to eight times the median. And in 2001, Pfizer's profits surpassed the profits of Fortune 500 companies in home building, apparel, railroad, and publishing industries combined."

Unintentional Inventions

As we have seen, accidental inventions have shaped modern sexuality in several ways. Professional men trying to improve their work efficiency promoted the vibrator, which revolutionized female masturbation. A heart medication inadvertently gave men erections, which led to Viagra as pharma companies medicalized and profited from impotence while reducing sexual physiological limitations in men. On the flip side, graham crackers and corn flakes show that sexually inspired products can wind up influencing nonsexual everyday activities.

It's relevant to examine the root of an invention and the usage of these items, because it was ultimately sex that inspired the invention or marketing of these products. Religious and Victorian attempts to eliminate any trace of natural sexual urges usually manifest themselves in moralizing lectures and spiritual movements. But sometimes that energy spills over into the mainstream culture by attaching itself to secular commodities. The impetus to profit off sex is obvious in prostitution, pornography, and contraception. But it's also prevalent in allegedly impartial areas like the medical field, where scientists and marketers profit from medicalizing sexual behavior. Sex can indirectly produce products that add nuance and enjoyment to our lives, all while powerful nonsexual forces imperceptibly shape society's sexual perception through commercialization.

the clerical closet

HOW THE CATHOLIC CHURCH INCENTIVIZES THE PRIESTHOOD FOR DEVOUT GAY MEN

S ince the founding of Christianity, there have always been sexually active priests. But until about a thousand years ago, clerical sex wasn't so secretive. For at least several hundred years, Roman Catholic priests openly had wives and children. The Church eventually outlawed priests from having spouses, which effectively made any clerical sex a grave sin. This change in discipline was partially carried out in response to medieval economic and political conditions to prevent clergymen from selling their office or passing church property to their sons.

Preventing priests from marrying altered the makeup of the priesthood over time, and unintentionally provided a shelter for some devout gay men to hide their sexual orientation. By continuing to disqualify women and married men, the priesthood attracts men who desire to forgo sex for the rest of their lives in an attempt to get closer to God. Unlike straight men, who are allowed to get married in the Church and have sexual relations with their spouses, gay men do not have a Church-approved outlet for their sexual desires. Because the Church denounces *all* homosexual sex, some devout gay men attempt to avoid sex at all costs, which leads some of these men to the celibate priesthood.

Many factors—a desire to help others, a connection to God, economic concerns, childhood upbringing, community and family pressure—influence a person's vocation, so it'd be too simplistic to say that sexuality alone leads these men to the priesthood. However, it'd also be intellectually dishonest to dismiss sexuality's ability to influence clerical demographics, given how many straight men have left the priesthood to marry and how many gay men remain clerics. Although the Catholic Church is often viewed as one the biggest opponents of gay marriage, the Church's hostility toward married clerics and homosexuality has helped make the Catholic priesthood disproportionately gay compared to the rest of the population.

Creating Clerical Celibacy

Catholic laypeople today expect their clergymen to be unmarried and sexually abstinent.[1]* But for about half of

---

*   Eastern Rite priests aren't prohibited from marrying. But the Latin Rite, the Western
      Church, makes up the vast majority of Catholics and their priests are celibate. However,

Christianity's existence, this wasn't the case. For centuries, it was accepted that priests would marry or take concubines, have sex, and have children. And it wasn't rare for the son of a priest to become a preacher himself, and take over his father's job. Several popes—Innocent I, Silverius, John XI—were sons of *popes*. Several other popes—Theodore I, Damasus I, Boniface I, Boniface VI, Felix III, Anastasius II, Agapetus, Marinus I, John XV, and Adeodatus I—were sons of lower-ranking clergy.[2]

Over time, the Church began increasingly penalizing clerical sex. The earliest known declarations against clerical sex come from the early fourth century when the Church's canon law instructed married clergymen to abstain from having sex with their wives.[3] Eventually, prospective priests were instructed to avoid marriage altogether; however for those who did choose to marry, their "illicit" marriages were still considered legally valid.[4] It wasn't until the eleventh

---

within the Western Church, there are *some* married priests, because former Protestant pastors who convert to Catholicism and become Catholic priests are allowed to retain their wives. (There are also former Catholic priests who left their church and became Protestant pastors so that they could marry.)

Among Latin Rite priests, there are also some strange exceptions, like that of priest-sexologist Robert Francoeur who became both ordained and married. Years after becoming a priest, he married a woman and fathered two children. The bishop of his diocese petitioned Rome to recognize Francoeur's marriage so Francoeur could still be allowed to function as a priest. To the surprise of Francoeur, Rome recognized his marriage. "The Vatican made a mistake," Francoeur told the *New York Times*. "The response came from Pope Paul VI rubber-stamped granted as requested. It was obviously a clerical error which they didn't want to call attention to, so I just fell through the cracks."

century that the Church really waged a fierce campaign to end clerical marriage, in a movement driven by doctrinal and economic considerations.[5]

Doctrinally, banning clerical marriage followed traditional theology that taught sex was impure and sinful, and that forgoing marriage and abstaining from sex could elevate one's holiness and bring a person closer to God.[6] Because Jesus never married or had sex, the Church has taught that clerical celibacy provides priests a better path to imitate Christ and dedicate themselves to the Church.[7]* What also may have influenced the glorification of celibacy was that several of the Church's first evangelizers, like St. Paul, often condemned sexual activity while displaying a lukewarm attitude toward marriage. But they did so under very specific contexts.

Scholars now believe that Paul and his followers were

---

*   The Catholic Church used to commission eunuch singers called castrati. In Italy, high voices were essential to opera and church music. Because women weren't allowed to participate in choirs, castrated men became integral performers. Composers took note. Handel, Mozart, and Monteverdi all wrote music intended for castrati. Under Pope Clement VII, the Sistine Chapel used castrati to serve the glory of God. It's estimated that the churches of Rome had about a hundred castrati by the late 1600s, and within a hundred years, the number doubled. The monastery of Monte Cassino even had its own castration center.

Although monasteries castrated men for the opera, the Church forbade that priests castrate themselves. In what might be the most peculiar "first order of business" to ever take place during a political assembly, the *first* canon from the Church's *first* ecumenical council (the famous First Council of Nicaea) banned those who castrated themselves from the priesthood. Which makes you wonder just how often devout fourth-century Catholic men were cutting off their junk.

influenced by their perception that the end of the world was near.[8] Paul denounced several sexual behaviors (and divorce), and implied that celibacy was superior to marriage.[9] But Paul also taught that slaves shall remain slaves and the unmarried shall remain unmarried because people should focus on preparing for the end of the world rather than wasting their energy on personal relationships.[10] In more recent centuries, Church leaders have praised marriage and celebrated the "gift of the sacrament of matrimony."[11] But for Paul, marriage was no gift at all. At best, it was a defense against desire.[12] "But I say to the unmarried and to widows that it is good for them if they remain [celibate] even as I. But if they do not have self-control, let them marry; for it is better to marry than to burn with passion," Paul wrote.[13]

Several of the early Church's most influential preachers held marriage in even greater contempt. Doctor of the Church St. John Chrysostom taught, "Matrimony is of much use to those still caught up in their passions, who desire to live the lives of swine and be ruined in brothels."[14] Another Doctor of the Church, St. Jerome, said, "Matrimony is always a vice. All that can be done is to excuse it and to sanctify it."[15] Unlike contemporary Christianity, which celebrates marriage, marriage wasn't a cornerstone of medieval Christian life. And for several centuries, the Church didn't recognize marriage as a sacrament.[16] According to Catholic theologian Rev. Edward Schillebeeckx, "The thought which lurked at the back of everyone's mind at this time was: how could marriage, which involves 'you know what' (!), be a sacramental source of salvation?"[17]* Historian John Boswell said the lack of marital sex surrounding Jesus's birth and life led early Christians to be skeptical of marriage. Which was "hardly surprising for a religion whose founder was supposed to have had no biological father, whose parents were not married at the time of His conception, who was believed to have had no siblings, who Himself never married, and whose followers—in direct opposition to those of Judaism and most pagan religions—considered celibacy the most virtuous lifestyle."[18]

Early Christians had further reason to be skeptical of marriage, because reproduction was a threat to their health. In the ancient Roman Empire, where Christianity initially prospered, sex and marriage placed incredible pressure on young women. Life expectancy in second-century Rome was fewer than twenty-five years, and the median age of marriage for Roman women may have been as low as fourteen.[19] Historian Peter Brown writes that "death fell savagely on the young," which was partially driven by maternal death. Through bachelor taxes and pro-natalist policies, the state pressured its citizens to bear more children to replace the dead, and each woman had to produce an average of five children in a primitive medical environment just to maintain population levels.[20] In this context, Paul's messages of sexual renunciation and virginal exaltation were likely quite appealing.

---

*   According to Schillebeeckx, "the reality of sex" was "really what prevented the full sacramental definition from being applied to marriage initially." He writes, "As a sacrament, marriage was seen to be a remedy for those who were unable to live in continence, and for this reason it had a purely negative significance with regard to grace."

Aside from the Church's initial general skepticism and even indifference toward marriage, the requirement of clerical celibacy also has roots in Jewish purity rituals.[21] Following in the tradition of the Levitical priesthood, early Christian theologians argued that by having sex, even if it was with a spouse, the priest contaminated his actions and the sacred position he held.[22] What began as sexual abstinence around the time of the Sabbath eventually evolved into a clerical marriage ban. But doctrine wasn't the sole driver of the priesthood's shift toward celibacy. Economics also played a large role.

Economic Reasons for Clerical Celibacy

Economically, married clergy were expensive to support. Aside from supporting the priest, the Church had to provide food and shelter for his spouse and children.[23] Richard Sipe, a psychotherapist and former Benedictine monk who writes extensively about clerical sexuality, says church leaders pushed for an unmarried clergy because "[e]conomic control of the single priest is simpler to regulate than that of a man engaged with the more elaborate network of a family."[24] Married clergy had the habit of treating their parish as if it were a family business by passing on their ecclesiastical offices to their sons.[25] Because this practice was common, "[t]he preservation of church property favored those who had no spouse or heirs," Sipe writes.[26]

Pope Gregory VII, who held the papacy from 1073 to 1085, wanted to end these dynasties and prevent the children of clergy members from inheriting church properties. Aside from limiting the power of sacerdotal dynasties, Gregory's reforms were also aimed at battling corruption. In medieval Europe, feudal lords were amassing vast amounts of land and appointing their own bishops, and in this context the selling of ecclesiastical offices (simony) became common, because the offices of high-ranking clerics were very valuable given the amount of land and power that was associated with them.[27]

By preventing clergy from marrying and ordering them to avoid sexual relations, Gregory's policies decreased the practice of priests passing property to their sons.[28] In declaring that only lifelong celibate men could become priests, Gregory significantly limited the priestly prospect pool, which limited the number of people who would be able to hold ecclesiastical offices, which reduced the demand for purchasing these offices.[29] To put an end to "the heresy of Simony" and to priests' families from claiming church holdings, Pope Gregory and his contemporaries took drastic action.[30] He declared that married clergy had to leave their wives or be deposed from office.[31] Other popes of the era forbade people to attend Mass conducted by married priests, and ordered the concubines of clerics to be forced into servitude as palace chattels.[32] Church reformers were often harsh to clerics' wives. Referring to the wives of priests, Saint Peter Damian, a cardinal and Doctor of the Church, stated, "The hands that touch the body and blood of Christ must not have touched the genitals of a whore."³³* The shift toward celibacy left many victims in its wake. Historian James Brundage writes:

> The frightened victims of the reformers' attacks on clerical marriage not only included clergymen, who were liable to be stripped of their positions and livelihoods, but also their wives and children... Women who had married clerics in good faith, women who were often themselves the daughters or granddaughters of priests or bishops, found themselves shorn of social position, driven from their homes, their marriages denounced as immoral from the pulpits, their honor ruined, their families broken, and their commitment to husband and children denounced as scurrilous and sinful. The children suffered a worse fate: their legitimacy was suspect, their capacity to inherit denied, their future clouded, and their very existence deplored by public authorities and spiritual

---

* In his crusade against clergy marriages, Damian stretched analogies incredible distances. He warned priests that fathers who seduce their daughters get excommunicated and sent to prison. Damian then added that laywomen are the priest's *spiritual* daughters, so to have sex with one of them is like committing spiritual incest. He claims priests having sex with laywomen (spiritual incest) is *worse* than ordinary incest. After accusing priests of committing incest with their spouses, he then asks, "If you commit incest with your spiritual daughter, how in good conscience do you dare perform the mystery of the Lord's body?" He added: "The day will come...when this impurity of yours will be turned into pitch on which the everlasting fire will feed, never to be extinguished in your very being; and with never-ending flames this fire will devour you, flesh and bones."

leaders. Reviled as the "cursed seed" of their fathers' lust, they were the innocent victims of high-minded idealists such as Peter Damian, Pope Gregory VII, and other reform leaders.[34†]

In banning married clergy, the Church no longer had to pay to support the families of priests. Mandatory clerical celibacy also reduced the practice of simony and prevented priests from having sons who would inherit church property. Another benefit to the Church was that unhinging priests from spouses and children allowed priests to further commit themselves solely to the Church.[35†] Priests could now devote

---

† Peter Damian had this to say about the *wives* of clergy: "I speak of you, female abodes of the ancient enemy, pick-axes, screech-owls, night-birds, she-wolves, blood suckers, crying 'Give, give, without ceasing.' Come and hear me, you garbage, prostitutes, puckered lips, pigsties for fat pigs, couches for foul spirits, nymphs, sirens, vampires, moon goddesses...you who through the allurements of your fake charm snatch away unfortunate men from ministry at the sacred altars where they are engaged, in order to strangle them in the slimy glue of your own passion."

† Priests certainly protested the prohibition of clerical marriage. According to Brundage, "The reaction of the lesser clergy to the imposition of reform was vigorous, sometimes violent. When the Bishop of Paris told his priests that they must give up their wives and children, they drove him from the church with jeers and blows, and he found it necessary to take refuge with the royal family in order to escape the wrath of his outraged clerics. Archbishop John of Rouen was stoned by his indignant clergy when he ordered them to abandon their concubines, while in northern Italy some bishops simply did not dare to publish the celibacy decrees for fear of their lives. Their misgivings were not unrealistic: in a letter to Bishop Josfried of Paris, Gregory VII reported in 1077 that a proponent of clerical celibacy had been burnt alive by the outraged clergy of Cambrai."

more time, energy, and resources to their spiritual and political ambitions.[36]

Sociologist David Greenberg writes that for "clear political and organizational reasons" Gregorian reformers were stricter about barring married clergy than they were about barring gay clergy. "Homosexual relationships did not result in progeny, and therefore did not threaten the preservation of church property," Greenberg writes, adding, "The more the church suppressed priestly marriage and concubinage, the stronger must have been the homosexual drive it aroused within its ranks."[37] While the Church gained several direct economic benefits through banning clerical marriage, it indirectly created an awkward social situation by creating a celibate homosocial power structure, which provided a closet for some gay Catholic men to hide in.[38]* But given that the Catholic Church has called gay sexual orientation an "objective disorder" and vocalizes its opposition to gay sex as "an intrinsic moral evil," why would a gay Catholic want to become a priest?[39]

Sexual Sublimation

One theory suggests that some devout gay Catholic men want to follow church teaching and sublimate their sexuality, and that sublimation nudges some men toward the priesthood. A

---

*   A gay priest told Jason Berry, "Religious life *attracts* [gay people]... And this doesn't have to be conscious or erotic, but if you're same-sex oriented, you're drawn to a life surrounded with guys."

gay priest told reporter Jason Berry, "Historically, I think a lot of gay men have gone into priesthood as a way of sublimating particular drives. The first time I went into a gay bar I saw four other priests: *here for the same reason I am*, I thought."[40] The Catechism of the Catholic Church encourages sublimation of homosexuality, as seen in its teaching, which states, "Homosexual persons are called to chastity. By the virtues of self-mastery that teach them inner freedom, at times by the support of disinterested friendship, by prayer and sacramental grace, they can and should gradually and resolutely approach Christian perfection."[41] The Church teaches that gay sex is a mortal sin, and that mortal sins are punishable by eternal hellfire unless the sinner confesses and is repentant. Because the Church opposes gay marriage, and only approves of sex within marriage, theoretically, the gravity of the sin isn't influenced by whether gay sex occurs casually or in a long-term relationship.[42†]

---

† Because the Church demands total abstinence from gay people, it can give the appearance of unintentionally "promoting promiscuity and humanly destructive and depersonalized sexual activity among Catholic homosexuals," wrote John McNeil. "A Catholic homosexual who confessed occasional promiscuity could receive absolution and be allowed to receive communion in good conscience. If, however, that person had entered into a genuine permanent love relationship, he or she would be judged in 'a state of sin,' and unless the person expressed a willingness to break off that relationship he or she would be denied absolution. Consequently, the traditional discipline unwittingly tended to undermine the development of healthy interpersonal relationships among homosexuals and gave the appearance that the Church disapproved more of the love between homosexuals than it did of their sexual activity as such."

Without any non-damnable sex acts available to them, some devout gay men attempt to bottle up their sexuality and avoid sex altogether. After the U.S. Conference of Catholic Bishops set up a National Review Board of lay members to investigate sex abuse in the Church, the Board reported, "Certain homosexual men appear to have been attracted to the priesthood because they mistakenly viewed the requirement of celibacy as a means of avoiding struggles with their sexual identities."[43] As gay former priest Christopher Schiavone put it, "I thought I would never need to tell another person my secret, because celibacy would make it irrelevant."[44]

The Board's findings were in line with what various Church observers had been saying for a while. Former priest and Boston College theology professor Thomas Groome writes, "Surely many good Catholic gay men, told by their church that their orientation is 'intrinsically disordered' and that they are 'called to chastity' for life, say to themselves, 'If I must be celibate, why not be a priest?'"[45] Priest-theologian Richard McBrien told the *Atlantic*, "Claiming celibacy is a wonderful cover for gays, and let's face it, the seminary presents a marvelous arena of opportunity for them."[46] These statements are echoed by what a gay priest told Sipe: "The church demands celibacy of homosexuals anyway. If I'm homosexual and I have to be celibate, I might as well be a priest and be useful."[47] Becoming a priest, a profession whose members are expected be lifelong sexually abstinent, gives some devout gay Catholic men more incentive to avoid sex with men, which can help them circumvent perceived damnation. But because empirical research on gay priests is scant, there's no way to tell if the sexually sublimating priests Berry, Sipe, and the National Review Board talked to represent the majority of gay priests, or if their conclusions come from viewing a nonrepresentative sample.

Another theory to explain the high numbers of gay priests is that as a discriminated-against minority, gay men may be more sensitive to empathize with people, and a strong desire to help others leads some of these men to the priesthood.[48] In an essay about gay priests, Rev. James Martin, a popular church commentator and an editor of the Jesuit magazine *America*, writes:

> Homosexuals are frequent targets of prejudice, ridicule, rejection from their own families and, sometimes, violence. Here, therefore, are men who understand suffering, stigma, and frustration, the very types of experiences that Christian theology teaches can lead one closer to companionship with the Christ who suffers. [...] Being schooled in this unique experience of suffering can result in a profound sense of compassion and identification with the most marginalized in society: the sick, the lonely, the refugee, the materially poor, the outcast, the least of my brothers and sisters.[49]*

---

*   Karen Lebacqz, a professor at the Pacific School of Religion, wrote, "Many gay Roman Catholics may indeed be attracted to the priesthood precisely because an active gay identity 'outside' is not respected but as a priest, the young man is offered a model of 'redemptive suffering' and avoidance of a disgraceful sexual identity."

Rev. Robert Nugent, cofounder of Catholic LGBT group New Ways Ministry, also believed that some gay clerics gain compassion and sympathy from their orientation. He wrote, "Gay clergy many times feel that their most effective ministerial gifts and talents flow from or are directly related to their experience of being homosexually oriented."[50] An anonymous gay cleric told Nugent that when he first became a priest, he thought, "Homosexuality was a curse to be escaped." But he eventually discovered that his "sexuality was the source of most of my personality traits that I valued and found effective in ministry."[51]

There are likely other reasonable theories that help explain why so many gay men become priests. However, sexual sublimation comes up the most when reviewing the existing literature. Instead of becoming priests, devout gay men could of course remain sexually abstinent as single laypeople. But eventually, they might have to explain to curious laypeople why they remain unmarried. People might get suspicious of a single older Catholic man in the congregation, but if the man forgoes a wife as part of his job requirements, then questions about his sexuality might be avoided.[52]* The National Review Board reported that for some gay men

---

* Law scholar Richard Posner theorized Catholic rituals might attract homosexuals. The adornment, theatrical expression, music, incense, and lavish garb might appeal more to a gay man than a straight man, he wrote. The idea gives a more thorough conceptualization to Steven Colbert's quip about Pope Francis's meager dress not fulfilling proper papal attire: "You're not really the head of the Catholic Church unless you look like you're in a Liberace cover band!"

the priesthood "provided them with a 'cover'—a ready explanation as to why they were not married."[53] Because celibacy can provide a cover for some gay men trying to conceal their sexuality, seminaries are "fraught with gays," McBrien told a reporter.[54†] Fran Ferder, a nun and clinical psychologist who has treated sexually abusive clergy members, told Berry, "I think some Catholic gay men delay it [dating] altogether and choose seminary as an acceptable way of not having to deal with sexuality. And then it comes out when they're in their twenties or thirties, emotionally at an age of fifteen or sixteen—a regressive homosexuality."[55†] While gay priests have been in the news a lot in the past few decades as sex abuse scandals and priests dying of AIDS garnered headlines, gay priests aren't a new phenomenon, as gay men have pursued the priesthood for centuries.

The Prevalence of Gay Priests

Writing a bishop friend in the eighth century, Saint Alcuin wrote, "I think of your love and friendship with such sweet memories, reverend bishop, that I long for that lovely time

---

†   Sociologist Dean Hoge found that more than half of U.S. priests believe there's a gay subculture in their diocese, and 41 percent said a gay subculture probably existed in their seminaries.

‡   Robert Nugent noticed a similar phenomenon in the early '80s. He wrote, "For many gay clergy, the process of self-discovery and self-acceptance often includes some overt homosexual behavior, usually combined with a strong affectivity, especially when this process has been bypassed in the usual course of sexual development."

when I may be able to clutch the neck of your sweetness with the fingers of my desires… [H]ow would I cover, with tightly pressed lips, not only your eyes, ears, and mouth but also your every finger and your toes, not once but many a time."[56] In 1145, Saint Bernard of Clairvaux told Pope Eugenius III, "Your brothers, the cardinals, must learn by your example not to keep young, long-haired boys and seductive men in their midst."[57] There isn't concrete evidence that the priests mentioned in this paragraph had gay sex, but their writings appear homoerotic even within the context of passionate medieval brotherhood. The further back in history you go, the more difficult identifying gay behavior in the priesthood becomes, especially because ancient societies didn't conceptualize a gay orientation as we do today. But what's easier to trace is the evidence of homosexuality in the priesthood today.

However, there still remain inherent difficulties in measuring the number of gay priests within the Catholic Church, and data on this topic tends to be American-centric. Catholic priests are a *global* brotherhood, so take caution when generalizing from studies on priest sex, because the majority are based on American samples. Another major limitation is that studies on clerical sexuality suffer from self-selection bias, because surveys without truly random samples tend to reflect the most vocal segment of a group rather than its general population.

People researching clerical sexuality aren't unscientific or lazy; it's just *really* difficult to get a random sampling from a large number of priests who are willing to discuss their sexuality. To procure a scientifically valid sample would require polling thousands of priests at random and obtaining their consent to use the collected data. Most studies on priests don't have the resources or connections to do this, so they use snowball and convenient samples, which generally estimate between 20 to 50 percent of Catholic priests to be gay.[58] In 1993 and 2002, the *Los Angeles Times* conducted the most generalizable studies on American priests' behavior and sexuality. The *Times* sent thousands of surveys to priests across the nation, and both of these projects garnered about 2,000 responses.[59] The study found about 15 percent of priests reported a homosexual orientation, and a little over a third of these priests report having engaged in sexual activity with another person after ordination.[60] Though the *Times'* numbers were more conservative than other studies, they still indicated the priesthood is disproportionately gay compared to the general population, which is estimated to be about 3.5 percent lesbian, gay, and bisexual.[61]

Surveys on priest sex should be viewed with skepticism, but they shouldn't be entirely dismissed. Real-world evidence backs up the estimates that the priesthood is disproportionately gay. In 1987, the *Atlantic*, the *Washington Post*, the *Chicago Tribune*, the *New York Times*, and the *Los Angeles Times* quoted health officials and AIDS counselors who recognized that some priests were part of the subgroup of the gay population that was at a high risk for contracting HIV.[62]* In 2000, the *Kansas City Star* ran an exposé on priests

---

*   In 1988, Damien Ministries held a conference for priests living with HIV. According to Jon Fuller, a Jesuit priest and physician who was the founding

dying of AIDS. After conducting interviews and examining death certificates, the *Star* estimated that at least 300 priests suffered AIDS-related deaths between the mid-1980s and 1999.[63] Because several states didn't disclose death records and some death certificates didn't accurately report AIDS deaths, the true number was likely even higher, the *Star* implied. The AIDS death rate for priests was at least four per 10,000, which was about double the adult male population rate and more than four times the general population rate, the *Star* claimed. One projection from the paper put the AIDS death rate for priests as high as seven per 10,000.[64]

Although *some* priests may have contracted HIV from blood transfusions or needle sharing in the early 1980s, those factors don't explain such a large discrepancy between a population allegedly refraining from sex and one dying of AIDS at a relatively high rate. Rather, obviously, most priests likely contracted HIV through having sex.[65] And much of that sex was with men. Because HIV spreads more quickly through anal than through vaginal sex, and because HIV was and is much more prevalent in the gay community in the U.S., priests who had gay sex were much more likely to acquire HIV than priests having straight sex. The high prevalence of AIDS within the priesthood wasn't the only tragic phenomenon that alerted the public that priests were having sex with other males.

---

president of the National Catholic AIDS Network, priests participating in the conference "felt so stigmatized and fearful of negative repercussions that they wore paper bags over their heads as they shared their experiences."

SUPERNATURAL SACRIFICES
AND EARTHLY INCENTIVES

It's likely that economic conditions influence seminary enrollment. A study in *Applied Economic Letters* examined how seminary enrollment (for all Christian denominations, not just Catholics) was affected by changes in unemployment and clergy salaries. The study found that people enroll in seminaries more often when unemployment and clergy salaries rise. A 1 percent increase in (lagged) unemployment was associated with a 3.5 percent increase in seminary enrollment. The study also found that for every $1,000 the average annual clergy salary exceeds the average salary for all occupations, seminary enrollments increase 2.7 percent.[66]

While the idea that economic conditions can influence how many people join the clergy is intriguing, there isn't much research on this topic. Most denominations are decentralized (meaning their congregations often lack a central governing body, unlike Catholicism, which has the Vatican), which makes accurate data gathering extremely difficult. Evidence of the economy's effect on clergy formation is typically anecdotal. One such example is a remark made by U.S. Conference of Catholic Bishops official Rev. David Toups: "Historically, times of challenge or crisis usually bring out the best in people. We saw a huge boon in candidates to the priesthood after the Great Depression and World War II."[67]

Toups's comment brings up another point. Even if economic conditions influence how many people join the clergy, the relationship may not be direct. As unemployment rises and people lose their jobs, the demand for social services that churches provide could also increase. Socially conscious, altruistic individuals already contemplating entering a seminary might be inspired to pursue clergyhood because of the increased demand for pastoral services. Of course, these theories are speculative, and there could be other extraneous variables influencing people to join the seminary beyond a "higher calling."

Sex Abuse Scandals

As early as the mid-1980s, reporters from outlets such as the *Times of Acadiana*, Cleveland's *Plain Dealer*, San Jose's *Mercury News*, and the *National Catholic Reporter* were publicly breaking stories on priests sexually abusing children and the subsequent cover-ups by Church officials.[68] Media coverage of clerical sex abuse scandals continued throughout the late 1980s and early 1990s, but after sex abuse accusations made against Chicago Cardinal Joseph Bernardin were withdrawn by the accuser in 1993, coverage of abuse scandals declined significantly.[69] "In a sense, the fiasco surrounding the Bernardin case gave newsrooms a rationalization to retreat from this kind of coverage," Jason Berry told NPR.[70] After the Bernardin case, much of the public failed to take serious notice of sex abuse within the Church until 2002, when the *Boston Globe* Spotlight team broke its Pulitzer-winning investigation. A string of lawsuits followed the *Globe* exposé, and dioceses began declaring bankruptcy during the 2000s.[71]

Theories behind what caused the sex abuse crisis are plentiful and politically charged. As priest-sociologist Andrew Greeley puts it, "Inside the Church the 'liberals' were blaming sexual abuse on celibacy, and the conservatives were blaming it on homosexuality, neither with much more in the way of evidence than strong personal opinions."[72] Reliable statistics for clerical sexual abuses are hard to come by, because so many dioceses have hidden and underreported abuse to civil authorities. The John Jay Report, commissioned by the U.S. Conference of Catholic Bishops in response to the scandals, relied on self-reported data from dioceses and found about 4 percent of American Catholic priests from 1950 to 2002 were accused of sexually abusing minors.[73]* But as Anne Barrett Doyle, codirector of the watchdog website BishopAccountability.org, points out, "There aren't many dioceses where prosecutors have gotten involved, but in every single instance there's a vast gap—a multiplier of two, three or four times—between the numbers of perpetrators that the prosecutors find and what the bishops released."[74]†

While the John Jay Report provides the most

---

*   Even among the accused, only 149 priests (or 3.5 percent of the 4.2 percent of priests that were accused of abuse) accounted for 26 percent of alleged abuses. That means just over 0.1 percent of priests accounted for more than a quarter of the abuses. On a broader scale, that would be like if Omaha accounted for a fourth of all sex crimes in the U.S.

†   According to the John Jay report, only "6% of all priests against whom allegations were made were convicted and about 2% received prison sentences to date."

comprehensive statistical profile of sexually abusive priests and is a somewhat transparent exercise from an institution that's often perceived as secretive, it's worth briefly mentioning at least four of the study's limitations before generalizing its results. First off, its figures for abusive priests may be too low for the reasons that Doyle mentioned. Second, as with any study of sexual abuse, abuse is likely underreported, and among victims who do report, there is often a time lag between when the abuse occurred and when the abuse was reported. Third, the report only looks at *American* abuse cases, while it's very evident that the sex abuse problem within the Church is a *global* phenomenon, which makes any of the report's conclusions about American culture contributing to the crisis *very* questionable.[75] Fourth, the study looks at the time frame of 1950–2002, but the problem of sexual abuse by priests and monks goes back well beyond 1950, as there are Church documents from the Middle Ages that address clerical sex abuse.[76]

Even within the U.S., it's pretty evident there were clerical sexual abuses prior to 1950. In recent years, elderly people have come forward about abuse that occurred when they were children.[77] And in 1947, Rev. Gerald Fitzgerald founded the Congregation of the Servants of the Paraclete to deal with priests' behavioral problems, which included pedophilia. Bishops sent the Paracletes so many sexually abusive priests that during the 1950s Fitzgerald searched for a private island that the Church could purchase to harbor and isolate clergy sex offenders from society. Although the island never came to be, Fitzgerald was so serious about secluding clerical pedophiles that he eventually made a $5,000 down payment on a $50,000 Caribbean island that he wanted his archdiocese to purchase.[78]

In line with modern psychological research, the John Jay Report found there was no correlation between priests having a gay identity and priests abusing minors, even though the vast majority of those abused were boys.[79] In her analysis of the John Jay Report, clinical psychologist Mary Gail Frawley-O'Dea writes in the *National Catholic Reporter*, "Sexual abuse is a crime of opportunity, not of sexual identity. In fact, the period of decline in priestly sexual abuse corresponds with both the gaying and graying of the priesthood... In any event, no Catholic pope, bishop, priest, or layperson can in good conscience identify gay priests as the primary source of sexual abuse, even of boys."[80] Frawley-O'Dea has a point, that it is far too simplistic to blame the pathology of abusive priests and the corruption of powerful officials on a gay orientation, and that opportunistic abusive priests had significantly greater access to boys than they did to girls given the homosocial structure of seminaries and the fact that boys made up the majority of altar servers.[81]*

But regardless of what the John Jay group or any other researchers find, the high number of abused boys will continue to drive many people to associate gay priests with

---

*   Psychologists have also found that many of the priests who molested boys self-identify as heterosexual. Aside from the higher access they had to boys, other reasons these men targeted more boys than girls included "pregnancy fears with female victims" and that they "more easily established trust" with boys.

sex abuse. Discussing either topic (gay priests *or* sex abuse in the Church) will likely remain contentious for some time. As investigative reporters Jason Berry and Gerald Renner point out, "The gay clergy issue cannot be easily reported without offending just about everyone. Many conservatives blame *'the gays'* for a crisis with many tangled roots; gay liberationists cry homophobia at any whisper of criticism."[82]* Because homosexuality can be such a hot-button topic in the Church, few gay priests publicly come out. For these men, the organization they've given their lives to produces mental anguish, as it condemns their sexuality and the way they're hardwired to express physical love.

The Cognitive Dissonance of Gay Priests

A 2016 *Washington Post* article stated that "the Catholic priesthood may be one of the last remaining closets—and it's a crowded one."[83] Because few gay priests publicly come out, positive visible role models remain hidden to congregants. Using a pseudonym, a gay cleric wrote in the Catholic magazine *Commonweal*:

---

*   They added, "There is a crucial distinction between homosexual priests who embody genuine Christian witness and the gay priest culture that arose in the 1970s, cynical about celibacy, riddled with hypocrisy and narcissistic behavior. We have not as a society come to terms with what it means when a victimized minority (*some* bishops and priests who are gay) gains power, creates cliques, and uses clericalism to harass heterosexual seminarians, cover up promiscuity, and extend its patterns of deception to blanket those who have sex with youths."

Gay priests like myself are caught in a double bind. If we speak the truth and discuss freely our existence in the church, and, more important, our experience of leading fulfilling lives as celibate men, we will be censured or removed from ministry. If we remain silent, though, we guarantee that the positive example of the celibate gay priest will remain hidden. Voiceless, the gay priest cannot defend himself within the church. Stereotyped, he cannot escape the suspicions of society at large. [...] I have long hoped to testify before my parish to this foundational experience of God's love in my life, but I am of course forbidden to do so.[84]

The Church has yet to come to terms with why this particular group of devout Catholics who've dedicated their lives to serving God feel the need to conceal part of their identity. James Martin writes, "The reason that you don't see any public models of healthy, mature, celibate gay priests to counteract the stereotype of the pedophile gay priest, is that they are forbidden to speak out publicly. Or they are simply afraid."[85†]

Surely, there are many gay priests who are comfortable with their sexuality.[86] But there are also many gay priests who

---

†   Richard Sipe writes, "If the Catholic Church were to excise from the list of its honored saints all men who had a homosexual orientation, the roles would be decimated. The list of outcasts would include apostles, martyrs, popes, bishops, and founders of religious orders."

face a disconnect between reconciling their sexual identity and their church's condemnation of homosexuality. Robert Mickens, a former Rome correspondent for the British Catholic magazine *The Tablet*, told *Frontline*, "[T]here's a lot of gay men in the Vatican who are very good people, who are celibate, who are not having sex, who are struggling to be good priests, to be good officials, to do their job well, to be compassionate men… But the culture itself mitigates against that. It's difficult to be good in the Vatican, because it is a hypocritical kind of culture."[87] Mickens says one of the "biggest problems" in the Catholic hierarchy is a "hypocritical presence of so many homosexuals, gay men, many of whom would not even classify themselves as gay men because they're so conflicted."[88]* The mental conflict of gay priests forms the basis of Richard Wagner's dissertation, *Gay Catholic Priests: A Study of Cognitive and Affective Dissonance*. Wagner, a sex therapist and gay former priest, concludes, "The dilemma of the gay priest, the cognitive and affective dissonance present in his life, is due in great measure to the confusion surrounding the issues of homosexuality and celibacy and their moral and theological implications."[89] In a later book, Wagner goes on to say:

---

*   Religion scholar Mark Jordan has written about modern clerics and seminarians who have gay sex but reject identifying as gay. "Homosexuality itself cannot be spoken, admitted, described," he writes. "So whatever happens cannot be homosexuality." In treating priest patients, Sipe notices, "An interesting subgroup of priests is marked by their fear of being homosexual. These men are conscientious and would identify themselves as gay if they could only resolve their internal conflict. But they cannot."

In fact, there is a sizable segment of the clergy population that is gay and who are forced to live duplicitous lives of repression and secrecy. This often creates an atmosphere of extreme isolation and loneliness that can and does drive these men to desperate measures to find emotional and moral support they should be receiving from their Church. These men love their Church, but hate what it is doing to them.[90]

In his survey of gay priests, sociologist James Wolf found that gay priests were more likely to have problems with "leading a celibate life" and "loneliness of the priesthood" compared to straight priests.[91] More than half of the gay priests Wolf surveyed said they struggled with the "relevance of certain church doctrine."[92] One respondent said:

If the parishioners found out, for example, that I am a homosexual, what would they do? This fear saddens me... I cannot let myself be known for who I truly am and be loved for who I truly am. So much of what is going on inside me I cannot share with people. There is such richness now in how I experience life and how I view the world, and I have to hold that back. To disclose my homosexual orientation to my parishioners would, to the best of my discernment, cause the following: polarization of the people for and against me; suspicion or accusation of immoral activities, especially with teens and children; a request for my removal; a need for the Ordinary [bishop] to make

some statement or take some action about me; a
witch-hunt for other closeted priests; and continued
fear in the young who are becoming aware of being
gay. The risk seems far too great.[93]

While the Church has traditionally declared gay sex
immoral, and there is no shortage of Vatican-issued statements that "progressive" people would call "homophobic,"
the writings of Joseph Ratzinger (Pope Benedict XVI) are
particularly interesting because his strict tone illustrates why
the gay priest Wolfe surveyed feared a "witch-hunt for other
closeted priests."

The Church's Recent Tone Change on Homosexuality

Before he became Pope Benedict XVI, Joseph Ratzinger
was a powerful theologian who served as Prefect of the
Congregation for the Doctrine of the Faith (CDF) from
1981 to 2005. The CDF was founded in 1542 to "defend
the Church from heresy" and to "promote and safeguard the
doctrine on the faith and morals throughout the Catholic
World."[94] The CDF's original name was the "Sacred
Congregation of the Universal Inquisition,"[95] but in 1908,
the Church changed the office's name, perhaps because being
associated with the human-rights abuses of the Inquisition
wasn't good for branding.

As head of the CDF, Ratzinger issued a 1986 letter to
bishops, "On the Pastoral Care of Homosexual Persons,"

which condemned gay sex *and* said having a gay orientation was "an objective disorder" that was "ordered toward an intrinsic moral evil." Ratzinger's letter said that "homosexual activity prevents one's own fulfillment and happiness" and that the Church "is really concerned" about the "pro-homosexual movement" and the people who've "been tempted to believe its deceitful propaganda."[96]

In another passage of the letter, Ratzinger seems concerned about discrimination against gay people. He states: "It is deplorable that homosexual persons have been and are the object of violent malice in speech or in action. Such treatment deserves condemnation from the Church's pastors wherever it occurs." However, in the next paragraph he blames gay-related hate crimes on *gay-rights laws.* "When homosexual activity is consequently condoned, or when civil legislation is introduced to protect behavior to which no one has any conceivable right, neither the Church nor society at large should be surprised when other distorted notions and practices gain ground, and irrational and violent reactions increase." He makes it clear that he does not want Church teaching to change: "With this in mind, this Congregation wishes to ask the Bishops to be especially cautious of any programmes which may seek to pressure the Church to change her teaching, even while claiming not to do so... No authentic pastoral programme will include organizations in which homosexual persons associate with each other without clearly stating that homosexual activity is immoral."[97]

The 1986 letter would not be the last time Ratzinger pushed to define a gay orientation as "disordered." In charge of preparing the 1997 edition of the Catechism of the Catholic Church, Ratzinger made "more than one hundred changes in wording," according to veteran Vatican insider John Thavis. One of the most significant changes, an edit of only a few words, came on an entry regarding homosexuality. The 1992 catechism stated: "The number of men and women who have deep-seated homosexual tendencies is not negligible. They do not choose their homosexual condition; for most of them it is a trial." Ratzinger changed the 1997 edition to say: "The number of men and women who have deep-seated homosexual tendencies is not negligible. This inclination, objectively disordered, is a trial for most of them."[98]

As Pope Benedict XVI, Ratzinger cited the wording change he placed in the 1997 catechism in a 2005 letter he approved that was intended to ban men with "deep-seated homosexual tendencies" from the priesthood.[99]* The letter was vague on how seminary directors were to carry out these orders. And when reporters pressed Church officials

---

*   Under Ratzinger, the CDF issued a 1992 letter that seemed to suggest that gay people should stay in the closet. It stated: "An individual's sexual orientation is generally not known to others unless he publicly identifies himself as having this orientation or unless some overt behavior manifests it. As a rule, the majority of homosexually oriented persons who seek to lead chaste lives do not publicize their sexual orientation. Hence the problem of discrimination in terms of employment, housing, etc., does not usually arise." A 2006 guideline from the United States Conference of Catholic Bishops also implied that gay people should conceal their sexual identity. It stated, "In the context of parish life, however, general public self-disclosures [of sexual orientation] are not helpful and should not be encouraged."

for details, their answers were unclear. When asked how he would identify gay candidates, the U.S. Conference of Catholic Bishops vocations director, Rev. David Toups echoed Justice Potter Stewart's description of pornography. "It's more like one of those things where it's hard to define," Toups said. "But 'I know it when I see it.'"[100] Among the many critics of the 2005 letter was James Martin, who wrote that weeding gay men out of seminaries "laid bare the cognitive dissonance that threatens a church that relies on celibate gay priests to carry out much of its ministerial work, and yet sets into place policies which would bar those same kinds of men from future ministry."[101†]

Although the 2005 letter received a lot of attention for attempting to rid seminaries of gays, it wasn't the first time the Vatican attempted to ban gay clerics.[102‡] A 1961 Church instruction stated, "Advancement to religious vows and ordination should be barred to those who are afflicted with

---

†   Religion scholar Mark Jordan told the *New York Times*, "And not the least irony here, is that these new regulations [to weed gay men out of seminaries] are being enforced in many cases by seminary directors who themselves are gay."

‡   After the 2005 letter came out, there was some confusion on whether it was really meant to ban all gay men from seminaries or if it just banned sexually active gay men. A 2008 Church guideline put an end to this confusion and made it clear that the Church intended to prevent anyone with a gay orientation from enrolling in a seminary. The 2008 letter stated, "It is not enough to be sure that he [a seminary applicant] is capable of abstaining from genital activity. It is also necessary to evaluate his sexual orientation… Chastity for the Kingdom, in fact, is much more than the simple lack of sexual relationships."

evil tendencies to homosexuality or pederasty."[103]* Given that many gay men still enrolled in seminaries after the 1961 edict, it's doubtful that Benedict's attempt to prevent gay men from becoming priests will work.[104]† While it's uncertain how the 2005 letter has impacted seminarian candidates, it is certain that Benedict's writings have upset many gay priests. One gay priest told *Frontline*, "I cannot understand this schizophrenic attitude of the hierarchy against gays when a lot of priests are gay."[105]

What makes Benedict's authoritative writings so interesting is that they contrast with how his successor, Pope Francis, presents himself. Although Pope Francis hasn't changed the Church's doctrine, and is very unlikely to make any changes to the Church's stance on gay marriage, his statements about homosexuality have been received much differently than Benedict's. In 2013, Francis garnered waves of international headlines when he answered a question about homosexuality in the Church with, "Who am I to judge them? They shouldn't be marginalized."[106] Soon after, he made more headlines when he told *America* magazine that the Church's obsession with gay marriage, abortion, and contraception needs to end; "otherwise the moral edifice of the church is likely to fall like a

---

*   The effort to ban gays from the seminaries really took off after the *Boston Globe*'s exposé brought sex abuse to people's attention. In 2002, the *New York Times* quoted a Vatican spokesperson who speculated that ordinations of even *current* gay priests might be declared invalid, just as a Catholic marriage can be annulled.

†   Sipe writes, "If the church today were to exclude all men of homosexual orientation from its celibate/sexual system, the church as we know it would cease to exist."

house of cards."[107] Francis also told *America*, "I used to receive letters from homosexual persons who are 'socially wounded' because they tell me that they feel like the church has always condemned them. But the church does not want to do this."[108] And in 2016, Francis sparked yet another round of headlines when he said that the Church should "say sorry to the person who is gay that it has offended."[109‡] Unlike Benedict's statements, Francis's remarks were well received by the media. Gay former priest Bill Dickinson exemplified the response of many outlets when he wrote in the *Daily Beast*, "Even in the absence of doctrinal change, promoting understanding, sensitivity, and proper language are acts of profound ministry."[110]

Many Church observers believe Francis will reform the Vatican. While there's no certainty to most Church speculation, especially regarding sexual topics, several of Francis's statements indicate that change is on the way. Benedict told bishops to be "especially cautious of any programmes which may seek to pressure the Church to change her teaching, even while claiming not to do so."[111] Francis has taken an approach opposite Benedict, and appears to embrace change. In his first year as pope, Francis told a group of religious pilgrims, "To be faithful, to be creative; we need to be able to change. To

---

‡   James Martin said the pope's comments were "groundbreaking." He writes, "No matter how many people tell you that this is nothing new, it's new. No pope has spoken like this regarding the LGBT community. Just a few years ago saying that the church should 'apologize' to gays and lesbians would have probably gotten a person censured, disciplined, or silenced. Why? Because a few years ago any call for an 'apology' would have been seen as a critique of church teaching on homosexuality."

change!"[112] A few years later, he told an audience of Italian bishops, "Before the problems of the church it is not useful to search for solutions in conservatism or fundamentalism, in the restoration of obsolete conduct and forms that no longer have the capacity of being significant culturally." He added, "Christian doctrine is not a closed system incapable of generating questions, doubts, interrogatives. But it is alive, knows being unsettled...it does not have a rigid face, it has a body that moves and grows."[113] In his first apostolic exhortation, he wrote that "the Church has rules or precepts which may have been quite effective in their time, but no longer have the same usefulness for directing and shaping people's lives."[114]

While Francis has drastically shifted the Church's tone on homosexuality, and his statements indicate he might reform aspects of the Church, Francis has also upheld Benedict's ban on gay seminarians, referred to gay marriage as "ideological colonization," and he quoted a group of bishops who wrote, "[A]s for proposals to place unions between homosexual persons on the same level as marriage, there are absolutely no grounds for considering homosexual unions to be in any way similar or even remotely analogous to God's plan for marriage and family."[115] When it comes to gay *marriage*, Francis's remarks have not been well received by the press. *National Catholic Reporter* editor Jamie Mason exemplifies the reaction of many media outlets when she writes, "The pope's brand of mercy suggests that LGBT Catholics should be tolerated by the church, but not embraced with genuine justice."[116]

There is a lot of noise when trying to decipher Francis's

intentions regarding LGBT-related policies. While his comments have prompted speculation that change is on the way, there are many others who insist that the Catholic Church cannot change and that discussion of reform is a moot point. Catholics and non-Catholics alike overstate the applicability of papal infallibility (a concept that wasn't invented until the nineteenth century)[117] and ignore the differences between things that cannot be changed (dogmatic faith-related declarations such as the resurrection of Christ) and things that can be changed (teachings on social issues, disciplines, customs). Before dismissing clerical celibacy or the Church's stance on homosexuality as immutable, it's worth taking a look at some of the changes the Church has made to its sexual teachings.

A Church that Can Change

Despite the common perception that the Catholic Church cannot change its rules, many of the Church's teachings and disciplines have changed considerably throughout its history. Just to name a few, the Church's stances on usury, slavery, the separation between church and state, freedom of the press, capital punishment, and religious freedom have all evolved throughout Church history.[118] The Church "often changed with the age," writes Pulitzer-winning historian Garry Wills. It "became Roman with the Roman Empire, shedding its Middle Eastern roots and adopting a Latin structure; became a super-monarchy in the age of monarchs; became super-ascetic in the age of Stoic contempt for the body; became misogynistic in the various patriarchies; became anti-Semitic when the world despised Jews."[119] As social contexts changed, the Church's original stance on certain social issues (like forbidding the lending of money with interest) eventually became untenable, which led to very gradual shifts in Church teaching.[120] As Wills puts it, "The church outlasted things that seemed to undermine it—not because it was unaffected by these transitory things, but because it joined them, drew on other sources, and lived to adopt different new things... There can be no history at all for those who just retroject the present into the past."[121] These gradual shifts in teaching also apply to sexuality.

Ancient Catholic theologians outlawed various sexual practices based on the reasoning that they perceived particular sexual practices were not "natural."[122] Saint Augustine argued that it was against nature to have sex for any reason other than procreation, which led him to conclude that sex during infertile periods was sinful.[123]* Which meant that it was sinful for even married people to have sex in old age, during pregnancy, and during particular points of a woman's monthly cycle.[124] According to judge and legal scholar John Noonan, the first recorded statement on contraception by a Catholic theologian came when Augustine condemned the

---

* Augustine, who had a child with a mistress before abandoning her, eventually became Christianity's most influential sexual philosopher. His writings were full of self-loathing, and he tended to view women as temptresses. He wrote, "There is nothing which degrades the manly spirit more than the attractiveness of female and contact with their bodies." And, "I fail to see what use woman can be to man, if one excludes the function of bearing children."

practice of having sex during infertile periods to avoid conception, which is noteworthy because in 1951, Pope Pius XII
officially approved the "rhythm method" as a "natural" form of
birth control for married couples.[125†] Noonan writes, "In the
history of the thought of theologians on contraception, it is,
no doubt, piquant that the first pronouncement on contraception by the most influential theologian teaching on such
matters [Augustine] should be such a vigorous attack on the
one method of avoiding procreation accepted by twentieth-
century Catholic theologians as morally lawful. History has
made doctrine take a topsy-turvy course."[126]

The "rhythm method" isn't the only sexual teaching the
Church has changed. While the Church is now agnostic
about which sexual positions married couples use, theologians used to obsess over the proper sexual position. Medieval
penitentials (handbooks for priests that aided them in hearing
confessions by listing penance suggestions for particular sins)
claimed it was against nature, and therefore sinful, to have
sex (again, even with one's spouse) "from the rear," and that
the only approved sexual style was the missionary position.[127‡]

[†] By approving the "rhythm method," the Church altered its reasoning for banning
contraception, according to Wills. "Before, it was the contraceptive *intent* that
was objected to," he wrote. "Now, people could space their sex acts with the
intent to avoid conception, so long as they did not interfere with 'the integrity
of the act'—which put a sacrosanct mechanics of sex above the motives of the
actors, reversing the normal priorities of moral reasoning. The mechanics of
killing a person, for instance, had not been considered the primary factor in
judging the morality of killing."

[‡] According to Brundage, medieval penitentials also "encouraged couples to have

Doggy-style coitus was deemed "unnatural" because it was common among animals and considered bestial and distasteful. However, for other types of sexual behavior, the behavior of animals determined what was "natural."[128] For example, Saint Thomas Aquinas declared that homosexuality was "unnatural" because he thought it *didn't* occur among animals.[129]* Although the Church has come around to allowing things like doggy-style entry and sex during infertile periods (which the Church actually *promotes* with variants of the "rhythm method"), it still maintains its bans on gay sex and clerical marriage, despite drastic shifts in the social contexts that inspired these teachings in the first place.

Bans on homosexual behavior were enacted at a time when the Church only allowed sex for procreative purposes.[130]†

---

sexual relations only at night and then to do so while at least partially clothed. One penitential stipulated that a husband should never see his wife naked."

* Thomas Aquinas also wrote, "In terms of nature's own operation, a woman is inferior and a mistake." He was also under the impression that females were "misbegotten males."

† Brundage points out that theorists who believed reproduction is the primary purpose of sex were almost always men. "Men are normally fertile from puberty to late old age, and male orgasm accompanies the emission of sperm. Thus the view that sex and reproduction are inextricably joined together reflects the experience of most men. Women experience sex differently. Females are fertile only for a fraction of their adult life, from puberty to menopause. The biological cycle of the human female, unlike that of most other mammals, does not involve a close link between ovulation and the female sex drive. Moreover, orgasm for women is primarily a function of the clitoris, which has no reproductive function at all. Thus the link between sexual satisfaction and reproduction is relatively weak from a woman's viewpoint. Reproductionist writers about sexual morality have historically rejected this point of view. Indeed, they have rarely even considered it."

While the Church still stresses that sex is ultimately intended for bearing children, Church officials no longer denounce sex among infertile people, and the Church now allows married couples to actively avoid conception with their version of the "rhythm method."[131†] John McNeil, a scholarly gay priest who was kicked out of the Jesuit order for refusing to quit his ministry to LGBT people, wrote, "From the moment the Church granted the morality of the rhythm method, for example, as a natural form of birth control, and justified sexual activity as still fulfilling the 'secondary' aims of mutual love and fulfillment, there was a serious reason to reconsider the traditional position that all homosexual activities are necessarily wrong on the ground that they cannot lead to procreation."[132]

Many contemporary theologians and high-ranking church officials have stressed the importance of the "unitive" (i.e., pair-bonding) aspect of sex.[133§] Pope Francis writes that Church members "need a healthy dose of self-criticism" when they "present marriage in such a way that its unitive meaning,

---

‡   It appears the Church is very subtly and very slowly altering its stance on condom usage. In recent years, Popes Benedict and Francis implied that it's OK for people in certain *rare* deadly situations to use condoms to avoid viruses like HIV and Zika.

§   John Paul II also shot down the idea that sex is inherently wrong, which previous theologians had implied. He wrote, "It is often necessary to relieve people of the widespread conviction that the sexual drive is something naturally bad which must be resisted in the name of the good. It is necessary to inculcate a conviction, in accordance with the proper conception of man, that sexual reactions are on the contrary perfectly natural, and have no intrinsic moral value. Morally they are neither good nor bad, but morally good or morally bad uses may be made of them."

its call to grow in love and its ideal of mutual assistance are overshadowed by an almost exclusive insistence on the duty of procreation."[134] Francis and his contemporaries recognize that sex holds importance beyond mere procreation, which is a drastically different sexual philosophy compared to that of the ancient theologians who originally banned gay sex largely based on its inability for procreation. A far cry from the teachings of prominent church figures such as Augustine and Peter Damian, who implied that sex was always sinful and that women were inferior and temptresses, John Paul II wrote that men should be less selfish in bed with their wives so that they could both orgasm. "The man must take this difference between male and female reactions into account, not for hedonistic, but for altruistic reasons," John Paul wrote. "There exists a rhythm dictated by nature itself which both spouses must discover so that climax may be reached both by the man and by the woman, and as far as possible occur in both simultaneously."[135]

What has also changed, aside from several Catholic sexual policies and the tone that Church leaders now apply, are the bureaucratic structures that originally influenced the celibacy discipline. One of the motives that led to clerical celibacy was that medieval popes felt they needed to end familial sacerdotal dynasties and the selling of church offices. Even if priests could marry and have children, it would be a logistical burden for them to pass power to their sons now that becoming a priest usually involves eight years of intensive education, positions are determined by bishops, priests receive meager compensation, and the selling of ecclesiastical positions is antiquated in today's world, because the Church has much less power than it used to. Even if priests had sons today, or had the power to sell their offices, there would be much less incentive for those sons and buyers to even pursue the priesthood. There would be less incentive because people no longer live in feudal societies where clergy hold much greater status than the working class, and clergymen have lost power since the Middle Ages because they are no longer among the only literate people in their congregations.[136] But medieval economic systems still retain influences in modern parishes, where priests remain celibate. Although the celibate condition is still in place, many people continue to challenge its merits in light of the flood of men who have left the priesthood in the past half-century.

The Heterosexual Clerical Exodus

Although research indicates there have been a disproportionate number of gay men in the priesthood for centuries, in the last half century there's been an increased "gaying of the priesthood" in the West, as many straight priests have left to marry.[137] Waves of priests left their positions while seminary enrollment fell off, leading to about a 35 percent decline in the total number of priests (a drop of roughly 20,000 people) in the U.S. from 1965 to 2015.[138] Throughout the 1970s, several hundred men left the priesthood each year, many of them leaving to marry.[139] Meanwhile, the number of permanent deacons, who can be married and can perform nearly every task required of a priest except consecrate the Eucharist or hear confessions, has soared since the 1970s, increasing by

nearly 17,000 people in the past forty years.[140] During this
time period, the "sexual revolution" evolved, women gained
more rights, and marriages shifted toward equality-based
partnerships and away from their patriarchal, breadwinner,
power-imbalanced past. The Church responded to these
changes by closing debate about the possibility of married
clergy, women priests, and gay marriages, and by banning
contraception, even though about 80 percent of Pope John
XXIII's Pontifical Commission on Birth Control approved
its usage for married couples.[141]*

As straight priests left the Church to marry, the proportion of remaining priests who were gay escalated. In the
Times data, 28 percent of priests between the ages of forty-six
and fifty-five were found to be gay.[142] This statistic was higher
than the percentages found in other age brackets and reflected
the outflow of heterosexual priests throughout the 1970s and
'80s.[143] In 2002, Bishop Wilton Gregory, then president of
the U.S. Conference of Catholic Bishops, complained about
an "ongoing struggle to make sure that the Catholic priesthood is not dominated by homosexual men."[144] Pope Benedict

---

*   The way many women use birth control is indirectly influenced by Catholic teach-
     ing. John Rock, coinventor of the Pill, was a devout Catholic who opened the first
     clinic in Boston that taught the Church-approved "rhythm method." Given the
     Church had already approved the "rhythm method," Rock built off its logic and
     designed the Pill around a twenty-eight-day cycle to mimic a woman's menstrual
     cycle in hopes of earning Church approval by aiming to make the contraceptive
     appear as "natural" as possible. Although the Church remains adamant in its stance
     against contraception, many of the Pill's consumers unintentionally follow Rock's
     appeal to Catholic theology.

told a reporter in 2010 that homosexuality in the priesthood was "one of the miseries of the church" and that the Church needed to "head off a situation where the celibacy of priests would practically end up being identified with the tendency to homosexuality."[145†] Regarding the rising proportion of priests who are gay, Wills quipped, "Many observers suspect that John Paul's real legacy to his church is a gay priesthood."[146]

While it's usually trivial to fret over the sexual habits of people in the public eye—politicians, athletes, celebrities—honestly examining what clergy do in their sex lives is important, because so many people base their sexual beliefs and behaviors on their pastors' recommendations. Given that clergymen are constantly lecturing everyone else on how and when people should have sex and threatening those who disobey their commands with damnation, it's not only fair for laypeople to be able to critique the sexual habits of clerics, it's necessary for an honest dialogue.

An Open Discussion of a Taboo Topic

Any conversation about priests having sex invites controversy because Roman Catholic clerical celibacy has been thoroughly enforced for about a millennium. With mandatory clerical celibacy, "every type of sexual union that they [priests] engaged in, no matter how stable or permanent,

---

†   According to John Thavis, "Never before had a Vatican official voiced so bluntly what so many of them feared privately: that the priesthood was turning into a gay ghetto."

became both a sin and a canonical crime," Brundage writes.[147] To maintain an appearance of adherence to this discipline and to avoid scandal, many high-ranking church officials have taken "vows of silence" to cover up any evidence that priests are having sex.[148] This culture of concealment led investigative reporters Jason Berry and Gerald Renner, who broke several stories about sex abuse in the Church, to conclude, "The Bishops were obsessed with secrecy because sexual intimacy was forbidden."[149] Despite efforts to hide this uncomfortable reality, it's quite clear there are priests having sex and that a fair amount of this sex is between males.

Roughly 16 percent of the world and 21 percent of the U.S. is Catholic, making it one of the largest religious denominations both in the world and in the U.S.[150] For many of these people, the teachings of the Church influence their opinions on sex, ethics, politics, and many other topics. Sipe recognizes the importance that clerical sex has on the world at large when he writes:

> The parameters of the conflict [between priests and their sexuality] are not limited to a relatively few men who may or may not practice the celibacy they profess. The power of Catholic priests and the sexual reasoning of Christian tradition have implications for life on this planet, including the issues of population growth, gender and racial equality, and understanding the nature of human sexuality. The salient questions are not about theoretical preferences, venerable traditions, or sacred opinions. The questions are practical

struggles for truth, which affect people's lives and the future of the planet.[151]

While the topic of clerical sex is important, we're not here to make any recommendations about what the Church should do. Though other denominations have shown that women, married men, and sexually active LGBT people can be entirely competent as pastors, for centuries the Catholic Church's model of relying on single, sexually abstinent men has generally served the institution well. Pope Gregory's clerical reforms helped put an end to corruption, simony, and nepotism. By not allowing priests to marry, the Church spent fewer of its resources on providing for its leaders, and because these leaders did not have families, they were able to devote more of their time and energy to the Church. Also, most priests are psychologically well-adjusted, altruistic, satisfied with their lives and occupation, and, according to some surveys, the majority have followed the Church's discipline by avoiding sex after ordination.[152] Although the declining number (and the rising median age) of priests in Western countries is a statistical fact, it won't necessarily lead to a drastic priest shortage that results in Catholics being deprived of Mass unless the priesthood is opened up to women and married men.[153] A priest shortage might be averted, because the reduction of priests runs alongside fewer Catholics attending Mass, fewer Catholics seeking Church sacraments, and deacons and laypeople providing more of the Church's services.[154]

This chapter isn't intended to spur change but rather intellectual honesty. Despite the entrenched idea among many people that the Catholic Church cannot change, history shows that many Church teachings have changed, including several related to sexuality. While it is uncertain whether the Church will change its teachings about homosexuality, it is certain that change within the Church on nondogmatic declarations is possible and that Pope Francis's comments about homosexuality display a remarkable shift in tone. It is not dishonest for the Church to maintain any of its policies, but it is dishonest to deny the possibility of change or the influence ancient social contexts and prejudices had on creating several of the Church's disciplines that are still in place.[155]* A large percentage of priests being gay doesn't intrinsically equate to a crisis. Rather, it denotes a complex phenomenon in the Church that makes many people uncomfortable, which illustrates how sexual regulations can produce ironic consequences.

In most cases it is a bit ahistorical to call thinkers from the eras of Augustine and Peter Damian prejudiced. But when social science is perpetually disregarded and the reasoning and edicts of medieval theologians are still upheld as sacrosanct, unadulterated criticism of medieval social expectations and biological knowledge is needed for sincere dialogue. For

---

*   The Church perpetually denies that past prejudices have influenced its teachings in any way. For example, a 1976 document from the CDF that reiterated that women can't be ordained priests stated, "It is true that in the writings of the Fathers one will find the undeniable influence of prejudices unfavourable to woman, but nevertheless, it should be noted that these prejudices had hardly any influence on their pastoral activity, and still less on their spiritual direction." According to this logic, a person's actions are not affected by their beliefs. Which is an interesting argument for a religious institution to make.

the most part, the Church continues to downplay shifting cultural contexts in favor of adhering to sexual renunciation laws developed by ancient eschatological communities and desert ascetics responding to an uncertain world.[156] The Church also continues to rely on clerical structures that were influenced by social and economic conditions from the Middle Ages. In doing so, the Church's hierarchy has contributed to a phenomenon it would rather have people ignore, which is that the Church's rigid policies on homosexuality and clerical celibacy have likely inadvertently driven many gay men toward the priesthood. "Bishops are caught in the middle and running scared," Richard McBrien told Berry. "They live in a church with a very hard-line policy on homosexuals, yet they realize they're drawing from that population well beyond its presence in society, by default."[157]

A paradox of this magnitude seems baffling. And it certainly is baffling for the gay priests who battle cognitive dissonance. But as an entry in *Human Sexuality in the Catholic Tradition* points out, "Christian faith proclaims its deepest truth in paradoxes."[158] Jesus was born of a virgin. He was both God *and* man. Though he was declared "King of Kings," he lived a modest life as a carpenter. Jesus said that a grain of wheat must die if it is to bear fruit, and that "the last shall be first, and the first last."[159] The contemporary Church's greatest paradox is that its positions of power and authority continue to be heavily represented by a population it declares "objectively disordered."

=10=

sex cells and religious pluralism

EXAMINING THE INTERFAITH DEPENDENCE OF MUSLIM WOMEN SEEKING REPRODUCTIVE ASSISTANCE

The necessity of religious pluralism can be found in the wombs of Middle Eastern Muslim women. Restrictions on assisted reproductive technologies (ARTs) in the Middle East show that religious factions sometimes need each other, as faith can bring people together even as it divides them. One major ART prohibition in the Middle East is that Sunni Muslims attempting to conceive a child are forbidden from using other people's eggs, sperm, and embryos (which are referred to as "donated gametes" or "third-party sex cells"). However, Shia Muslims are not forbidden from using third-party sex cells. These restrictions present dilemmas for infertile couples in Sunni-majority countries, where societies place cultural pressure on women to have their own children, and the consequences of failing these cultural expectations can be socially devastating.

Sunni couples who seek reproductive help through other people's gametes make trade-offs between adhering to religious rules and fulfilling societal obligations. For those who value having their own children over their religion's code, religious pluralism becomes beneficial in a very practical way.

Denominational Differences

Restrictions on ARTs can be confusing because they vary by country and denomination.[1]* While Sunnis in places such as Egypt can use their own gametes for things like artificial insemination or in-vitro fertilization, third-party sperm or egg donation and surrogates are prohibited by a 1980 fatwa that declared reproduction should only take place between husband and wife. According to Shereen El Feki in *Sex and*

---

*   Some Middle Eastern countries also have confusing rules regarding homosexuality and transgenderism. For example, in Iran, homosexuality can be punishable by death. However, Iranian clerics believe that people can be trapped in a body of the wrong sex, so the country allows for sex reassignment surgery. In some cases the government will give people loans if they can't afford the procedure and will coerce gay people into having the surgery. Sometimes gay people in Iran (who *aren't* suffering from gender dysphoria) will actually seek out these surgeries themselves in order to avoid potential execution for their homosexual behavior.

the Citadel: Intimate Life in a Changing Arab World, using donor gametes would be sinful and would produce illegitimate children.[2] Only married couples are allowed to use any sort of ARTs, and they are restricted to using their own gametes when they do so.

According to Yale anthropologist Marcia Inhorn, the ban on third-party gametes among Sunnis affects about 80 to 90 percent of the world's 1.6 billion Muslims.[3] However, some Shiites, on the other hand, have recently seen a change in decree. As new reproductive technologies sprang up throughout the 1990s, several Shia jurists (whose opinions were key to the legitimization of third-party donation) resorted to interpreting the Qur'an to decide on the permissibility of third-party gamete donation.[4] In doing so, the interpretations of these jurists differed and, at times, were even contradictory, with some allowing third-party donation and others rejecting it. In Shia Islam, the opinions of senior jurists are equally valid, and one does not rule out the other, as each jurist has his own followers.[5] "The contradictions between the jurists leaves wide gaps, blurs the lines, and allows room for manipulation by all concerned," Oxford anthropologist Soraya Tremayne says.[6]

Medical practitioners relied on the rulings of jurists that approved outside donors and set up clinics that practiced third-party gamete donation. Some of these clinics even framed the fatwas that approved of third-party donation, and placed the framed documents on their mantelpieces so they could "carry on without any possible objection," Tremayne says.[7] Clinics that practice third-party donation are only allowed in Shia-majority countries, so Muslims in Sunni-majority countries who seek third-party donation must venture into Shia-dominated areas to get the reproductive assistance they desire.

As the demand for reproductive assistance rose, Shia-majority Iran and Lebanon became the only two Muslim-majority countries in the world to allow infertile couples to purchase donor sex cells, making these two countries hubs for Middle Eastern "reproductive travelers" of many faiths—such as Shia Muslims, Sunni Muslims, Druzes, and Christians.[8] Most Sunnis support their denomination's third-party ban.[9]* However, in Muslim societies, parenthood is expected, and childlessness is socially stigmatized. With the intense pressure to have children, the outlawing of reproductive technologies that increase chances of conception poses ethical dilemmas for infertile Sunni couples. Regarding the millions of infertile Muslim couples, Inhorn states, "Infertility may ruin their reputations, their marriages, their livelihoods, their physical health, and their long-term security in ways that are truly disastrous. Indeed, infertility is a particularly pernicious form of reproductive disruption, one that engulfs whole lives in endless circles of treatment-seeking and human suffering."[10] Sunnis who feel that the importance of having their own children outweighs breaking religious law venture into Shia

---

* According to Inhorn, the majority of Sunni Muslims support the ban on third-party gamete donation for three main reasons: "(1) the moral implications of third-party donation for marriage, (2) the potential for incest, and (3) the moral implications of donation for kinship and family life."

territory to become reproductive travelers by journeying to other countries for the purpose of accessing reproduction-related technologies and resources.[11]*

This form of reproductive travel is only incentivized when countries ban acquiring sex cells. The bans on sex cell donation are partially inspired by beliefs about sexual sin, but they are also related to lineage, paternity, descent, and inheritance.[12] Sunnis are concerned about producing a "stranger's child" if they accept sperm donation.[13] And they are concerned about having their "own child" being given to someone else if they decide to donate their sex cells. Many Middle Eastern societies are patrilineal, meaning that kinship and ancestry are traced through the father's bloodline. To avoid confusing the lines of descent and inheritance, formal adoption and certain ARTs are prohibited, because paternal bloodlines carry significant cultural significance. According to El Feki, adherence to the paternal bloodline "determines everything from whom a woman can sit with unveiled to rights of inheritance. As a consequence, such techniques [artificial insemination, in-vitro fertilization] are for married people only—a widow, for example, wanting to use her dead husband's frozen sperm or their embryos from earlier cycles of IVF, can have a hard time arguing her case."[14] Sunnis aren't unique in their strict rules regarding reproduction, because in many religious denominations,

---

*   Inhorn notes that for centuries people have been traveling to "saints' tombs, herbalists, healers, and holy men" in hopes of improving their chances at conception. She says that, in a way, reproductive travel is "as old as conception itself."

adherence to detail is often strongest in sexual matters.[15†] But for some Sunni women, these rules can create dissonance, especially for those living in highly infertile areas where adoption is frowned upon.

Adoption and Infertility

If childlessness is frowned upon in these societies, why don't infertile couples address their issues with adoption? That's a fair question, especially given adoption's social acceptance in the West. But in places such as Egypt, the Western conceptualization of adoption is forbidden by the Qur'an, and adopted children in Egypt aren't supposed to claim the last name of their adoptive father, nor do they inherit their adoptive parents' wealth.[16] In Egypt, adoption is more like fostering an orphan. And while this is allowed, and even seen as a good

---

† El Feki notes that while Muslim-majority countries may be perceived to be sexually strict by modern Westerners, that hasn't always been the case, because attitudes and stereotypes have changed. "The Arab world, once famous in the West for sexual license, envied by some but despised by others, is now widely criticized for sexual intolerance. It's not just Western liberals who hold this view. It has also become a keynote in some of the 'Islamophobic' discourse of conservatives in America and Europe, the self-proclaimed last stand in the battle between 'Western' values and the depredations of 'radical' Islam, particularly as they relate to the rights of women. And the West, once praised by some in the Arab world for its hard line on same-sex relations, is now seen by many as a radiating source of sexual debauchery from which the region must be shielded. Perceptions, however flawed, are shaped by position. Western views of Arab sexuality, and vice versa, have shifted in part because attitudes within their respective societies have also changed."

deed, it's an unpopular practice, especially among the wealthy. As an Egyptian woman told Inhorn:

> If the family is poor, no one will care [if they "adopt" an orphan]. But, for the rich who can afford adoption, adoption is seen as no way at all, because all the sisters and brothers and aunts and uncles will resent that this amount of money [spent on raising the child] is going to an "outsider." So, it's very complicated.[17]

Adoption stigmas are a big deal in countries with sizable Muslim populations, partly because there are high rates of infertility in many of these areas. Of the 50 million to 80 million people worldwide estimated to be infertile, it's estimated more than half are Muslim.[18] Many Muslims live in an "infertility belt" in sub-Saharan Africa, where infertility rates reach up to 32 percent, affecting about one-third of couples.[19] Some major factors contributing to the high infertility rates include untreated STDs, poor medical care, and female circumcision.[20] Although male infertility is quite common in these regions, infertility is often perceived as a "woman's problem."[21] With adoption an unacceptable avenue for growing a family, overcoming infertility becomes a huge issue in countries where having children is a social obligation. Tremayne noted:

> What is emerging strongly from this analysis is the interface between reproduction as a means of personal achievement and love of one's own biological child,

against one's sense of social identity as a member of the social group. Clearly, the importance of reproducing socially is paramount for individuals, who are prepared to go to any length to demonstrate that they have fulfilled their reproductive duties and to secure their rightful place in society.[22]

In many of these countries, such as Egypt, women are continuously blamed for infertility, even though male infertility is often the main cause leading childless couples to in-vitro fertilization (IVF) clinics.[23] According to the account of an Egyptian woman who married a divorced man:

> Here in Egypt, if a man knows he doesn't get his wife pregnant, he's always upset. And if you're pushing him all the time, and he's the reason for the problem, he feels like giving up [on the marriage], because there are no children to keep in the house. In my husband's case, he preferred to divorce her [his first wife] because their relationship became bad. They had different attitudes and behaviors, and in this case, the major reason for the divorce was that he knows he's the reason for no pregnancy. He's very kind, and she's very nervous and always asking too many questions. So my husband asked for divorce because their marriage became bad.[24]

In promoting awareness about reproduction-related discoveries, some researchers have overstated the reach of new technologies.[25] There is even a scholarly book, *Infertility in the Modern World: Present and Future Prospects*, which claims, "Modern technology can provide genetically related offspring to 80 percent of couples seeking treatment, and pregnancy to a further 10–15 percent using donated gametes."[26] While *Infertility in the Modern World* had a specific scholarly audience, there are other times the overoptimistic comments of researchers reach the mass media, who then broadcast the message to the masses. In a 2001 PBS special, "Eighteen Ways to Make a Baby," Princeton molecular biologist Lee Silver said, "What IVF does is it takes the process of reproduction out of the darkness of the womb, into the light of the laboratory. And all of the sudden you can do anything you want with these human embryos and eggs, which couldn't be done before."[27] Although there have been remarkable developments in reproductive technology in recent history, comments like "you can do anything you want with these human embryos and eggs" overlook that attempts at producing test-tube babies fail 70 to 80 percent of the time, even in Western medical centers.[28] New ARTs may not be the technological saviors they're sometimes made out to be. But for some infertile couples seeking reproductive assistance, they can indeed be a godsend.[29]*

---

*   While some Muslim couples have called these donor technologies a "marriage savior" that helps them avoid "marital and psychological disputes," research from Soraya Tremayne shows that donor children sometimes aren't treated as well as biological children, and anecdotally they can fall victim to overbearing fathers. Also, the life quality of donor children sometimes depends on whether they come from sperm or egg donation. There are tendencies for fathers to be more hostile toward children who came from sperm donation than from egg donation.

TILL THE CONTRACT
ENDS, DO US PART

One way some Muslims sidestep lineage conundrums in utilizing third-party gametes or engaging in nonmarital sex without technically breaking rules is through entering temporary marriages. A mut'a marriage is time-limited and can range from hours to years.[30] Divorce isn't necessary here, because the time-limited element is the point of these unions. They simply expire, sort of like a driver's license or cable subscription.

Similar to third-party gamete donation, mut'a marriages are practiced by some Shiites but not by Sunnis.[31] (Although some Sunnis practice other forms of informal marriages, such as 'urfi and misyar marriages, these informal marriages are not viewed as socially legitimate for Sunnis as mut'a marriages are for Shiites.[32]) In some instances, temporary marriages go hand in hand with gamete donation because they allow donors to become "spouses," which means the conception *technically* happens within the confines of marriage. For example, if a married man is infertile, his wife can "divorce" him, "marry" the donor, receive the sperm while "married" to the donor, and then "remarry" her original husband after her "marriage" to the sperm donor expires.[33]

Temporary marriages can also give a religious cover to sexual pleasures that otherwise would be sinful. AIDS epidemiologist Elizabeth Pisani says that because of these temporary marriages, she has met prostitutes who have been married hundreds of times. "Good Muslim clients perform the wedding ceremony for themselves before starting in on the girl," Pisani writes. "An hour later, they divorce her. Since they were married while they were having sex, they have not sinned."[34] Young people looking to fool around, or married or divorced adults looking to pick up a brief lover, can enter a temporary marriage, do their business, let the marriage expire, and avoid committing nonmarital-sexual transgressions. Surely there are jealous Christians out there who wish their religious leaders had thought of and approved these rules.

Interfaith Dependence

Infertile Muslim couples in the Middle East generally face four tough options. They can remain together without children. They can foster an orphan. They can add more partners to their marriage, and pursue polygamy rather than monogamy in hopes of increasing their reproductive probabilities. Or they can divorce so they can attempt to have children with other partners.[35] All of these options present potential stigma.[36]* But for Shiites who have the money to do so, third-party sex cell donation gives them another option

---

*   Regarding the stigmatization of sex, an Egyptian gynecologist told El Feki, "In
        the Arab world, sex is the opposite of sport. Everyone talks about football, but
        hardly anyone plays it. But sex—everyone is doing it, but nobody wants to talk
        about it."

that in some ways is more socially desirable, because it doesn't involve sex with new partners, adoption, or divorce.[37] While most infertile Muslim couples cannot treat their reproductive difficulties with expensive ARTs, those who can do so can prevent their reputations, marriages, and livelihoods from being damaged due to an inability to meet social expectations through procreation.[38] This option is also available to Sunnis who want to circumvent religious rules in favor of producing their own offspring. But to do this, Sunnis will need assistance that comes from outside their religious branch.

Sunnis seeking reproductive assistance aren't alone in relying on outside religious denominations to maneuver around the confines of their own denomination. For centuries, people have benefitted from those of different faiths.[39] The reliance upon people of different faiths ranges from simple things such as avoiding Sabbath work commandments[†] to loopholing around complex religious guidelines, such as when Orthodox Jews sell chametz during Passover. Chametz are leavened foods that Orthodox Jews aren't allowed to eat, or even possess, during Passover. So sometimes Jews "sell" their chametz to a non-Jew with the understanding that their non-Jewish acquaintance will "sell" the chametz right back after Passover.[40] For private households, this merely

---

[†]   It's interesting that preachers tell laity to avoid working on the Sabbath. Yet the preacher's main job is usually to provide a weekend worship service. And it is during this weekend service, while the preacher is at work, that the preacher tells followers that *they* shouldn't work. If everyone literally obeyed Sabbath work commandments, theoretically, ceremonies dedicated to their holiness could be halted.

curtails a small inconvenience. But for Jewish grocers, this
practice prevents a traditional custom from derailing livelihoods. While the exchange process is often done with an
acquaintance, there are also online markets for the Passover
exchange. And interreligious reliance isn't limited to Sabbaths
and holidays. All year long, the preservation of the burial site
of Christ (The Holy Sepulchre) relies on religious cooperation. Because tensions build between Christian denominations over who controls the area, Muslims guard the site to
prevent violence.[41]

But of all these pluralistic examples, Muslim women
seeking reproductive assistance present the most interesting trade-offs. In the example of Sunnis seeking third-
party reproductive assistance, religious prohibitions lead to
behavioral adaptations that result in an interfaith exchange
of economic resources for sexual cooperation. This practice
of one denomination relying upon another for reproductive assistance illustrates conflict between religion, science,
modernity, tradition, and social expectations. Muslim reproductive practices show religious diversity isn't *just* ideal. For
many laypeople, sometimes it's necessary.

afterword

As we have seen, sexuality manifests itself throughout society and impacts culture, tradition, and ultimately behavior, through political, economic, and religious forces. Although he laid it on a bit thick, the influential sexologist Magnus Hirschfeld had a point when he wrote: "Let us admit once and for all that sex is the basic principle around which all the rest of human life, with all its institutions, is pivoted."[1]

Much of the influence of sex in our society is accidental, as sexuality has inadvertently influenced several household products from VCRs to corn flakes. But there are also deliberate controls placed on passion that produce unintended effects. For example, most people in the West idealize sticking to one sexual partner at a time because Greco-Roman emperors made calculated decisions to nudge their constituents toward monogamy. But consequences of these policies can extend beyond their forecasted impact, as when China's

one-child policy began altering savings rates. And there are
other times when altogether unforeseen effects pop up in
response to sexuality. Gays who felt outcast congregated
together and helped rebuild city cores. Fatwas outlawing
third-party reproductive assistance led to Sunni Muslims
relying on people of different religious faiths. Instances
of risk compensation, vendor lock-in, path dependence,
network effects, accidental inventions, and externalities show
that sex effects follow their own "rules" and are riddled with
irregularities.

Predicting or tracing the influence of pleasure becomes
puzzling, because there are no hard rules that apply to every
situation. Sure, reducing sexual regulations often turns out
to be relatively harmless or even works in society's favor, as
became evident in the process of legalizing pornography or
loosening rules on sexual orientation in the military. But
on the other hand, denouncing restrictions on sex can be
problematic. Promoting condoms as a Band-Aid solution
to AIDS epidemics may have cost lives that could've been
spared through a stronger emphasis on partner reduction
and circumcision.

Despite its prevalence and how much people obsess over
it, society knows comparatively little about sex from a social-
science perspective. For something that affects the growth
and decline of countries and is a major provider of pleasure
and pain, both individually and institutionally, sex rarely
garners our best intellectual efforts. Instead, its study is often
relegated to magazine advice columns, television gossip, and
"sexperts" with "doctorates" from unaccredited universities.

Due to an overworked media where cable news churns 24/7 and online outlets expect multiple stories daily from each writer, information gatekeepers rely on poor information because it's easily accessible. This is particularly troublesome with a topic such as sex, because the public's fixation on sex makes it an easy target for ratings surges, which are sorely needed in a struggling media climate. Broadcasting without proper investigation misleads the sexually polarized public further, which is how you end up with so many Americans who believe that divorces, rape, STDs, and teenage births are rising, even though all are actually relatively stable or in decline. And it's how fifteen-year-old studies from Pfizer consultants are *still* being used, usually without question, to prop up the necessity of sexual dysfunction products.

America's puritanical knee-jerk relationship with sex narcotizes analysis. As long as discussions on the issue are led by polarizing free-love advocates and conservative prudes, society's common knowledge on sexual matters will face uphill battles. In their book chronicling America's sexual history, historians John D'Emilio and Estelle Freedman conclude, "[S]exuality has come to occupy a prominent place in our economy, our psyches, and our politics. For this reason, it is likely to stay vulnerable to manipulation as a symbol of social problems and to be the subject of efforts to maintain social hierarchies. As in the past, sex will remain a source of both deep personal meaning and heated political controversy."[2]

The drive for a rational sexual dialogue is also hampered by institutional review boards, which often squash the ability of researchers to venture into this important and practical field. Proposals on sex research must be cleverly cloaked to get by these bureaucrats, who, in trying to prevent their university from being sued, effectively prevent anything useful or interesting from being found out about one of life's most basic and necessary functions.[3] These restrictions aren't without consequence.

When AIDS broke out in the U.S. in the 1970s and '80s, it was concentrated among gay men. And epidemiologists had no clue how to predict and best curtail the disease, because no one knew how many gay men were in the U.S., because nobody had really studied the topic much since Kinsey. And even if they had found out where gay men resided, epidemiologists had no clue about their sexual behaviors, because most research on studying homosexuality had been shunned.[4] Openly discussing and studying sex is important because expanding our knowledge will likely be one of the best defenses in combatting future sex-related epidemics, regardless of whether the fight is against rape, disease, unwanted pregnancies, etc. But rather than honest and thorough conversation, society typically follows this cycle in its sexual discussions:

> A quack who sounds the alarm and who, finding no serious scientific obstacles in his way, achieves some degree of success; a famous physician who, echoing the quack, supports the warning with the weight of his authority and thereupon builds a theory; a society that discovers in the theory an answer to some of its questions and so adopts it; a long period during

which this theory reigns, with hardly any detractors, and spreads a climate of fear... Then opponents, rare at first, then numerous, who make no scientific discoveries but who simply note, one after another, that the theory doesn't hold water; now a reversal of opinions, first partial, then total; the acknowledgment that what had been taken as abnormal was in fact normal.[5]

The above sequence from Jean Stengers and Anne Van Neck summarizes Western society's tumultuous history with masturbation. Similar responses are happening right now as the public overreacts to new sexual issues. At this point, we're far from collectively exceeding our capacity for reckless reactions, as seen in responses to politician sex scandals.

And it's a shame because, overall, sex is inherently more interesting than orgasms, guilt, or boner pills. It's a powerful and pervasive force penetrating personalities deeper than any other act. While the act itself warrants obvious attention, what's much more intriguing is everything that surrounds and coincides with it. Understanding these social effects facilitates better understanding of human environments and behavior. The examples here only scratch the surface. Surely more lies underneath.

notes

Introduction

1   Richard Dawkins, *The Selfish Gene* (Oxford: Oxford University Press, 1976).

2   Frank Fasick, "On the 'Invention' of Adolescence," *Journal of Early Adolescence* 14, no. 1 (1994): 6–23, doi:10.1177/0272431694014001002.

3   Dawkins, *The Selfish Gene.*

4   Helen Epstein, "God and the Fight against AIDS," *New York Review of Books*, April 28, 2005, http://www.nybooks.com/articles/2005/04/28/god-and-the-fight-against-aids/.

Chapter 1

1   John Witte, *The Western Case for Monogamy over Polygamy* (New York: Cambridge University Press, 2015), 16–17.

2   Patrick Gray, "Ethnographic Atlas Codebook," *World Cultures* 10, no. 1 (1998): 86–136, http://eclectic.ss.uci.edu/~drwhite/worldcul/Codebook4EthnoAtlas.pdf.

3   Michael Price, "Alexander's Theory of the Political Advantages of Monogamy: Empirical Support and Evolutionary Psychological Aspects," Department of Anthropology, Center for Evolutionary Psychology, University of California, Santa Barbara, (unpublished manuscript, March, 1999), PDF; Helen Fisher, *Anatomy of Love: The Natural History of Monogamy, Adultery, and Divorce* (New York: W. W. Norton, 1992), 69.

4   Kyle Harper, "The Case of Monogamy," Oklahoma University, TEDx video, 19:01, accessed January 15, 2016, https://www.youtube.com/watch?v=rTH-8g6ZrF4.

5   Harper, "The Case of Monogamy."

6   David Barash, *Out of Eden: The Surprising Consequences of Polygamy* (New York: Oxford University Press, 2015), 57; David Barash, "Sex at Dusk," *Chronicle of Higher Education*, July 21, 2012, http://chronicle.com/blogs/brainstorm/sex-at-dusk-2/50099; Michael Price, "Was Monogamy Established for the Benefit of Women?," *Psychology Today*, September 11, 2011, https://www.psychologytoday.com/blog/darwin-eternity/201109/was-monogamy -established-the-benefit-women-0.

7   Lynn Saxon, *Sex at Dusk: Lifting the Shiny Wrapper from Sex at Dawn*, (CreateSpace Independent Publishing Platform, 2012), 44.

8   Richard Jones and Kristin Lopez, *Human Reproductive Biology* (San Diego: Academic Press, 2013), 140; Helen Fisher, *Anatomy of Love: The Natural History of Monogamy, Adultery, and Divorce* (New York: W. W. Norton, 1992), 68; Maia Szalavitz, "When Men Stop Seeking Beauty and Women Care Less about Wealth," *Time*, September 12, 2012, http://healthland .time.com/2012/09/07/when-men-stop-seeking-beauty-and-women-care-less-about

-wealth/; Meg Sullivan, "Near Ovulation, Your Cheatin' Heart Will Tell on You, Find UCLA, University of New Mexico Researchers," *UCLA Newsroom*, January 4, 2006, http://newsroom .ucla.edu/releases/Near-Ovulation-Your-Cheatin-Heart-6713?RelNum=6713.

9   David Buss, "Sex Differences in Human Mate Preferences: Evolutionary Hypotheses Tested in 37 Cultures," *Behavioral and Brain Sciences* 12, no. 01 (1989): 1–14, doi: 10.1017 /S0140525X00023992; Steven Gangestad, Randy Thornhill, and Christine Garver -Apgar, "Women's Sexual Interests across the Ovulatory Cycle Depend on Primary Partner Developmental Instability," *Proceedings of the Royal Society of London B: Biological Sciences* 272, no. 1576 (2005): 2023–2027, doi: 10.1098/rspb.2005.3112; David Barash and Judith Lipton, *The Myth of Monogamy: Fidelity and Infidelity in Animals and People* (New York: Henry Holt and Co., 2001), 78. Footnote information found in Kristina Durante, Norman Li, and Martie Haselton, "Changes in Women's Choice of Dress across the Ovulatory Cycle: Naturalistic and Laboratory Task-Based Evidence," *Personality and Social Psychology Bulletin* 34, no. 11 (2008): 1451–1460, doi:10.1177/0146167208323103; Sullivan, "Near Ovulation Your Cheatin' Heart Will Tell on You"; Robert Burriss, "The Face of Fertility: Why Do Men Find Women Who Are Near Ovulation More Attractive?" *Independent*, July 2, 2015, http://www .independent.co.uk/life-style/health-and-families/features/the-face-of-fertility-why-do-men -find-women-who-are-near-ovulation-more-attractive-10359906.html; Nicolas Guéguen, "Makeup and Menstrual Cycle: Near Ovulation, Women Use More Cosmetics," *Psychological Record* 62, no. 3 (2012): 541–548; Martie Haselton et al., "Ovulatory Shifts in Human Female Ornamentation: Near Ovulation, Women Dress to Impress," *Hormones and Behavior* 51, no. 1 (2007): 40–45, doi:10.1016/j.yhbeh.2006.07.007; James Kohl and Robert Francoeur, *The Scent of Eros: Mysteries of Odor in Human Sexuality* (Lincoln, NE: IUniverse, 2002), 149; Daniel Denoon, "Women Risk Risky Sex at Worst Time," *WebMD Health News*, November 7, 2007, http://www.webmd.com/sex-relationships/news/20071107/women-risk-risky-sex -at-worst-time; Jamie Wilson, "Ovulation Turns on Desire for Sex," *Guardian*, June 9, 2004, http://www.theguardian.com/society/2004/jun/10/health.medicineandhealth.

10   Harper, "The Case of Monogamy."

11   Kevin MacDonald, "The Establishment and Maintenance of Socially Imposed Monogamy in Western Europe," *Politics and the Life Sciences* 14, no. 1 (1995): 3–23.

12   Walter Scheidel, "A Peculiar Institution? Greco-Roman Monogamy in Global Context," *History of the Family* 14, no. 3 (2009): 280–291, doi: 10.1016/j.hisfam.2009.06.001.

13   Price, "Alexander's Theory"; Fisher, *Anatomy of Love*, 69; Laura Betzig, "Means, Variances, and Ranges in Reproductive Success: Comparative Evidence," *Evolution and Human Behavior* 33, no. 4 (2012): 309–317, doi: 10.1016/j.evolhumbehav.2011.10.008.

14   Michael Price, email interview, September 25, 2015.

15   Barash, "Sex at Dusk."

16   Robert Wright, *The Moral Animal: The New Science of Evolutionary Psychology* (New York: Pantheon, 1994), 66–67.

17   David Buss, *The Dangerous Passion: Why Jealousy Is as Necessary as Love and Sex* (New York: Simon & Schuster, 2000), 57–60.

18   David Buss, "Sexual Jealousy," *Psychological Topics* 22, no. 2 (2013): 155–182, https ://static1.squarespace.com/static/53cfd5dbe4b085d58f30791c/t/53d2bcebe4b04e06965 ed06f/1406319851957/sexual-jealousy.pdf; David Buss, Randy Larsen, Drew Westen, and Jennifer Semmelroth, "Sex Differences in Jealousy: Evolution, Physiology, and Psychology," *Psychological Science* 3, no. 4 (1992): 251–255, doi: 10.1111/j.1467–9280.1992.tb00038.x; Barash, "Sex at Dusk."

19   Price, "Alexander's Theory"; Harper, "The Case of Monogamy." Footnote information in Witte, *The Western Case for Monogamy*, 108.

20   Witte, *The Western Case for Monogamy*, 102.

21   Ibid., 102–03.

22   Ibid., 110.

23   Ibid., 55.

24   Ibid., 108.

25   Laura Betzig, "Roman Polygyny," *Ethology and Sociobiology* 13, no. 5 (1992): 309–349, doi:10.1016/0162-3095(92)90008-R; Laura Betzig, "Roman Monogamy," *Ethology and Sociobiology* 13, no. 5 (1992): 351–383, doi: 10.1016/0162-3095(92)90009-S.

26   Richard Alexander, *The Biology of Moral Systems* (New York: Transaction Publishers, 1987), 71; Harper, "The Case of Monogamy."

27   Michael Price, "Why We Think Monogamy Is Normal." *Psychology Today*, September 9, 2011, https://www.psychologytoday.com/blog/darwin-eternity/201109/why-we-think-monogamy-is-normal. Footnote information in Melvin Konner, *Women After All: Sex, Evolution, and the End of Male Supremacy* (New York: W. W. Norton & Company, 2015), 182.

28   Harper, "The Case of Monogamy."

29   Price, "Alexander's Theory." Footnote information in Witte, *The Western Case for Monogamy*, 114; Harper, "The Case of Monogamy."

30   Witte, *The Western Case for Monogamy*, 124, 141.

31   Eugene Hillman, *Polygamy Reconsidered: African Plural Marriage and the Christian Churches* (Maryknoll, NY: Orbis Books, 1975), 17.

32   John Witte, "Why Two in One Flesh? The Western Case for Monogamy over Polygamy," *Emory Law Journal* 64 (2014): 1675–1746, http://law.emory.edu/elj/_documents/volumes/64/6/witte.pdf.

33   Hillman, *Polygamy Reconsidered.*

34   Witte, *The Western Case for Monogamy*, 103.

35   Scheidel, "A Peculiar Institution"; Harper, "The Case of Monogamy"; Price, "Why We Think Monogamy Is Normal."

36   Scheidel, "A Peculiar Institution"; MacDonald, "The Establishment and Maintenance of Socially Imposed Monogamy in Western Europe"; Harper, "The Case of Monogamy."

37   Joseph Henrich, Robert Boyd, and Peter Richerson, "The Puzzle of Monogamous Marriage," *Philosophical Transactions of the Royal Society B: Biological Sciences* 367, no. 1589 (2012): 657–669, doi: 10.1098/rstb.2011.0290.

38   A. J. Jacobs, *The Know-It-All: One Man's Humble Quest to Become the Smartest Person in the World* (New York: Simon & Schuster, 2004), 130.

39   Nicholas Dima, *Culture, Religion, and Geopolitics* (Bloomington, IN: Xlibris Corporation, 2010), 79–80.

40   Pascale Harter, "Mauritania's 'Wife-Fattening' Farm," *BBC News*, January 26, 2004, http://news.bbc.co.uk/2/hi/3429903.stm.

41   Harrison Jacobs, "Tanned Skin Is So Frowned Upon in China That Women Wear These Crazy Face Masks to the Beach," *Business Insider*, August 6, 2014, http://www.businessinsider.com/chinese-beach-face-maskes-2014-8; John Glionna, "In South Korea, Beachgoers Stay Out of the Sun," *Los Angeles Times*, August 14, 2011, http://articles.latimes.com/2011/aug/14/world/la-fg-south-korea-beach-20110814.

42   Thomas Fuller, "A Vision of Pale Beauty Carries Risks for Asia's Women," *New York Times*, May 14, 2006, http://www.nytimes.com/2006/05/14/world/asia/14thailand.html?_r=3.

43   Michael Castleman, "How Women Really Feel about Penis Size," *Psychology Today*, November 1, 2014, https://www.psychologytoday.com/blog/all-about-sex/201411/how-women-really-feel-about-penis-size.

44   John Boswell, *Same-Sex Unions in Premodern Europe* (New York: Villard Books, 1994), 114–115.

45   John Boswell, *Christianity, Social Tolerance, and Homosexuality: Gay People in Western Europe from the Beginning of the Christian Era to the Fourteenth Century* (Chicago: University of Chicago Press, 1980), 116.

46   Roy Baumesiter and Brad Bushman, *Social Psychology and Human Nature* (Belmont, CA: Cengage Learning, 2013), 425; Marina Adhsade, *Dollars and Sex: How Economics Influences Sex and Love* (San Francisco: Chronicle, 2013), 68.

47   Jennifer Steinhauer, "Studies Find Big Benefits in Marriage," *New York Times*, April 10, 1995, http://www.nytimes.com/1995/04/10/us/studies-find-big-benefits-in-marriage.html; Noam Shpancer, "Sexual Satisfaction: Highly Valued, Poorly Understood," *Psychology Today*, February 16, 2014, https://www.psychologytoday.com/blog/insight-therapy/201402/sexual -satisfaction-highly-valued-poorly-understood; Robert Regoli, John Hewitt, and Matt DeLisi, *Delinquency in Society: The Essentials* (Burlington, MA: Jones & Bartlett Learning, 2011), 254; Adshade, *Dollars and Sex*, 68.

48   Mark Regnerus and Jeremy Uecker, *Premarital Sex in America: How Young Americans Meet, Mate, and Think about Marrying* (New York: Oxford University Press, 2010), 175.

49   Henrich, Boyd, and Richerson, "The Puzzle of Monogamous Marriage."

50   David Herlihy, *Medieval Households* (Cambridge, MA: Harvard University Press, 1985), 78.

51   Henrich, Boyd, and Richerson, "The Puzzle of Monogamous Marriage."

52   Ibid.

53   Rose McDermott and Jonathan Cowden, "Polygyny and Violence against Women," *Emory Law Journal* 64 (2014): 1767–1814, http://law.emory.edu/elj/_documents/volumes/64/6 /mcdermott-cowden.pdf.

54   Price, "Alexander's Theory."

Chapter 2

1   Jon Stewart et al., *America (The Book): A Citizen's Guide to Democracy Inaction* (New York: Grand Central Pub, 2004), 54.

2   "The Last Temptation of Homer," *The Simpsons*, Fox, December 9, 1993.

3   Larry Flynt and David Eisenbach, *One Nation under Sex: How the Private Lives of Presidents, First Ladies, and Their Lovers Changed the Course of American History* (New York: Macmillan, 2011).

4   Shelly Kirkpatick and Edwin Locke, "Leadership: Do Traits Matter?," *Executive* 5, no. 2 (1991): 48–60, doi:10.5465/AME.1991.4274679; Michael McCormick, "Self-Efficacy and Leadership Effectiveness: Applying Social Cognitive Theory to Leadership," *Journal of Leadership & Organizational Studies* 8, no. 1 (2001): 22–33, doi:10.1177/107179190100800102.

5   Amy Brunell et al. "Leader Emergence: The Case of the Narcissistic Leader," *Personality and Social Psychology Bulletin* 34, no. 12 (2008): 1663–1676, doi:10.1177/0146167208324101; Michael Maccoby, "Narcissistic Leaders: The Incredible Pros, the Inevitable Cons," *Harvard Business Review*, January 2004, https://hbr.org/2004/01/narcissistic-leaders-the-incredible -pros-the-inevitable-cons; Seth Rosenthal and Todd Pittinsky, "Narcissistic Leadership," *Leadership Quarterly* 17, no. 6 (2006): 617–633, doi:10.1016/j.leaqua.2006.10.005; Emily Grijalva et al., "Narcissism and Leadership: A Meta-analytic Review of Linear and Nonlinear Relationships," *Personnel Psychology* 68, no. 1 (2014): 1–47, doi:10.1111/peps.12072; Peter Harms, Seth Spain, and Sean Hannah, "Leader Development and the Dark Side of Personality," *Leadership Quarterly* 22, no. 3 (2011): 495–509, doi:10.1016/j.leaqua.2011.04.007.

6   Roy Baumeister, Kathleen Catanese, and Harry Wallace, "Conquest by Force: A Narcissistic Reactance Theory of Rape and Sexual Coercion," *Review of General Psychology* 6, no. 1 (2002): 92–135, doi:10.1037/1089-2680.6.1.92; Brad Bushman et al., "Narcissism, Sexual Refusal, and Aggression: Testing a Narcissistic Reactance Model of Sexual Coercion," *Journal of Personality and Social Psychology* 84, no. 5 (2003): 1027–1040, doi:10.1037/0022-3514.84.5.1027.

7   Paul Piff et al., "Higher Social Class Predicts Increased Unethical Behavior," *Proceedings of the National Academy of Sciences* 109, no. 11 (2012): 4086–4091, doi:10.1073/pnas.1118373109.

8   Mary Carmichael, "The Cheating Man's Brain," *Newsweek*, March 11, 2008, http://www.newsweek.com/cheating-mans-brain-83569.

9   Irving Weiner and W. Edward Craighead, eds., *The Corsini Encyclopedia of Psychology* Volume 4 (New York: John Wiley & Sons, 2010), 1471.

10   Marvin Zuckerman, "Are You a Risk Taker?," *Psychology Today*, November 1, 2000, https://www.psychologytoday.com/articles/200011/are-you-risk-taker.

11   Helen Fisher, *Anatomy of Love: The Natural History of Monogamy, Adultery, and Divorce* (New York: W. W. Norton & Co., 1992), 172; Carmichael, "The Cheating Man's Brain."

12   Marvin Zuckerman, *Behavioral Expressions and Biosocial Bases of Sensation Seeking* (New York: Cambridge University Press, 1994), 27.

13   Zuckerman, "Are You a Risk Taker?"; Yoon-Mi Hur and Thomas Bouchard, "The Genetic Correlation Between Impulsivity and Sensation Seeking Traits," *Behavior Genetics* 27, no. 5 (1997): 455–463, doi:10.1023/A:1025674417078; Marvin Zuckerman and David Kuhlman, "Personality and Risk-Taking: Common Biosocial Factors," *Journal of Personality* 68, no. 6 (2000): 999–1029, doi:10.1111/1467–6494.00124; David Fulker, Sybil Eysenck, and Marvin Zuckerman, "A Genetic and Environmental Analysis of Sensation Seeking," *Journal of Research in Personality* 14, no. 2 (1980): 261–281, doi:10.1016/0092–6566(80)90033–1.

14   Rick Hoyle, Michele Fejfar, and Joshua Miller, "Personality and Sexual Risk Taking: A Quantitative Review," *Journal of Personality* 68, no. 6 (2000): 1203–1231, http://www.columbia.edu/cu/psychology/courses/3615/Readings/Hoyle_2000.pdf; Jonathan Roberti, "A Review of Behavioral and Biological Correlates of Sensation Seeking," *Journal of Research in Personality* 38, no. 3 (2000): 256—279, doi:10.1016/S0092–6566(03)00067–9; Camille Lalasz and Daniel Weigel, "Understanding the Relationship Between Gender and Extradyadic Relations: The Mediating Role of Sensation Seeking on Intentions to Engage in Sexual Infidelity," *Personality and Individual Differences* 50, no. 7 (2011): 1079–1083, doi:10.1016/j.paid.2011.01.029.

15   Marvin Zuckerman, *Sensation Seeking and Risk* (Washington DC: American Psychological Association, 2007); Carmichael, "The Cheating Man's Brain."

16   Flynt and Eisenbach, *One Nation Under Sex*, 258.

17   Justin Garcia et al., (2010). "Associations Between Dopamine D4 Receptor Gene Variation with Both Infidelity and Sexual Promiscuity," *PLoS One* 5, no. 11 (2010), doi:10.1371/journal.pone.0014162.

18   Gail Glover, "Study: Propensity for Infidelity, One-Night Stands Could be Genetic," *Binghamton University*, December 7, 2010, http://www.binghamton.edu/inside/index.php/inside/story/731/study-suggests-that-propensity-for-infidelity-one-night-stands-could-be-gen/.

19   Philip Sherwell, "The World According to Henry Kissinger," *Telegraph*, May 21, 2011, http://www.telegraph.co.uk/news/worldnews/us-politics/8528270/The-world-according-to-Henry-Kissinger.html.

20   Angela Serratore, "Alexander Hamilton's Adultery and Apology," *Smithsonian*, July 25, 2015, http://www.smithsonianmag.com/history/alexander-hamiltons-adultery-and-apology-18021947/.

21   Homer Calkin, "Pamphlets and Public Opinion during the American Revolution," *Pennsylvania Magazine of History and Biography* (1940): 22–42, https://journals.psu.edu/pmhb/article/viewFile/29581/29336.

22   Andrew Glass, "Thomas Jefferson Accused of Affair, Oct. 19, 1796," *Politico*, October 19, 2011, http://www.politico.com/story/2011/10/thomas-jefferson-accused-of-affair-oct-19-1796-066263.

23   Cali Williams Yost, "American Revolution's Pamphleteers, Today's Bloggers and Twitterers for Change," *Fast Company*, July 10, 2009, http://www.fastcompany.com/1306652/american -revolutions-pamphleteers-todays-bloggers-and-twitterers-change.

24   Flynt and Eisenbach, *One Nation under Sex*, 262.

25   Ibid, 22–23.

26   Fawn Brodie, (1974). *Thomas Jefferson: An Intimate History* (New York: W. W. Norton & Co., 1974); Robert Watson, *Affairs of State: The Untold History of Presidential Love, Sex, and Scandal, 1789–1900* (Lanham MD: Rowman & Littlefield Publishers, 2012), 144–153, 163–165.

27   Flynt and Eisenback, *One Nation under Sex*, 22–25.

28   Ibid., 38.

29   Ibid., 225.

30   Barton Bernstein, "The Road to Watergate and Beyond: The Growth and Abuse of Executive Authority Since 1940," *Law and Contemporary Problems* (1976): 58–86, doi:10.2307/1191371; Kate Doyle, "The End of Secrecy: US National Security and the Imperative for Openness," *World Policy Journal* 16, no. 1 (1999): 34–51, http://www.jstor.org/stable/40209610.

31   Flynt and Eisenbach, *One Nation under Sex*, 170.

32   Lina Lotridge Levin, *The Making of FDR: The Story of Stephen T. Early, America's First Modern Press Secretary* (New York: Prometheus Books, 2008), 232; Joseph Persico, *Franklin and Lucy: President Roosevelt, Mrs. Rutherfurd, and the Other Remarkable Women in His Life* (New York: Random House, 2008), 188.

33   Russell Baker, "The Charms of Eleanor," *New York Review of Books*, June 9, 2011, http://www .nybooks.com/articles/2011/06/09/charms-eleanor-roosevelt/; Persico, *Franklin and Lucy*, 200–214.

34   Persico, *Franklin and Lucy*, 188.

35   Charles McGrath, "No End of the Affair," *New York Times*, April 20, 2008, http://www .nytimes.com/2008/04/20/weekinreview/20mcgrath.html.

36   Nicholas Lemann, "Ronald Reagan's Performance," *New York Times*, June 26, 1983, http ://www.nytimes.com/1983/06/26/books/ronald-reagan-s-performance.html.

37   Persico, *Franklin and Lucy*, 125.

38   Flynt and Eisenbach, *One Nation Under Sex*, 105–106.

39   Persico, *Franklin and Lucy*, 165–166.

40   Franklin D. Roosevelt Presidential Library and Museum, "Biography of Eleanor Roosevelt," accessed February 20, 2016, http://www.fdrlibrary.marist.edu/education/resources/bio _er.html; Maureen Dowd, "E.R.," *New York Times*, July 4, 1999, http://www.nytimes.com /books/99/07/04/reviews/990704.704dowdt.html.

41   Persico, *Franklin and Lucy*, 200–214; Robert Aldrich and Garry Wotherspoon, eds., *Who's Who in Gay and Lesbian History: From Antiquity to World War II* (New York: Routledge, 2002), 450; Baker, "The Charms of Eleanor"; Flynt and Eisenbach, *One Nation under Sex*, 101.

42   Andrew Sullivan, "The First Gay President," *Newsweek*, May 21, 2012.

43   Jim Loewen, "Our Real First Gay President," *Salon*, May 14, 2012, http://www.salon .com/2012/05/14/our_real_first_gay_president/.

44   Flynt and Eisenbach, *One Nation under Sex*, 50.

45   Katherine Cooney, "Who Was Our First Gay President?," *Time*, May 17, 2012, http ://newsfeed.time.com/2012/05/17/who-was-our-first-gay-president/.

46   George Ticknor Curtis, *Life of James Buchanan: Fifteenth President of the United States* Volume 1 (New York: Harper & Brothers, 1883), 519.

47   Tom Geoghegan, "James Buchanan: Worst US President?," *BBC News*, July 2, 2013, http ://www.bbc.com/news/magazine-22946672.

48   Flynt and Eisenbach, *One Nation under Sex*, 180, 213.

49 Robert Miraldi, *Seymour Hersh: Scoop Artist* (Lincoln, NE: University of Nebraska Press, 2013), 290.

50 Flynt and Eisenbach, *One Nation under Sex*, 170.

51 Ibid., 133–135.

52 David Garrow, "The FBI and Martin Luther King," *Atlantic*, July/August 2002, http://www.theatlantic.com/magazine/archive/2002/07/the-fbi-and-martin-luther-king/302537/.

53 Beverly Gage, "What an Uncensored Letter to M.L.K. Reveals," *New York Times Magazine*, November 11, 2014, http://www.nytimes.com/2014/11/16/magazine/what-an-uncensored-letter-to-mlk-reveals.html.

54 Flynt and Eisenbach, *One Nation under Sex*, 191.

55 John Meroney, "What Really Happened Between J. Edgar Hoover and MLK Jr.," *Atlantic*, November 11, 2011, http://www.theatlantic.com/entertainment/archive/2011/11/what-really-happened-between-j-edgar-hoover-and-mlk-jr/248319/.

56 Athan Theoharis, *From the Secret Files of J. Edgar Hoover* (Chicago: Ivan R. Dee, 1993), 103.

57 Flynt and Eisenbach, *One Nation under Sex*, 143–167.

58 Janet Hook, "Crime Drop a Boost for Clinton, a Challenge for GOP," *Los Angeles Times*, May 7, 1996, http://articles.latimes.com/1996-05-07/news/mn-1399_1_crime-issue.

59 Steve Schifferes, "Bill Clinton's Economic Legacy," *BBC News*, January 15, 2001, http://news.bbc.co.uk/2/hi/business/1110165.stm.

60 The Associated Press, "Lewinsky and the First Lady," *USA Today*, March 19, 2008, http://usatoday30.usatoday.com/news/politics/2008-03-19-852575883_x.htm.

61 Kenneth Starr, *The Starr Report: The Findings of Independent Counsel Kenneth W. Starr on President Clinton and the Lewinsky Affair* (New York: PublicAffairs, 1998), 325.

62 Flynt and Eisenbach, *One Nation under Sex*, 249–250, 255–256.

63 Monica Lewinsky, "Shame and Survival," *Vanity Fair*, June 2014, https://www.vanityfair.com/style/society/2014/06/monica-lewinsky-humiliation-culture.

Chapter 3

1 Pope Benedict XVI, "Interview of the Holy Father Benedict XVI During the Flight to Africa," *Vatican*, March 17, 2009, http://w2.vatican.va/content/benedict-xvi/en/speeches/2009/march/documents/hf_ben-xvi_spe_20090317_africa-interview.html.

2 The New York Times Editorial Board, "The Pope on Condoms and AIDS," *New York Times*, March 17, 2009, http://www.nytimes.com/2009/03/18/opinion/18wed2.html.

3 Ben Goldacre, "Pope's Anti-Condom Message Is Sabotage in Fight Against AIDS," *Guardian*, September 11, 2010, http://www.theguardian.com/commentisfree/2010/sep/11/bad-science-pope-anti-condom.

4 Edward Green, "Condoms, HIV-AIDS and Africa—The Pope Was Right," *Washington Post*, March 29, 2009, http://www.washingtonpost.com/wp-dyn/content/article/2009/03/27/AR2009032702825.html.

5 Edward Green, *Broken Promises: How the AIDS Establishment Has Betrayed the Developing World* (Sausalito CA: PoliPointPress, 2011), xiv–xv.

6 Ibid., 34.

7 Rand Stoneburner and Daniel Low-Beer, "Population-Level HIV Declines and Behavioral Risk Avoidance in Uganda," *Science* 304, no. 5671 (2004): 714–718, doi:10.1126/science.1093166.

8 James Shelton et al., "Partner Reduction Is Crucial for Balanced 'ABC' Approach to HIV Prevention," *British Medical Journal* 328, no: 7444 (2004): 891.doi:10.1136/bmj.328.7444.891.

9 Edward Green and Kim Witte, "Can Fear Arousal in Public Health Campaigns Contribute to the Decline of HIV Prevalence?," *Journal of Health Communication* 11, no. 3 (2006): 245–259, doi:10.1080/10810730600613807.

10   Ibid.

11   Gary Slutkin et al., "How Uganda Reversed Its HIV Epidemic," *AIDS and Behavior* 10, no. 4 (2006); 351–360, doi:10.1007/s10461–006–9118–2.

12   Craig Timberg and Daniel Halperin, *Tinderbox: How the West Sparked the AIDS Epidemic and How the World Can Finally Overcome It* (New York: Penguin, 2012), 5.

13   Arvis, Tom, *Captain Condom and Lady Latex at War with the Army of Sex Diseases* (Washington DC: Program for Appropriate Technology in Health, 1991).

14   Green and Witte, "Can Fear Arousal," 245–259.

15   J. Genuis and S. K. Genuis, "HIV/AIDS Prevention in Uganda: Why Has It Worked?," *Postgraduate Medical Journal* 81, no. 960 (2005): 615–617., doi:10.1136/pgmj.2005.034868; Daniel Low-Beer and Rand Stoneburner, "AIDS Communications through Social Networks: Catalyst for Behavior Changes in Uganda," *African Journal of AIDS Research* 3, no. 1 (2004): 1–13, doi:10.2989/16085900409490313; Timberg and Halperin, *Tinderbox*; Edward Green et al., "Uganda's HIV Prevention Success: The Role of Sexual Behavior Change and the National Response," *AIDS and Behavior* 10, no. 4 (2006): 335–346, doi:10.1007/s10461–006–9073–y; Helen Epstein, *The Invisible Cure: Why We Are Losing the Fight Against AIDS in Africa* (New York: Picador, 2008).

16   Green et al., "Uganda's HIV Prevention Success."

17   Norman Hearst and Sanny Chen, "Condom Promotion for AIDS Prevention in the Developing World: Is it Working?, *Studies in Family Planning* 35, no. 1 (2004); 39–47, doi: 10.1111/j.17284465.2004.00004.x; Stoneburner and Low-Beer, "Population-Level HIV Declines," 714–718. Footnote information in Kirby, "Changes in Sexual Behaviour"; Peter Doskoch, "In Uganda, Fewer Partners and More Condom Use Were Key to Drop in HIV," *International Family Planning Perspectives* 34, no. 4 (2008): 201202, doi:10.2307/27642890.

18   Douglas Kirby, "Changes in Sexual Behavior Leading to the Decline in the Prevalence of HIV in Uganda: Confirmation from Multiple Sources of Evidence," *Sexually Transmitted Infections* 84, supplement 2 (2008): ii35–ii41, doi: 10.1136/sti.2008.029892. Footnote information in Shelton, Halperin, and Wilson, "Has Global HIV Incidence Peaked?"

19   Timothy Hallett et al., "Declines in HIV Prevalence Can Be Associated with Changing Sexual Behavior in Uganda, Urban Kenya, Zimbabwe, and Urban Haiti," *Sexually Transmitted Infections* 82, supplement 1 (2006): i1–i8, doi:10.1136/sti.2005.016014; A. H. Kilian et al., "Reductions in Risk Behavior Provide the Most Consistent Explanation for Declining HIV-1 Prevalence in Uganda," *AIDS* 13, no. 3 (1999): 391–398, doi:10.1097/00002030–199902250–00012.

20   Yoweri Museveni, *What Is Africa's Problem?* (Minneapolis: University of Minnesota Press, 2000), 252.

21   Edward Green et al., "The Need to Reemphasize Behavior Change for HIV Prevention in Uganda: A Qualitative Study," *Studies in Family Planning* 44, no. 1 (2013): 25–43, doi: 10.1111/j.17284465.2013.00342.x.

22   David Hunter, "AIDS in Sub-Saharan Africa: The Epidemiology of Heterosexual Transmission and the Prospects for Prevention," *Epidemiology* 4, no. 1 (1993): 63–72.

23   Epstein, *Invisible Cure*, 145; Matthew Connelly, *Fatal Misconception: The Struggle to Control World Population* (Cambridge, MA: Harvard University Press, 2009).

24   UNAIDS, UNFPA, WHO, and UNAIDS: Position Statement on Condoms and the Prevention of HIV, Other Sexually Transmitted Infections and Unintended Pregnancy," July 7, 2015, http://www.unaids.org/en/resources/presscentre/featurestories/2015 /july/20150702_condoms_prevention.

25   PEPFAR, "Implementing the ABC Approach," accessed January 7, 2016, http://www.pepfar .gov/reports/guidance/75852.htm. The PEPFAR website still features the same language found in the following policy document that was issued when PEPFAR first began: PEPFAR,

"ABC Guidance #1 for United States Government In-Country Staff and Implementing Partners Applying the ABC Approach to Preventing Sexually-Transmitted HIV Infections within the President's Emergency Plan for AIDS Relief," accessed January 7, 2016, http ://www.state.gov/documents/organization/57241.pdf.

26   Helen Epstein, interview, October 12, 2015; James Chin, *The AIDS Pandemic: The Collision of Epidemiology with Political Correctness* (Oxford: Radcliffe Publishing, 2007), 1–2, 165.

27   Joanne van Harmelen et al., "An Association Between HIV-1 Subtypes and Mode of Transmission in Cape Town, South Africa," *AIDS* 11, no. 1 (1997): 81–87, doi:10.1097/00002030–199701000–00012; Carolyn Williamson et al., "HIV-1 Subtypes in Different Risk Groups in South Africa," *Lancet* 346, no. 8977 (1995): 782, doi: 10.1016/ S0140–6736(95)91543–5.

28   Green, *Broken Promises*, 179.

29   Helen Epstein, "God and the Fight against AIDS," *New York Review of Books*, April 28, 2005, http ://www.nybooks.com/articles/2005/04/28/god-and-the-fight-against-aids/; Helen Epstein, "There Is No Room for Sexual Morality in an Honest Conversation about AIDS," *Guardian*, August 8, 2007, http://www.theguardian.com/commentisfree/2007/aug/09/comment.health.

30   Josh Kron, "In Uganda, an AIDS Success Story Comes Undone," *New York Times*, August 2, 2012, http://www.nytimes.com/2012/08/03/world/africa/in-uganda-an-aids-success-story -comes-undone.html.

31   Ministry of Health, "Uganda AIDS Indicator Survey 2011," August 2012, 105, http://health .go.ug/docs/UAIS_2011_REPORT.pdf.

32   UNAIDS, "The HIV and AIDS Uganda Country Progress Report 2014," June 15, 2015, 11, http://www.unaids.org/sites/default/files/country/documents/UGA_narrative _report_2015.pdf; UNAIDS, "The Gap Report," July 16, 2014, 30–31, http ://www.unaids.org/sites/default/files/en/media/unaids/contentassets/documents /unaidspublication/2014/UNAIDS_Gap_report_en.pdf; UNAIDS, "HIV Estimates with Uncertainty Bounds 1990–2013," accessed January 7, 2016, http://www.unaids.org /en/resources/campaigns/2014/2014gapreport/gapreport/; AVERT, "HIV and AIDS in Uganda," accessed January 7, 2016, http://www.avert.org/professionals/hiv-around-world /sub-saharan-africa/uganda; PEPFAR, "Uganda Operational Plan Report FY 2013," January 14, 2014, 143, http://www.pepfar.gov/documents/organization/222185.pdf; Danida, "Strengthening Uganda's Response to HIV/AIDS 2007–2010," May 2007, 6, http://uganda .um.dk/en/~/media/Uganda/Documents/English%20site/The%20new%20Danida%20 HIV%20AIDS%20Programme%20for%20Uganda.pdf.

33   Ministry of Health, "Uganda AIDS Indicator Survey," 4; UNAIDS, "HIV and AIDS Uganda Country Progress Report; 2013," March 31, 2014, 15, https://www.uhasselt.be/Documents /UHasselt/onderwijs/internationaal/noord-zuid_2015/HIV_and_AIDS_Uganda _Country_Progress_Report_2013.pdf; statistics accessed January 7, 2016, http://legacy .statcompiler.com/.

34   Alex Opio et al., "Trends in HIV-Related Behaviors and Knowledge in Uganda, 1989– 2005: Evidence of a Shift Toward More Risk-Taking Behaviors," *Journal of Acquired Immune Deficiency Syndromes*, 49, no. 3 (2008): 320–326, doi: 10.1097/QAI.0b013e3181893eb0. Footnote information in Epstein, *Invisible Cure*, 183.

35   Green et al., "The Need to Reemphasize Behavior Change"; Timberg and Halperin, *Tinderbox*, 368.

36   Statistics accessed January 7, 2016, http://legacy.statcompiler.com/.

37   James Shelton, Daniel Halperin, and David Wilson, "Has Global HIV Incidence Peaked?," *Lancet* 367, no. 9517 (2006): 1120–1122, doi: 10.1016/S0140–6736(06)68436–5.

38   Green et al., "The Need to Reemphasize Behavior Change."

39   Eileen Stillwaggon, "AIDS and Poverty in Africa," *The Nation*, May 21, 2001, http://www
      .thenation.com/article/aids-and-poverty-africa/; Joan Smith, "HIV-AIDS Has Mutated
      into a Disease of Poverty," *Independent*, November 30, 2013, http://www.independent.co.uk
      /voices/comment/hiv-aids-has-mutated-into-a-disease-of-poverty-8975000.html.

40   Green, *Broken Promises*, 178. Footnote information in Halperin and Epstein, "Why Is HIV
      Prevalence So Severe in Southern Africa?"; Chin, *AIDS Pandemic*, 68–69; Helen Epstein,
      interview, October 12, 2015; Statistics accessed January 7, 2016, http://legacy.statcompiler
      .com/.

41   Lucia Corno and Damien de Walque, "Mines, Migration, and HIV/AIDS in Southern Africa,"
      Journal of African Economies 21, no. 3 (2012): 465–498, doi: 10.1093/jae/ejs005; Belinda
      Beresford, "AIDS Takes an Economic and Social Toll," *Africa Recovery*, June 2001, 19–23,
      http://www.un.org/en/africarenewal/vol15no1/15no1pdf/151aids9.pdf; Daan Brummer,
      Labor Migration and HIV/AIDS in Southern Africa (Pretoria South Africa: International
      Organization for Migration Regional Office for Southern Africa, 2002).

42   Leickness Simbayi et al., *South African National HIV Prevalence, Incidence, and Behavior Survey,*
      2012, Pretoria South Africa: Human Sciences Research Council 2014), 86–96; Leigh Johnson
      et al., "Sexual Behavior Patterns in South Africa and Their Association with the Spread of
      HIV: Insights from a Mathematical Model," *Demographic Research* 21 (2009): 289–339,
      doi:10.4054/DemRes.2009.21.11.

43   Leigh Johnson and Peter White, "A Review of Mathematical Models of HIV/AIDS
      Interventions and Their Implications for Policy," *Sexually Transmitted Infections* 87, no. 7
      (2011): 629–634, doi:10.1136/sti.2010.045500.

44   Douglas Kirby, B. A. Laris, and Lori Rolleri, "Sex and HIV Education Programs: Their Impact
      on Sexual Behaviors of Young People Throughout the World," *Journal of Adolescent Health*
      40, no. 3 (2006): 206–217, doi:10.1016/j.jadohealth.2006.11.143; Gina Wingood et al.,
      "Efficacy of an HIV Intervention in Reducing High-Risk Human Papillomavirus, Nonviral
      Sexually Transmitted Infections, and Concurrency among African American Women:
      A Randomized-Controlled Trial," *Journal of Acquired Immune Deficiency Syndromes* 63,
      supplement 1 (2013): s36–43, doi:10.1097/QAI.0b013e3182920031. Footnote information
      in Kirby, Laris, and Rolleri, "Sex and HIV Education Programs"; David Ross, Bruce Dick,
      and Jane Ferguson, eds., "Preventing HIV/AIDS in Young People: A Systematic Review of
      the Evidence from Developing Countries," *World Health Organization Technical Report Series*,
      no. 938 (2006): 136, http://www.unicef.org/aids/files/PREVENTING_HIV_AIDS_IN
      _YOUNG_PEOPLE__A_SYSTEMATIC_REVIEW_OF_THE_EVIDENCE
      _FROM_DEVELOPING_COUNTRIES_WHO 2006.pdf; "Long-Term Evaluation of
      the MEMA kwa Vijana Adolescent Sexual Health Programme in Rural Mwanza, Tanzania:
      A Randomized Controlled Trial," *MEMA kwa Vijana Programme Technical Briefing Paper*,
      no. 7, November 2008, http://r4d.dfid.gov.uk/PDF/Outputs/ReproHealthHIV_RPC
      /MkVtechnicalbrief.pdf; Helen Epstein, "AIDS Education Programs Miss Target," *AIDS* 24,
      no. 13 (2010): 2140, doi:10.1097/QAD.0b013e32833c872f.

45   Daniel Halperin and Helen Epstein, "Concurrent Sexual Partnerships Help to Explain Africa's
      High HIV Prevalence: Implications for Prevention," *Lancet* 364, no. 9428 (2004), 4–6,
      doi:10.1016/S0140–6736(04)16606–3.

46   Christopher Hudson, "Concurrent Partnerships Could Cause AIDS Epidemics," *International
      Journal of STD & AIDS* 4, no. 5 (1993): 249–253, doi:10.1177/095646249300400501;
      Christopher Hudson, "AIDS in Rural Africa: A Paradigm for HIV-1 Prevention," *International
      Journal of STD & AIDS* 7, no. 4 (1996): 236–243, doi: 10.1258/0956462961917906; Martina
      Morris and Mirjam Kretzschmar, "Concurrent Partnerships and Transmission Dynamics
      in Networks," *Social Networks* 17 (1995): 299–318, doi: 10.1016/0378–8733(95)00268-S;

Martina Morris and Mirjam Kretzschmar, "Concurrent Partnerships and the Spread of HIV," *AIDS* 11, no. 5 (1997): 641–648, doi:10.1097/00002030–199705000–00012.

47   Halperin and Epstein, "Concurrent Sexual Partnerships."

48   Epstein, *Invisible Cure*, 85.

49   Darlene Taylor et al., "Probability of a False-Negative HIV Antibody Test Result During the Window Period: A Tool for Pre- and Post-Test Counseling," *International Journal of STD & AIDS* 26 no. 4 (2015): 215–224, doi:10.1177/0956462414542987; AIDS Foundation of Chicago, "Facts about HIV/AIDS," accessed January 8, 2016, http://www.aidschicago.org /page/about-hiv/facts-about-hivaids; Elizabeth Pisani, *The Wisdom of Whores: Bureaucrats, Brothels, and the Business of AIDS* (New York: W. W. Norton & Company, 2008), 35.

50   Morris and Kretzschmar, "Concurrent Partnerships"; Halperin and Epstein, "Concurrent Sexual Partnerships"; Helen Epstein and Martina Morris, "Concurrent Partnerships and HIV: An Inconvenient Truth," *Journal of the International AIDS Society* 14, no. 1 (2011): 13, doi:10.1186/1758–2652–14–13; Hudson, "Concurrent Partnerships Could Cause AIDS Epidemics,"; Frank Tanser et al., "Effect of Concurrent Sexual Partnerships on Rate of New HIV Infections in a High-Prevalence, Rural South African Population: A Cohort Study," *The Lancet* 387, no. 9787 (2011): 247–255, doi:10.1016/S0140–6736(11)60779–4. Footnote information in Halperin and Epstein, "Concurrent Sexual Partnerships"; Epstein, *Invisible Cure*, 51.

51   Green, "The Pope Was Right."

52   Green, *Broken Promises*, 52–53.

53   Timberg and Halperin, *Tinderbox*, 148–149.

54   World Health Organization, "Male Circumcision for HIV Prevention," accessed January 8, 2016, http://www.who.int/hiv/topics/malecircumcision/en/.

55   Timberg and Halperin, *Tinderbox*, 201; Nico Nagelkerke et al., "Modeling the Public Health Impact of Male Circumcision for HIV Prevention in High Prevalence Areas in Africa," *BMC Infectious Diseases* 7, no. 1 (2007): 16, doi: 10.1186/1471–2334–7-16.

56   Timberg and Halperin, *Tinderbox*, 105.

57   Godfrey Kigozi, "Foreskin Surface Area and HIV Acquisition in Rakai, Uganda (Size Matters)," *AIDS* 23, no. 16 (2009): 2209–2213, doi: 10.1097/QAD.0b013e328330eda8.

58   Epstein, *Invisible Cure*, 37; Pisani, *Wisdom of Whores*, 133.

59   Pisani, *Wisdom of Whores*, 136; Timberg and Halperin, *Tinderbox*, 249.

60   Don Boroughs, "What Botswana's Teen Girls Learn in 'Sugar Daddy' Class," *NPR*, July 20, 2015, http://www.npr.org/sections/goatsandsoda/2015/07/30/419565650/how-to -convince-teen-girls-to-stay-away-from-sugar-daddies.

61   Edward Green, "New Evidence Guiding How We Conduct AIDS Prevention," Presentation to the Manhattan Institute, New York, January 9, 2008, http://newparadigmfund.org/APRP /docs/green-manhattan-institute-lecture-010908.pdf.

62   Daniel Halperin et al., "Surprising Prevention Success: Why Did the HIV Epidemic Decline in Zimbabwe?" *PLoS Medicine* 8, no. 2 (2011): e1000414. doi:10.1371/journal.pmed.1000414.

63   Ibid.

64   Erika Check, "HIV Infection in Zimbabwe Falls at Last," *Nature*, February 2, 2006, http ://www.nature.com/news/2006/060130/full/news060130-9.html.

65   James Kirchick, "Do or Dybul," *New Republic*, March 11, 2009, https://newrepublic.com /article/62374/do-or-dybul; Michelle Goldberg, "Ending the Compromise Era on AIDS," *American Prospect*, February 11, 2009, http://prospect.org/article/ending-compromise-era-aids.

66   Pisani, *Wisdom of Whores*, 28; UNAIDS, "AIDS Epidemic Update," *UNAIDS*, December 1998, http://data.unaids.org/Publications/IRC-pub06/epiupdate98_en.pdf.

67   Pisani, *Wisdom of Whores*, 28.

68   Ibid., 95. Footnote information in "The Not-So-Fair Sex: Women May Be More Responsible

for Spreading HIV than Has Been Suspected," *The Economist*, June 28, 2007, http://www
.economist.com/node/9401560.

69   Timberg and Halperin, *Tinderbox*, 150.

70   Steven Levitt and Stephen Dubner, *Freakonomics: A Rogue Economist Explores the Hidden Side
of Everything* (New York: HarperCollins, 2005), 92.

71   Denis Campbell, "UN Overstated AIDS Risk, Says Specialist," *Guardian*, June 7, 2008, http
://www.theguardian.com/world/2008/jun/08/aids.health.

72   Green, *Broken Promises*, 197; Timberg and Halperin, *Tinderbox*, 249–250.

73   Timberg and Halperin, *Tinderbox*, 251.

74   Peter Piot, "AIDS: A Global Response," *Science* 272, no. 5270 (1996), 1855, doi:10.1126
/science.272.5270.1855.

75   Chin, *AIDS Pandemic*, 174.

76   Peter Piot, "AIDS and the Way Forward: A World AIDS Day Address," Lecture, Woodrow
Wilson International Center for Scholars, Washington DC, November 30, 2004, http://data
.unaids.org/media/speeches02/sp_piot_wilsoncenter_30nov04_en.pdf. Footnote information
in Timberg and Halperin, *Tinderbox*, 139.

77   Timberg and Halperin, *Tinderbox*, 138–142, 297–298, 368.

78   Peter Piot et al., "A Global Response to AIDS: Lessons Learned, Next Steps," *Science* 304, no.
5679 (2004): 1909–1910, doi:10.1126/science.1101137. Footnote information in Timberg
and Halperin, *Tinderbox*, 237.

79   Timberg and Halperin, *Tinderbox*, 198.

80   Green, *Broken Promises*, 198–200; Timberg and Halperin, *Tinderbox*, 297–298; UNAIDS,
"AIDS Epidemic Update 2007," November 15, 2007, 1, http://data.unaids.org/pub
/EPISlides/2007/2007_epiupdate_en.pdf.

81   UNAIDS, "UNAIDS Annual Report 2007: Knowing Your Epidemic," March 2008, 31,
http://www.unaids.org/sites/default/files/media_asset/jc1535_annual_report07_en_1.pdf.

82   Peter Piot, *No Time to Lose: A Life in Pursuit of Deadly Viruses* (New York: W. W. Norton &
Co., 2012), 338.

83   Shelton, Halperin, and Wilson, "Has Global HIV Incidence Peaked?"; Daniel Halperin,
interview, October 7, 2015; Edward Green, email interview, May 10, 2015; Gabriel Rotello,
email interview, September 24, 2015.

84   Gabriel Rotello, *Sexual Ecology: AIDS and the Destiny of Gay Men* (New York: Dutton, 1998),
127–130.

85   Chin, *AIDS Pandemic*, 136, 152.

86   UNAIDS, "AIDS Epidemic Update," December 2005, 5, http://data.unaids.org/Publications
/IRC-pub06/epi_update2005_en.pdf.

87   UNAIDS, "AIDS by the Numbers 2013," accessed January 15, 2016, 8, http://www.unaids
.org/sites/default/files/media_asset/JC2571_AIDS_by_the_numbers_en_1.pdf. Footnote
information in UNAIDS, "World AIDS Day Report 2012," 35.

88   Timberg and Halperin, *Tinderbox*, 297–298.

89   UNAIDS, "Fast-Track: Ending the AIDS Epidemic by 2030," 9, 26.

90   UNAIDS, "World AIDS Day Report 2012," November 20, 2012, 9, http://www.unaids.org
/sites/default/files/media_asset/JC2434_WorldAIDSday_results_en_1.pdf.

91   Timberg and Halperin, *Tinderbox*, 301–302. Footnote information in Green and Ruark,
"AIDS in South Africa."

92   Ibid., 302.

93   Epstein, "There Is No Room"; Green et al., "The Need to Reemphasize Behavior Change."

94   Epstein, *Invisible Cure*, 176. Footnote information in UNAIDS, "World AIDS Day Report
2012," 36.

95   Victoria Fan et al., "The Financial Flows of PEPFAR: A Profile," *Center for Global Development Policy Paper* 27 (2013): 1–28, http://www.cgdev.org/publication/financial-flows-pepfar -profile.

96   Timberg and Halperin, *Tinderbox*, 131; Halperin, email interview.

97   Green, *Broken Promises*, xiv, 34.

98   Timberg and Halperin, *Tinderbox*, 201.

99   Daniel Halperin and Helen Epstein, "Why Is HIV Prevalence So Severe in Southern Africa? The Role of Multiple Concurrent Partnerships and Lack of Male Circumcision: Implications for HIV Prevention," *Southern African Journal of HIV Medicine* 26 (2007): 19–23, http ://newparadigmfund.org/APRP/docs/halperin_epstein-why-is-hiv-prevalence-so-severe.pdf.

100   Timberg and Halperin, *Tinderbox*, 204–205.

101   UNAIDS, "How AIDS Changed Everything, Millennium Development Goal 6: 15 Years, 15 Lessons of Hope from the AIDS Response," July 2, 2015, 112, http://www.unaids. org/sites/default/files/media_asset/MDG6Report_en.pdf; AIDS.gov, "How We're Spending," accessed January 8, 2016, https://www.aids.gov/federal-resources/funding-opportunities/how-were-spending/; AVERT, "Funding for HIV and AIDS," accessed January 8, 2016, http://www.avert.org/professionals/hiv-around-world/global-response/ funding#footnoteref2_k7ssepz. Footnote information in UNAIDS, "World AIDS Day Report 2012," 22.

102   UNFPA, "Contraceptives and Condoms"; UNFPA, "Donor Support for Contraceptives."

103   UNFPA, "Contraceptives and Condoms for Family Planning and STI & HIV Prevention: External Procurement Support Report 2013," December 2014, https://www.unfpa.org/sites /default/files/pub-pdf/UNFPA%20donor%20support%20report%202013%20web_4_5 .pdf; UNFPA, "Donor Support for Contraceptives and Condoms for Family Planning and STI/HIV Prevention 2010," August 2011, http://www.unfpa.org/sites/default/files/pub -pdf/FINAL%20Donor%20Support%202010-2.pdf.

104   James Shelton, "ARVs as HIV Prevention: A Tough Road to Wide Impact," *Science*, 334, no. 6063 (2011): 1645–1646, doi:10.1126/science.1212353.

105   The Henry J. Kaiser Family Foundation, "The U.S. President's Emergency Plan for AIDS Relief (PEPFAR)," November 5, 2015, http://kff.org/global-health-policy/fact-sheet/the-u -s-presidents-emergency-plan-for/; Rene Bonnel et al., *Funding Mechanisms for Civil Society: The Experience of the AIDS Response* (Washington DC: World Bank Publications, 2013), 44.

106   Timberg and Halperin, *Tinderbox*, 211–212.

107   Kaiser Foundation, "PEPFAR."

108   Michael Bernstein and Sarah Jane Hise, "PEPFAR Reauthorization: Improving Transparency in U.S. Funding for HIV/AIDS," *Center for Global Development*, November 12, 2007, http://www .cgdev.org/publication/pepfar-reauthorization-improving-transparency-us-funding-hivaids.

109   Fan et al., "The Financial Flows of PEPFAR."

110   Ibid.

111   Curt Tarnoff and Marian Leonardo Lawson, "Foreign Aid: An Introduction to US Programs and Policy," *Congressional Research Service*, February 10, 2011, https://www.fas.org/sgp/crs /row/R40213.pdf.

112   Pisani, *Wisdom of Whores*, 283–284.

113   Annamaria La Chimia, *Tied Aid and Development Aid Procurement in the Framework of EU and WTO Law: The Imperative for Change* (Oxford: Bloomsbury Publishing, 2013), 40; Annamarie Bindenagel Sehovic, *HIV/AIDS and the South African State: Sovereignty and the Responsibility to Respond* (Burlington, VT: Ashgate Publishing Co., 2014), 130. Footnote information in Donald Berwick, "'We All Have AIDS': Case for Reducing the Cost of HIV Drugs to Zero," *British Medical Journal* 324, no. 7331 (2002): 214–218, doi:10.1136/bmj.324.7331.214; Rachel

Swarns, "Free AIDS Drugs in Africa Offer Dose of Life," *New York Times*, February 8, 2003, http://www.nytimes.com/2003/02/08/world/free-aids-drugs-in-africa-offer-dose-of-life. html?pagewanted=all; Ed Vulliamy, "How Drug Giants Let Millions Die of AIDS," *Observer*, December 18, 1999, https://www.theguardian.com/uk/1999/dec/19/theobserver.uknews6.

114   Tarnoff and Lawson, "Foreign Aid"; data from OECD via email, accessed August 25, 2015.

115   Data from OECD via email, accessed October 29, 2016.

116   Celia Dugger, "U.S. Jobs Shape Condoms' Role in Foreign Aid," *New York Times*, October 29, 2006, http://www.nytimes.com/2006/10/29/world/29condoms.html?_r=1.

117   Tarnoff and Lawson, "Foreign Aid"; Nicola Bulled, *Prescribing HIV Prevention: Bringing Culture into Global Health Communication* (Walnut Creek, CA: Left Coast Press, 2014), 212.

118   Fan et al., "The Financial Flows of PEPFAR."

119   Green, *Broken Promises*, 115–117.

120   Timberg and Halperin, *Tinderbox*, 225.

121   Green, *Broken Promises*, 115–117.

122   Epstein, *Invisible Cure*, 146.

123   Tshireletso Motlogelwa, "PSI Pulls Out Controversial Condoms Adverts," *Mmegi Online*, May 10, 2007, http://www.mmegi.bw/index.php?sid=1&aid=34&dir=2007/may/Thursday10.

124   Green, *Broken Promises*, 115–117.

125   Phoebe Kajubi et al., "Increasing Condom Use without Reducing HIV Risk: Results of a Controlled Community Trial in Uganda," *Journal of Acquired Immune Deficiency Syndromes* 40, no. 1 (2005): 77–82, doi:10.1097/01.qai.0000157391.63127.b2; Michael Cassell et al., "Risk Compensation: The Achilles' Heel of Innovations in HIV Prevention?," *British Medical Journal* 332, no. 7541 (2006): 605–607, doi:10.1136/bmj.332.7541.605.

126   Wiel Janssen, "Seat-Belt Wearing and Driving Behavior: An Instrumented-Vehicle Study," *Accident Analysis & Prevention* 26, no. 2 (1994): 249–261, doi:10.1016/0001-4575(94)90095-7.

127   William Ecenbarger, "Buckle Up Your Seatbelt and Behave," *Smithsonian*, April 2009, http://www.smithsonianmag.com/science-nature/buckle-up-your-seatbelt-and-behave -117182619/?no-ist.

128   Rotello, *Sexual Ecology*, 186–187.

129   Green, *Broken Promises*, 115–117.

130   Ibid., 130.

131   Timberg and Halperin, *Tinderbox*, 286–287.

132   Ibid., 131.

133   Epstein, "God and the Fight against AIDS."

134   Enrique Seoane-Vazquez et al., "Incentives for Orphan Drug Research and Development in the United States," *Orphanet Journal of Rare Disease* 3, no. 33 (2008), doi: 10.1186/1750-1172-3-33; Christopher Anderson and Ying Zhang, "Security Market Reaction to FDA Fast Track Designations," *Journal of Health Care Finance* 37, no. 2 (2009): 27–48, http://people. ku.edu/~cwanders/FDA_fasttrack.pdf; U.S. Food and Drug Administration, "Fast Track," accessed January 8, 2016, http://www.fda.gov/ForPatients/Approvals/Fast/ucm405399.htm.

135   Pisani, *Wisdom of Whores*, 165–166.

136   Oluwafemi Oguntibeju, "Quality of Life of People Living with HIV and AIDS and Antiretroviral Therapy," *HIV/AIDS* 4 (2012): 117–124, doi:10.2147/HIV.S32321.

137   Nicole Dukers et al., "Sexual Risk Behavior Relates to the Virological and Immunological Improvements During Highly Active Antiretroviral Therapy in HIV-1 Infection," *AIDS* 15, no. 3 (2001): 369–378.

138   Sam Ruteikara, "Let My People Go, AIDS Profiteers," *Washington Post*, June 30, 2008, http ://www.washingtonpost.com/wp-dyn/content/article/2008/06/29/AR2008062901477.html.

139   World Health Organization, "HIV/AIDS Key Facts," accessed January 8, 2016, http://www
        .who.int/mediacentre/factsheets/fs360/en/.

140   Edward Green and Allison Ruark, "AIDS in South Africa," *National Review,* August 29, 2014,
        http://www.nationalreview.com/article/386574/aids-south-africa-edward-c-green-allison-ruark.

141   UNAIDS, "Fast-Track: Ending the AIDS Epidemic by 2030," November 18, 2014, http://www.unaids
        .org/sites/default/files/media_asset/JC2686_WAD2014report_en.pdf. Footnote information in The
        New York Times Editorial Board, "The World Could End AIDS if It Tried," The New York Times,
        June 13, 2016, http://www.nytimes.com/2016/06/13/opinion/the-world-could-end-aids-if-it-tried
        .html?_r=0; VICE Special Report: Countdown to Zero, December 1, 2015, HBO.

142   Eric Elfman, "8 Brilliant Scientific Screw-Ups," *Mental Floss,* October 19, 2014, http
        ://mentalfloss.com/article/21135/8-brilliant-scientific-screw-ups.

143   Andrew Francis-Tan, "The Wages of Sin: How the Discovery of Penicillin Reshaped Modern
        Sexuality," *Archives of Sexual Behavior* 42, no. 1 (2013): 5–13, doi: 10.1007/s10508–012–0018–4.

144   Ibid.

145   Ibid.

146   Dukers et al., "Sexual Risk Behavior"; Lisa Eaton and Seth Kalichman, "Risk Compensation
        in HIV Prevention: Implications for Vaccines, Microbicides, and Other Biomedical HIV
        Prevention Technologies," *Current HIV/AIDS Reports* 4, no. 4 (2007): 165–172, doi:10.1007/
        s11904–007–0024–7; Ineke Stolte et al., "Homosexual Men Change to Risky Sex When
        Perceiving Less Threat of HIV/AIDS Since Availability of Highly Active Antiretroviral
        Therapy: A Longitudinal Study," *AIDS* 18, no. 2 (2004): 303–309, doi:10.1097/00002030–
        200401230–00021; Green et al., "The Need to Reemphasize Behavior Change"; Rebecca Bunnell,
        et al., "Changes in Sexual Behavior and Risk of HIV Transmission after Antiretroviral Therapy
        and Prevention Interventions in Rural Uganda," *AIDS* 20, no. 1 (2006): 85–92, doi:10.1097/01.
        aids.0000196566.40702.28; Mead Over et al., *HIV/AIDS Treatment and Prevention in India:
        Modeling the Costs and Consequences* (Washington DC: World Bank Publications, 2004), xix.

147   Jimmy Volmink et al., "Antiretrovirals for Reducing the Risk of Mother-to-Child Transmission
        of HIV Infection," *Cochrane Database of Systematic Reviews* (2007), doi:10.1002/14651858.
        CD003510.pub2.

148   Timberg and Halperin, *Tinderbox,* 286–287.

149   Jon Cohen, "Two Hard-Hit Countries Offer Rare Success Stories: Thailand & Cambodia,"
        Science 301, no. 5640 (2003): 1658—1662, doi:10.1126/science.301.5640.1658.

150   Ellen Setsuko Hendriksen et al., "Predictors of Condom Use among Young Adults in South
        Africa: The Reproductive Health and HIV Research Unit National Youth Survey," *American
        Journal of Public Health* 97, no. 7 (2007): 1241–1248, doi:10.2105/AJPH.2006.086009;
        Green, *Broken Promises,* 56; Audrey Pettifor, A., et al., "Young People's Sexual Health in South
        Africa: HIV Prevalence and Sexual Behaviors from a Nationally Representative Household
        Survey," *AIDS* 19, no. 14 (2005): 1525–1534, doi:10.1097/01.aids.0000183129.16830.06;
        Brooke Grundfest Schoepf, "AIDS, Sex and Condoms: African Healers and the Reinvention
        of Tradition in Zaire," *Medical Anthropology* 14, no. 2–4 (1992): 225–242, doi:10.1080/014
        59740.1992.9966073; James Shelton, "Ten Myths and One Truth About Generalized HIV
        Epidemics," *Lancet* 370, no. 9602 (2007): 1809–1811, doi:10.1016/S0140–6736(07)61755–3.

151   Timberg and Halperin, *Tinderbox,* 4.

152   Shelton et al., "Partner Reduction Is Crucial"; David Wilson, "Partner Reduction and the
        Prevention of HIV/AIDS: The Most Effective Strategies Come from Within Communities,"
        British Medical Journal 328, no. 7444 (2004): 848–849, doi:10.1136/bmj.328.7444.848;
        Epstein, *Invisible Cure,* 175–176.

153   Epstein, *Invisible Cure,* 178–179.

154   Chin, *AIDS Pandemic,* 171.

155   Randy Shilts, *And the Band Played On: Politics, People, and the AIDS Epidemic* (New York: St. Martin's Press, 1987), 301, 315, 480.

156   Michael Fumento, "A Myth that Kills," *New York Post*, July 3, 2008, http://nypost .com/2008/07/03/a-myth-that-kills/; Footnote information in Piot, *No Time to Lose*, 353.

157   Timberg and Halperin, *Tinderbox*, 140, 342; Edward Maswanya et al., "Drivers of HIV/AIDS Epidemics in Tanzania Mainland: Case Study of Makete, Temeke, Geita, Lindi, Kigoma & Meru Districts," Tanzania National Institute for Medical Research, July 2010, http://www. tanzania.go.tz/egov_uploads/documents/Drivers_of_HIV-AIDS_epidemics_in_Tanzania_ Mainland_sw.pdf.

158   Pisani, *Wisdom of Whores*, 311.

159   Shilts, *And the Band Played On*, 315.

160   Green, *Broken Promises*, 98.

Chapter 4

1   Angela Serratore, "The Curious Case of Nashville's Frail Sisterhood," *Smithsonian*, July 8, 2011, http://www.smithsonianmag.com/ist/?next=/history/the-curious-case-of-nashvilles-frail -sisterhood-7766757/.

2   Ibid.

3   James Ciment, ed. *Social Issues in American: An Encyclopedia* (New York: Routledge, 2015), 1404; Lisa Tendrich Frank, ed., *The World of the Civil War: A Daily Life Encyclopedia* (Santa Barbara, CA: Greenwood, 2015), 176. Footnote information in Frederick Lane, *Obscene Profits: Entrepreneurs of Pornography in the Cyber Age* (New York: Routledge, 2001), 44.

4   Vern Bullough, *Science in the Bedroom: A History of Sex Research* (New York: Basic Books, 1995), 107.

5   Thomas Fleming, *The Illusion of Victory: America in World War I* (New York: Basic Books, 2004), 217.

6   Andrea Tone, *Devices and Desires: A History of Contraceptives in America* (New York: Macmillan, 2002), 99, 110; Allan Brandt, *No Magic Bullet: A Social History of Venereal Disease in the United States Since 1880* (New York: Oxford University Press, 1987), 77.

7   Brandt, *No Magic Bullet*, 77.

8   Tone, *Devices and Desires*, 99.

9   Ibid., 99.

10   United States Army Center of Military History, "United States Army in the World War, 1917–1919: General Orders, GHQ, AEF," *United States Army Center of Military History*, 16, (1992): 71, http://www.history.army.mil/html/books/023/23-22/CMH_Pub_23-22.pdf.

11   Ibid., 144–145.

12   Charles Reynolds, "Prostitution as a Source of Infection with the Venereal Diseases in the Armed Forces," *American Journal of Public Health*, 30, no. 11 (1940): 1276–1282, http://ajph .aphapublications.org/doi/pdf/10.2105/AJPH.30.11.1276.

13   Ibid.

14   Lynne Haney and Lisa Pollard, eds., *Families of a New World: Gender, Politics, and State Development in a Global Context* (New York: Routledge, 2014), 50–52.

15   Reynolds, "Prostitution as a Source of Infection."

16   Nathaniel Frank, *Unfriendly Fire: How the Gay Ban Undermines the Military and Weakens America* (New York: St. Martin's Press, 2009), 1.

17   Steve Estes, email interview, September 29, 2015; Steve Estes, *Ask and Tell: Gay and Lesbian Veterans Speak Out* (Chapel Hill, NC: University of North Carolina Press, 2009).

18   Frank, *Unfriendly Fire*, xviii.

19   Steve Estes, email interview, September 29, 2015.

20   Randy Shilts, *Conduct Unbecoming: Gays and Lesbians in the U.S. Military* (New York: Macmillan, 1994), 15.

21   Michel Foucault, *The History of Sexuality, Volume 1: An Introduction*, trans. Robert Hurley (New York: Vintage, 1978), 43, 101.

22   Ibid,, 15. Footnote information in Gary Lehring, *Officially Gay: The Political Construction of Sexuality* (Philadelphia: Temple University Press, 2010), 80–81.

23   Lawrence Murphy, *Perverts by Official Order: The Campaign Against Homosexuals by the United States Navy* (New York: Routledge, 1988), 16.

24   Jeff Pearlman, "'Y.M.C.A.' (an Oral History)," *Spin*, May 27, 2008, http://www.spin.com/2008/05/ymca-oral-history/.

25   Murphy, *Perverts by Official Order*, 25.

26   Ibid., 22–25.

27   Shilts, *Conduct Unbecoming*, 16.

28   Ibid., 16; The New York Times, "Lay Navy Scandal to F. D. Roosevelt," *New York Times*, July 20, 1921.

29   Shauna Miller, "50 Years of Pentagon Studies Support Gay Soldiers," *Atlantic*, October 20, 2009, http://www.theatlantic.com/politics/archive/2009/10/50-years-of-pentagon-studies-support-gay-soldiers/28711/; Allan Bérubé, *Coming Out under Fire: The History of Gay Men and Women in World War II* (New York: Free Press, 1990), 277–78.

30   Miller, "50 Years of Pentagon Studies." Footnote information in Bérubé, *Coming Out under Fire*, 277–279.

31   Rhonda Evans, "U.S. Military Policies Concerning Homosexuals: Development, Implementation, and Outcomes," *Law & Sexuality: Rev. Lesbian, Gay, Bisexual, and Transgender Legal Issues*, 11, (2002): 113. https://escholarship.org/uc/item/2wv6s1qb#page-1.

32   Allan Bérubé, *My Desire for History: Essays in Gay, Community, and Labor History* (Chapel Hill, NC: University of North Carolina Press, 2011), 128.

33   Wilbur Scott and Sandra Carson Stanley, eds., *Gays and Lesbians in the Military: Issues, Concerns, and Contrasts* (New York: Aldine Transaction, 1994), 19.

34   Doyle McManus, "Challenge to Military's Anti-Gay Stance Found in Report Dismissed by Pentagon," *Los Angeles Times*, October 23, 1989, http://articles.latimes.com/1989-10-23/news/mn-464_1_homosexuals.

35   Scott and Stanley, *Gays and Lesbians in the Military*, 26.

36   Gary Gates, "Lesbian, Gay, and Bisexual Men and Women in the U.S. Military: Updated Estimates," The Williams Institute (2010), http://williamsinstitute.law.ucla.edu/wp-content/uploads/Gates-GLBmilitaryUpdate-May-20101.pdf. Footnote information in Timothy Lynch et al., eds., *Oxford Encyclopedia of American Military and Diplomatic History* (New York: Oxford University Press, 2013), 481.

37   Frank, *Unfriendly Fire*, 3.

38   Randy Shilts, *The Mayor of Castro Street: The Life and Times of Harvey Milk* (New York: Macmillan, 1982), 50–52; Bérubé, *Coming Out Under Fire*, 139–141.

39   Bérubé, *Coming Out Under Fire*, 152–153.

40   Ibid., 152–153.

41   Newsweek, "Homosexuals in uniform," *Newsweek*, June 9, 1947, http://www.leonardmatlovich.com/images/Newsweek_6-9-47_Homosexuals_in_Uniform-s.pdf.

42   Shilts, The Mayor of Castro Street, 50.

43   Gary Gates, "How Many People are Lesbian, Gay, Bisexual and Transgender?," The Williams Institute (2011), http://williamsinstitute.law.ucla.edu/wp-content/uploads/Gates-How-Many-People-LGBT-Apr-2011.pdf.

44   D'Emilio, *Sexual Politics*, 24.

45   Bullough, *Science in the Bedroom*, 296.

46   Shilts, *Conduct Unbecoming*, 96; Anne-Marie O'Connor, "A Woman's Place," *Los Angeles Times*, April 13, 2003, http://articles.latimes.com/2003/apr/13/entertainment/ca-oconnor13.

47   Shilts, *Conduct Unbecoming*, 67.

48   Jack Beatty, "Vietnam: Sorrow, Rage, and Remembrance," *Washington Post*, June 3, 1984, https://www.washingtonpost.com/archive/entertainment/books/1984/06/03/vietnam -sorrow-rage-and-remembrance/ca669d48-0358-4a4b-8e3e-7a1ae00e3cf7/; EJ Dickson, "The Faulty Test Used to Punish Sex Offenders," Vice, June 7, 2016, https://www.vice.com /en_us/article/jmk8w3/the-faulty-test-used-to-punish-sex-offenders.

49   Ibid., 67.

50   Frank, *Unfriendly Fire*, 11.

51   Bérubé, *Coming Out under Fire*, 255–257.

52   Ibid, 228–249.

53   Ibid., 248.

54   Ibid., 33.

55   Ibid., 262.

56   Bullough, *Science in the Bedroom*, 166.

57   John D'Emilio, *Sexual Politics, Sexual Communities: The Making of a Homosexual Minority in the United States, 1940–1970* (Chicago: University of Chicago Press, 1983), 22

58   Shilts, *Conduct Unbecoming*, 140.

59   Shilts, *The Mayor of Castro Street*, 50.

60   Bullough, *Science in the Bedroom*, 166.

61   Donald Webster Cory, *The Homosexual in America: A Subjective Approach* (New York: Greenberg, 1951), 107–108; Bérubé, *Coming Out under Fire*, 117.

62   Bérubé, *Coming Out under Fire*, 248–257. Footnote information in Rhonda Rivera, review of *Sexual Politics, Sexual Communities: The Making of a Homosexual Minority in the United States 1940– 1970*, by John D'Emilio, *University of Pennsylvania Law Review* 132, no, 191 (1984): 391419, http ://scholarship.law.upenn.edu/cgi/viewcontent.cgi?article=4629&context=penn_law_review.

63   Bullough, *Science in the Bedroom*, 298.

64   Bérubé, *Coming Out under Fire*, 249; Raymond Smith and Donald Haider-Markel, *Gay and Lesbian Americans and Political Participation: A Reference Handbook* (Westport, CT: ABC-CLIO, 2002), 73; Ronald Bayer, *Homosexuality and American Psychiatry: The Politics of Diagnosis* (Princeton: Princeton University Press, 1987), 69.

65   Bérubé, *Coming Out under Fire*, 276.

66   Associated Press, "Gay Activist Who Battled Air Force Dies," *Los Angeles Times*, June 23, 1988, http://articles.latimes.com/1988-06-23/news/mn-7479_1_air-force.

67   Alfonso Narvaez, "Gay Airman Who Fought Ouster Dies from AIDS," *New York Times*, June 24, 1988, http://www.nytimes.com/1988/06/24/us/gay-airman-who-fought-ouster-dies-from-aids.html.

68   The New York Times, "Lesbian Struggles to Serve in Army," *New York Times*, August 10, 1989, http://www.nytimes.com/1989/08/10/us/lesbian-struggles-to-serve-in-army.html.

69   *New York Times*, "Lesbian Struggles to Serve in Army."

70   Margo Huston, "Gay Woman Fights Army Dismissal," *Milwaukee Journal*, January 28, 1976, https://news.google.com/newspapers?nid=1499&dat=19760128 &id=pgcvAAAAIBAJ&sjid=IikEAAAAIBAJ&pg=7381,3310453&hl=en.

71   Linda Greenhouse, "Supreme Court Roundup; Justices Refuse to Hear Challenge to Military Ban on Homosexuals," *New York Times*, February 27, 1990, http://www.nytimes .com/1990/02/27/us/supreme-court-roundup-justices-refuse-hear-challenge-military-ban -homosexuals.html.

72   Vicki Eaklor, *Queer America: A GLBT History of the 20th Century* (Westport, CT: ABC-CLIO, 2008), 200.

73   David Dunlap, "Perry Watkins, 48, Gay Sergeant Won Court Battle with Army," *New York Times*, March 21, 1996, http://www.nytimes.com/1996/03/21/nyregion/perry-watkins-48-gay-sergeant-won-court-battle-with-army.html.

74   Clifford Levy, "Thousands March in a Celebration of Gay Pride," *New York Times*, June 28, 1993, http://www.nytimes.com/1993/06/28/nyregion/thousands-march-in-a-celebration-of-gay-pride.html.

75   Shilts, *The Mayor of Castro Street*, 50–51. Footnote information in D'Emilio, *Sexual Politics*.

76   BBC News, "U.S. Military Pondered Love Not War," *BBC News*, January 15, 2005, http://news.bbc.co.uk/2/hi/4174519.stm.

77   Hank Plante, "Pentagon Confirms It Sought to Build a 'Gay Bomb,'" *CBS 5 Berkeley*, June 8, 2007, https://web.archive.org/web/20071104162113/http://cbs5.com/topstories/local_story_159222541.html.

78   Mary Roach, *Grunt: The Curious Science of Humans at Ware* (New York: W. W. Norton & Co., 2016), 15.

79   FoxNews, "Air Force Considered Gay 'Love Bomb' Against Enemies," *FoxNews*, June 12, 2007, http://www.foxnews.com/story/2007/06/12/air-force-considered-gay-love-bomb-against-enemies.html.

80   BBC News, "'Gay Bomb' Scoops Ig Nobel Award," *BBC News*, October 4, 2007, http://news.bbc.co.uk/2/hi/science/nature/7026150.stm.

81   Elizabeth Bumiller, "Obama Ends 'Don't Ask, Don't Tell' Policy," *New York Times*, July 22, 2011, http://www.nytimes.com/2011/07/23/us/23military.html.

82   Ernesto Londoño, "Pentagon Removes Ban on Women in Combat," *Washington Post*, January 24, 2013, https://www.washingtonpost.com/world/national-security/pentagon-to-remove-ban-on-women-in-combat/2013/01/23/6cba86f6–659e-11e2–85f5-a8a9228e55e7_story.html.

83   Mark Thompson, "Women in Combat: Why the Pentagon Chief Overruled the Marines," *Time*, December 3, 2015, http://time.com/4135583/women-combat-marines-ash-carter/.

84   Walbert Castillo, "Sexual Orientation Added to Military's Equal Opportunity Policy," *CNN*, June 9, 2015, http://www.cnn.com/2015/06/09/politics/carter-sexual-orientation-policy/.

85   Andrew Tilghman, "Here are the New Rules for Transgender Troops," *Military Times*, June 30, 2016, http://www.navso.org/news/here-are-new-rules-transgender-troops.

86   Merrit Kennedy, "2 Lawsuits Challenge Trump's Ban on Transgender Military Service," NPR, August 28, 2017, http://www.npr.org/sections/thetwo-way/2017/08/28/546731931/2-lawsuits-challenge-trumps-ban-on-transgender-military-service.

87   Amanda Kerri, "The End of the Trans Military Ban: Details, Baby, Details," *Advocate*, July 5, 2016, http://www.advocate.com/commentary/2016/7/05/end-trans-military-ban-details-baby-details.

88   Halimah Abdullah and Courtney Kube, "Eric Fanning, First Openly Gay Army Secretary, Confirmed by U.S. Senate," NBC News, May 18, 2016, http://www.nbcnews.com/news/us-news/first-openly-gay-army-secretary-confirmed-n575661.

89   John D'Emilio, *Sexual Politics, Sexual Communities: The Making of a Homosexual Minority in the United States, 1940–1970* (Chicago: University of Chicago Press, 1983), 24

Chapter 5

1   Steve Neavling, "'Bring on More Gentrification,' Declares Detroit's Economic Development Czar," *Motor City Muckraker*, May 16, 2013, http://motorcitymuckraker.com/2013/05/16/bring-on-more-gentrification-declares-detroits-economic-development-czar-george-jackson/.

2   Richard Florida and Gary Gates, "Technology and Tolerance: The Importance of Diversity to High-Technology Growth," The Brookings Institution, June 2001, http://www.brookings.edu/~/media/research/files/reports/2001/6/technology-florida/techtol.pdf.

3   Lei Ding, Jackelyn Hwang, and Eileen Divringi, "Gentrification and Residential Mobility in Philadelphia," Federal Reserve Bank of Philadelphia, December 2015; Gillespie, "How Gentrification May Benefit the Poor."

4   Khalil AlHajal, "Detroit Blight Task Force Counts Nearly 80,000 Abandoned Structures, Proposes 5-Year Solution," MLive Detroit, May 27, 2014, http://www.mlive.com/news/detroit/index.ssf/2014/05/detroit_blight_task_force_coun.html; Steve Neavling, "'Bring on More Gentrification,' Declares Detroit's Economic Development Czar," Motor City Muckraker, May 16, 2013, http://motorcitymuckraker.com/2013/05/16/bring-on-more-gentrification-declares-detroits-economic-development-czar-george-jackson/.

5   Gary Gates, "Same-Sex and Different-Sex Couples in the American Community Survey: 2005–2011," Williams Institute, February 2013, http://williamsinstitute.law.ucla.edu/wp-content/uploads/ACS-2013.pdf; Gary Gates, "LGBT Parenting in the United States," Williams Institute, February 2013, http://williamsinstitute.law.ucla.edu/wp-content/uploads/LGBT-Parenting.pdf.

6   Danielle Kurtzleben, "Gay Couples More Educated, Higher-Income Than Heterosexual Couples," U.S. News & World Report, March 1, 2013, http://www.usnews.com/news/articles/2013/03/01/gay-couples-more-educated-higher-income-than-heterosexual-couples.

7   Ghaziani, There Goes the Gayborhood, 288, 308; Ghaziani, email interview.

8   Neal Rubin, "Graffiti a Sign of Widening Divide in Detroit Neighborhood," Detroit News, August 1, 2013, https://web.archive.org/web/20130801141331/http://www.detroitnews.com/article/20130801/METRO01/308010039/Graffiti-sign-widening-divide-Detroit-neighborhood?odyssey=tab%7Ctopnews%7Ctext%7CFRONTPAGE.

9   MC Slim JB, "The South End Is So Over," Boston Magazine, November 2007, http://www.bostonmagazine.com/2007/10/the-south-end-is-so-over/.

10   Col Flyn, "YUPPIES OUT! Living on the Front Line of Gentrification in Brixton," New Statesman, July 16, 2013, http://www.newstatesman.com/politics/2013/07/yuppies-out-living-front-line-gentrification-brixton.

11   Amin Ghaziani, There Goes the Gayborhood? (Princeton, NJ: Princeton University Press, 2014), 218–219.

12   Patrick Sharkey, Stuck in Place: Urban Neighborhoods and the End of Progress toward Racial Equality (Chicago: University of Chicago Press, 2013), 162–163; Patrick Gillespie, "How Gentrification May Benefit the Poor," CNN Money, November 12, 2015, http://money.cnn.com/2015/11/12/news/economy/gentrification-may-help-poor-people/.

13   Kelefa Sanneh, "Is Gentrification Really a Problem?," New Yorker, July 11, 2016, http://www.newyorker.com/magazine/2016/07/11/is-gentrification-really-a-problem.

14   Rubin, "Graffiti a Sign."

15   Megan Smith et al., eds., Let's Go: Boston, 4th ed. (New York: St. Martin's Press, 2003), 92.

16   Ibid., 92.

17   BU Today Staff, "Getting to Know Your Neighborhood: The South End," BU Today, January 15, 2015, http://www.bu.edu/today/2015/getting-to-know-your-neighborhood-the-south-end/.

18   Zillow, "South End Boston Real Estate," accessed February 28, 2016, http://www.zillow.com/south-end-boston-ma/.

19   Jeff Dickey and Jules Brown, The Rough Guide to Washington DC (New York: Rough Guides, 2008), 197; Nastaran Zandian, Bridging the Worlds through Art and Culture: An Iranian Cultural Center in Washington DC (College Park, MD: University of Maryland, 2007), 22–23; Sarah Shoenfield et al., Hub, Home, Heart: Greater H Street NE Heritage Trail (Washington

DC: Cultural Tourism DC, 2011); Harry Jaffe, "The Insane Highway Plan That Would Have Bulldozed DC's Most Charming Neighborhoods," *Washingtonian*, October 21, 2015, http://www.washingtonian.com/2015/10/21/the-insane-highway-plan-that-would-have-bulldozed-washington-dcs-most-charming-neighborhoods/.

20   Dickey and Brown, *The Rough Guide*, 197.

21   Marisa Kashino and Harrison Smith, "These 19 Washington Zip Codes Are in High Demand," *Washingtonian*, April 22, 2015, http://www.washingtonian.com/2015/04/22/these-19-zip-codes-are-in-high-demand/.

22   Kevin Davis, "Catching up with Tom Tunney," *Crain's Chicago Business*, January 9, 2013, http://www.chicagobusiness.com/article/20130109/SPOTLIGHT/130109928/catching-up-with-tom-tunney; Alby Gallun, "Tunney Closing Ann Sather Restaurant in Andersonville," *Crain's Chicago Business*, August 14, 2013, http://www.chicagobusiness.com/realestate/20130814/CRED03/130819895/tunney-closing-ann-sather-restaurant-in-andersonville.

23   Tom Tunney, interview, December 10, 2013.

24   Tracy Baim, "The Daley Dynasty to End," *Windy City Times*, November 17, 2010, http://www.windycitymediagroup.com/APParticle.php?AID=29481.

25   Ibid.

26   Jessica Seigel, "Daley's Support is Inspiration to Gay Pride Parade," *Chicago Tribune*, June 26, 1989, http://articles.chicagotribune.com/1989-06-26/news/8902120552_1_gay-pride-parade-gay-rights-movement-mayor-richard-daley.

27   Josh Noel, "Gay Games a Test for Olympics, Daley Says," *Chicago Tribune*, July 11, 2006, http://articles.chicagotribune.com/2006-07-11/news/0607110108_1_gay-games-chicago-gay-community-mayor-richard-daley.

28   Itay Hod, "Let the Gay Games Begin," *Daily Beast*, October 2, 2009, http://www.thedailybeast.com/articles/2009/10/02/let-the-gay-games-begin.html. Footnote information in Victor Matheson, "LeBron and the $500M Lie: How Sports Economic-Impact Studies Trick You," *Deadspin*, November 14, 2014, http://regressing.deadspin.com/lebron-and-the-500m-lie-how-sports-economic-impact-st-1658861205; Jim Buzinski, "Cleveland Pledges $700,000 for 2014 Gay Games," *Outsports*, September 15, 2009, http://www.outsports.com/2009/9/15/4048626/cleveland-pledges-700000-for-2014-gay-games.

29   Windy City Times, "Remarks from Chicago Mayor Richard M. Daley, Gay Games VII Opening Ceremony," *Windy City Times*, August 16, 2006, http://www.windycitymediagroup.com/lgbt/Remarks-from-Chicago-Mayor-Richard-M-Daley-Gay-Games-VII-Opening-Ceremony-July-15-2006-Soldier-Field/12374.html.

30   Tunney, interview.

31   Ibid.

32   Tracy Baim, interview, December 12, 2013.

33   Advocate, "Unsung Chicago LGBT Heroes," *Advocate*, accessed March 7, 2016, http://www.advocate.com/pride/2015/9/22/unsung-chicago-lgbt-heroes.

34   Associated Press, "Chicago Hopes to Become Gay Destination," *NBC News*, June 22, 2007, http://www.nbcnews.com/id/19374590/ns/travel-destination_travel/t/chicago-hopes-become-gay-destination/#.VtNz-fkrLIU.

35   Aamer Madhani, "LGBT-Friendly Senior Housing Opening across U.S. Cities," *USA Today*, October 6, 2014, http://www.usatoday.com/story/news/nation/2014/10/06/chicago-minneapolis-philadelphia-senior-lgbt-housing/16115641/.

36   Ross Levitt, "Ex-Detroit Mayor Kilpatrick Gets 28 Years in Prison," *CNN*, October 10, 2013, http://www.cnn.com/2013/10/10/justice/detroit-kilpatrick-sentencing/.

37   Jason Michael, "Detroit Mayor Denounces Marriage Equality for Gays on National Television,"

Pridesource, March 4, 2004, http://www.pridesource.com/article.html?article=6715. Footnote information in Corey Dade and Patricia Montemurri, "Kilpatrick Adamant in His Stand on Gays," Detroit Free Press, May 31, 2001, https://web.archive.org/web/20040604024658/http://www.freep.com/news/ politics/gay31_20010531.htm.

38   Wendy Case, "Affirming Ferndale," *Detroit Metro Times*, May 30, 2007, http://www.metrotimes.com/detroit/affirming-ferndale/Content?oid=2187417.

39   Greg Tasker, "Funky Ferndale: Cool Vibe Draws Shop Owners to Nine Mile," *Detroit News*, May 15, 2007, http://web.archive.org/web/20150625172839/http://www.detroitnews.com /article/20070515/metro/108010011/Funky-Ferndale.

40   Newport and Gates, "San Francisco Metro Area Ranks Highest."

41   Gary Gates, "How Many People Are Lesbian, Gay, Bisexual, and Transgender," Williams Institute, April 2011, http://williamsinstitute.law.ucla.edu/wp-content/uploads/Gates-How -Many-People-LGBT-Apr-2011.pdf.

42   Frank Newport, "Americans Greatly Overestimate Percent Gay, Lesbian in U.S.," *Gallup*, May 21, 2015, http://www.gallup.com/poll/183383/americans-greatly-overestimate-percent-gay -lesbian.aspx.

43   Garance Franke-Ruta, "Americans Have No Idea How Few Gay People There Are," *Atlantic*, May 31, 2012, http://www.theatlantic.com/politics/archive/2012/05/americans-have-no -idea-how-few-gay-people-there-are/257753/.

44   NPR Staff, "Can Detroit Return to Its Former Glory?," *NPR*, March 23, 2013, http://www .npr.org/2013/03/23/175138306/can-detroit-return-to-its-former-glory.

45   Joe Posch, interview, October 3, 2013.

46   Posch, interview.

47   Posch, "On Gayborhoods."

48   Richard Florida, *The Rise of the Creative Class: And How It's Transforming Work, Leisure, Community, and Everyday Life* (New York: Basic Books, 2002), 243–245.

49   Richard Florida, *Who's Your City: How the Creative Economy Is Making Where to Live the Most Important Decision of Your Life* (New York: Basic Books, 2008), 135.

50   Erik Bottcher, interview, October 7, 2013.

51   Frank Newport and Gary Gates, "San Francisco Metro Area Ranks Highest in LGBT Percentage," *Gallup*, March 20, 2015, http://www.gallup.com/poll/182051/san-francisco -metro-area-ranks-highest-lgbt-percentage.aspx.

52   Jan Stevenson, "Michigan Must Get Cool About Gays," *Pridesource*, December, 18, 2003, http://www.pridesource.com/article.html?article=5832.

53   Ibid.

54   Sharon Gittleman, "Gay 'Brain Drain,'" *Pridesource*, January 12, 2006, http://www.pridesource .com/article.html?article=17169.

55   Edward Glaeser, review of *The Rise of the Creative Class*, by Richard Florida, *Regional Science and Urban Economics* 35, no. 5 (2005): 593–596, doi:10.1016/j.regsciurbeco.2005.01.005; Amin Ghaziani, email interview, November 2, 2015.

56   Bottcher, interview.

57   Curtis Lipscomb, multiple interviews, 2013–2015.

58   Ghaziani, *There Goes the Gayborhood*, 88.

59   Ibid., 167; World Values Survey, Wave 6: 2010–2014, statistics accessed July 5, 2016, http ://www.worldvaluessurvey.org/WVSOnline.jsp.

60   Florida, *Who's Your City*, 178.

61   Ghaziani, *There Goes the Gayborhood*, 135.

62   Ibid., 135.

63   Pew Research Center, "A Survey of LGBT Americans: Attitudes, Experiences and Values

in Changing Times," *Pew Research Center*, June 13, 2013, http://www.pewsocialtrends
.org/2013/06/13/a-survey-of-lgbt-americans/.

64　　Mike Wilkinson, "Tax Reform for Detroit Residents Needed for Economics Development,"
Bridge Magazine, July 24, 2014, http://www.mlive.com/news/detroit/index.ssf/2014/07
/giving_detroiters_a_tax_break.html.

65　　Posch, interview.

66　　Joe Posch, "Mike Duggan's Small Mention of Detroit's Gay Community Is a Huge Deal,"
Detroit Free Press, November 8, 2013, https://web.archive.org/web/20140219040902/http
://www.freep.com/article/20131107/OPINION05/311070113/.

Chapter 6

1　　Lee Rainwater, ed., *Social Problems and Public Policy: Deviance and Liberty* (Chicago: Aldine
Publishing Company, 1974), 143.

2　　Ibid., 143.

3　　Gay Talese, *Thy Neighbor's Wife* (New York: Harper Perennial, 1981), 375–378; Kenneth
Maxwell, *A Sexual Odyssey: From Forbidden Fruit to Cybersex* (New York: Springer, 1996), 262.

4　　Richard Nixon, "Statement about the Report on the Commission on Obscenity and
Pornography," *The American Presidency Project*, October 24, 1970, http://www.presidency
.ucsb.edu/ws/?pid=2759.

5　　Richard Nixon, "Special Message to the Congress on Obscene and Pornographic Materials," *The
American Presidency Project*, May 2, 1969, http://www.presidency.ucsb.edu/ws/?pid=2032.

6　　Philip Shenon, "Justice Dept. Pornography Study Finds Material Is Tied to Violence,"
New York Times, May 14, 1986, http://www.nytimes.com/1986/05/14/us/justice-
dept-pornography-study-finds-material-is-tied-to-violence.html; E. Edward Bruce,
"Prostitution and Obscenity: A Comment upon the Attorney General's Report on
Pornography," *Duke Law Journal* (1987): 123–139, http://scholarship.law.duke.edu/
cgi/viewcontent.cgi?article=2975&context=dlj. Footnote information in Kauffman,
Bad Girls, 235–236; Edwin McDowell, "Some Say Meese Report Rates an 'X,'" *New
York Times*, October 21, 1986, http://www.nytimes.com/1986/10/21/books/some-say
-meese-report-rates-an-x.html.

7　　Linda Kauffman, *Bad Girls and Sick Boys: Fantasies in Contemporary Art and Culture*
(Berkeley, CA: University of California Press, 1998), 236.

8　　Ronald Ostrow, "Meese Panel Asks Porn Crackdown: Sexually Violent Materials and Actions
Connected, Commission Concludes," *Los Angeles Times*, July 10, 1986, http://articles.latimes
.com/1986-07-10/news/mn-22453_1_sexual-violence/2; Carol Tarvis, "The Illogic of Linking
Porn and Rape: Meese Commission Overlooks Proper Reasoning in Findings," *Los Angeles Times*,
July 7, 1986, http://articles.latimes.com/1986-07-07/local/me-20516_1_commission-members.

9　　Kauffman, *Bad Girls*, 236.

10　　Ibid., 236.

11　　Ibid., 237.

12　　Eric Schlosser, *Reefer Madness: Sex, Drugs, and Cheap Labor in the American Black Market*
(Boston: Houghton Mifflin Company, 2003), 111, 200.

13　　Robin Morgan, *Going Too Far: The Personal Chronicle of a Feminist* (New York: Random House,
1977), 169; Eric Hoffman, "Feminism, Pornography, and Law," *University of Pennsylvania Law
Review* 133, no. 497 (1985): 497–534, http://scholarship.law.upenn.edu/cgi/viewcontent
.cgi?article=4030&context=penn_law_review.

14　　Havana Marking, "The Real Legacy of Andrea Dworkin," *Guardian*, April 15, 2005, http
://www.theguardian.com/world/2005/apr/15/gender.politicsphilosophyandsociety.

15　　Rebecca Kaplan, "Santorum Says Obama Not Enforcing Internet Porn Laws," *CBS News*,

March 16, 2012, http://www.cbsnews.com/news/santorum-says-obama-not-enforcing
-internet-porn-laws/.

16   Anthony D'Amato, "Porn Up, Rape Down," *Northwestern Public Law Research Paper* (2006),
        doi:10.2139/ssrn.913013.

17   Todd Kendall, "Pornography, Rape, and the Internet," Clemson University Department of
        Economics (2006), http://idei.fr/sites/default/files/medias/doc/conf/sic/papers_2007
        /kendall.pdf.

18   Christopher Ferguson and Richard Hartley, "The Pleasure is Momentary...the Expense
        Damnable? The Influence of Pornography on Rape and Sexual Assault," *Aggression and Violent
        Behavior* 14 (2009): 323–329, doi:10.1016/j.avb.2009.04.008.

19   Milton Diamond, "Pornography, Public Acceptance, and Sex Related Crime: A Review,"
        International Journal of Law and Psychiatry 32 (2009): 304–314, doi:10.1016/j.ijlp.2009.06.004.

20   D'Amato, "Porn Up, Rape Down."

21   Steven Landsburg, "How the Web Prevents Rape," *Slate*, October 30, 2006, http://www.slate
        .com/articles/arts/everyday_economics/2006/10/how_the_web_prevents_rape.single.html.

22   Donald Symons, *The Evolution of Human Sexuality* (New York: Oxford University Press,
        1979), 282–283.

23   Nancy Gertner, "Sex, Lies, and Justice," *American Prospect*, Winter 2015, http://prospect.org
        /article/sex-lies-and-justice.

24   Danielle Teller and Astro Teller, "The 50% Divorce Rate Stat Is a Myth, So Why Won't It Die?,"
        Quartz, December 4, 2014, http://qz.com/306166/the-divorce-star-that-just-keeps-cheating-50/;
        Dan Hurley, "Divorce Rate: It's Not as High as You Think," *New York Times*, April 19, 2005, http
        ://www.nytimes.com/2005/04/19/health/divorce-rate-its-not-as-high-as-you-think.html.

25   Clair Cain Miller, "The Divorce Surge Is Over, But the Myth Lives On," *New York Times*,
        December 2, 2014, http://www.nytimes.com/2014/12/02/upshot/the-divorce-surge-is
        -over-but-the-myth-lives-on.html.

26   Ibid.

27   Teller and Teller, "The 50% Divorce Rate."

28   CDC, "Health, United States, 2014: With Special Feature on Adults Aged 55–64," US
        Department of Health and Human Services, May 2015, 147, http://www.cdc.gov/nchs/data
        /hus/hus14.pdf#037.

29   Karen Kaplan, "Abortion Falls to Record Low in the U.S., CDC Says," *Los Angeles Times*,
        December 11, 2015, http://www.latimes.com/science/sciencenow/la-sci-sn-us-pregnancy
        -rate-abortion-record-low-20151210-story.html.

30   Kimberly Leonard, "Teen Birth Rate, Multiple Births Reach Historic Low," *U.S. News
        & World Report*, December 23, 2015, http://www.usnews.com/news/blogs/data-mine
        /articles/2015-12-23/teen-birth-rate-multiple-births-reach-historic-low.

31   Heather Boonstra, "What Is Behind the Declines in Teen Pregnancy Rates?," *Guttmacher Policy
        Review* 17, no. 3 (2014): 15–21, http://www.guttmacher.org/pubs/gpr/17/3/gpr170315.pdf;
        U.S. Department of Health & Human Services, "Contraceptive and Condom Use," accessed
        February 29, 2016, http://www.hhs.gov/ash/oah/adolescent-health-topics/reproductive
        -health/contraceptive-use.html.

32   Kimberly Leonard, "Teens Today Have Less Sex Than Their Parents Did," *U.S. News & World
        Report*, July 22, 2015, http://www.usnews.com/news/blogs/data-mine/2015/07/22/cdc
        -report-shows-declines-in-teen-sexual-activity-pregnancies.

33   Christopher Ingraham, "Teen Drug and Alcohol Use Continues to Fall, New Federal Data
        Show," *Washington Post*, September 16, 2014, https://www.washingtonpost.com/news/wonk
        /wp/2014/09/16/teen-drug-and-alcohol-use-continues-to-fall-new-federal-data-show/;
        Kimberly Leonard, "Teen Drinking Continues to Decline in the U.S.," *U.S. News & World*

Report, December 16, 2014, http://www.usnews.com/news/blogs/data-mine/2014/12/16/teen-drinking-continues-to-decline-in-the-us.

34   Patchen Barss, *The Erotic Engine: How Pornography Has Powered Mass Communication, from Gutenberg to Google* (Toronto: Anchor Canada, 2011), 3–4.

35   Stephanie Condon, "ABC v. Aereo: Will the Supreme Court Change the Way We Watch TV?," *CBS News*, April 22, 2014, http://www.cbsnews.com/news/abc-v-aereo-will-the-supreme-court-change-the-way-we-watch-tv/.

36   Derek Khanna, "A Look Back at How the Content Industry Almost Killed Blockbuster and Netflix (And the VCR)," *Tech Crunch*, December 27, 2013, http://techcrunch.com/2013/12/27/how-the-content-industry-almost-killed-blockbuster-and-netflix/; Robert Schwartz, "It's the 30th Anniversary of the Supreme Court's Monumental Decision about Betamax," *Slate*, January 17, 2014, http://www.slate.com/blogs/future_tense/2014/01/17/betamax_supreme_court_opinion_anniversary_the_decision_has_had_long_reaching.html; Jane Ginsburg, "Secondary Liability for Copyright Infringement in the U.S.: Anticipating the Après-Grokster," *Columbia Law School*, March 2006, https://www.law.columbia.edu/law_school/communications/reports/winter06/facforum1.

37   Schwartz, "It's the 30th Anniversary"; Eduardo Porter, "Copyright Ruling Rings with Echo of Betamax," *The New York Times*, March 26, 2013, http://www.nytimes.com/2013/03/27/business/in-a-copyright-ruling-the-lingering-legacy-of-the-betamax.html?_r=0; Los Angeles Times Editorial Board, "What the 1984 Betamax Ruling Did for Us All," *Los Angeles Times*, January 17, 2014, http://articles.latimes.com/2014/jan/17/opinion/la-ed-betamax-ruling-anniversary-20140117.

38   Frederick Wasser, *Veni, Vidi, Video: The Hollywood Empire and the VCR* (Austin: University of Texas Press, 2002), 19.

39   Frederick Wasser, email interview, October 15, 2015.

40   Wasser, *Veni, Vidi, Video*, 94; Frederick Lane, *The Decency Wars: The Campaign to Cleanse American Culture* (Amherst NY: Prometheus, 2006), 138.

41   Jack Schofield, "Why VHS Was Better Than Betamax," *Guardian*, January 24, 2003, http://www.theguardian.com/technology/2003/jan/25/comment.comment; Barss, *Erotic Engine*, 101.

42   Frederick Lane, email interview, February 14, 2016.

43   Barss, *Erotic Engine*, 97.

44   Ibid., 91–92.

45   Ibid., 92.

46   Jonathan Coopersmith, "Pornography, Technology, and Progress," *ICON* 4 (1998): 94–125, http://www.jstor.org/stable/23785961.

47   History Channel, "The Invention of the Internet," *History*, accessed February 29, 2016, http://www.history.com/topics/inventions/invention-of-the-internet.

48   Keenan Mayo and Peter Newcomb, "How the Web Was Won," *Vanity Fair*, July 2008, http://www.vanityfair.com/news/2008/07/internet200807.

49   Ibid.

50   Barss, Erotic Engine, 118.

51   Ibid., 118.

52   Anthony Lane, "'Lo and Behold' and 'Mia Madre' Reviews," *New Yorker*, August 29, 2016, http://www.newyorker.com/magazine/2016/08/29/lo-and-behold-and-mia-madre-reviews.

53   Frederick Lane, *Obscene Profits: The Entrepreneurs of Pornography in the Cyber Age* (New York: Routledge. 2001), 115.

54   Ibid., 114–115.

55   Patchen Barss, email interview, October 16, 2015.

56   Lane, *Obscene Profits*, 89, 220–225; Barss, *Erotic Engine*, 171–173.

57   Barss, *Erotic Engine*, 171–173. Footnote information in Eric Schlosser, "The Business of Pornography," *U.S. News & World Report*, February 10, 1997; Timothy Egan, "Wall Street Meets Pornography," *New York Times*, October 23, 2000, http://www.nytimes.com/2000/10/23 /technology/23PORN.html?pagewanted=all.

58   Lane, *Obscene Profits*, 70, 181. Footnote information in Lubove, "See No Evil."

59   Ibid., 115.

60   Matt Richtel and John Schwartz, "Credit Cards Seek New Fees on Web's Demimonde," *New York Times*, November 18, 2002, http://www.nytimes.com/2002/11/18/technology/18PORN .html?pagewanted=all.

61   Seth Lubove, "See No Evil," *Forbes*, September 17, 2001, http://www.forbes.com /forbes/2001/0917/068.html.

62   Barss, *Erotic Engine*, 249, 255.

63   Ibid., 187.

64   Ibid.

65   Mike Musgrove, "Technology's Seamier Side," *Washington Post*, January 21, 2006, http://www .washingtonpost.com/wp-dyn/content/article/2006/01/20/AR2006012001888.html; Doug Gross, "In the Tech World, Porn Quietly Leads the Way," *CNN*, April 23, 2010, http ://www.cnn.com/2010/TECH/04/23/porn.technology/.

66   Barss, *Erotic Engine*, 199.

67   Ibid., 69.

68   Congress.gov, "H.R. 1786—Telephone Decency Act," accessed February 29, 2016, https ://www.congress.gov/bill/100th-congress/house-bill/1786.

69   Associated Press, "Justices Reject Total Ban on 'Dial-a-Porn' Messages," *Los Angeles Times*, June 25, 1989, http://articles.latimes.com/1989-06-25/news/mn-6190_1_dial-a-porn-messages -indecent-messages-dial-a-porn-industry.

70   Lane, *Obscene Profits*, 155.

71   Michel Marriott, "Virtual Porn: Ultimate Tease," *New York Times*, October 4, 1995, http ://www.nytimes.com/1995/10/04/garden/virtual-porn-ultimate-tease.html?pagewanted=all.

72   Jonathan Lyons, "All Men Watch Porn, Scientists Find," *Telegraph*, December 2, 2009, http ://www.telegraph.co.uk/women/sex/6709646/All-men-watch-porn-scientists-find.html.

73   Peter Rubin, "Virtual-Reality Porn Is Coming, and Your Fantasies May Never Be the Same," *Wired*, February 15, 2015, http://www.wired.com/2015/02/vr-porn/.

74   Barss, *Erotic Engine*, 286–288.

75   Annalee Newitz, "Sorry You Can't Have Any More Sex Toys Because of This Patent," *Gizmodo*, July 23, 2015, http://gizmodo.com/sorry-you-cant-have-any-more-sex-toys-because-of-this -p-1719816692.

76   Barss, *Erotic Engine*, 281–285.

77   Lulu Chang, "Will Lovely, the Wearable for Your Penis, Enhance Your Sex Life?," *Digital Trends*, June 11, 2015, http://www.digitaltrends.com/wearables/lovely-wearable-sex-toy/; Barss, *Erotic Engine*, 281–285.

78   Barss, *Erotic Engine*, 281–285; Helen Croydon, "Get in the Mood for Teledildonics: The App that Logs Your Orgasms and Turns Your Phone into a Vibrator," *Metro*, November 25, 2015, http ://metro.co.uk/2015/11/25/get-in-the-mood-for-teledildonics-the-app-that-logs-your-orgasms -and-turns-your-phone-into-a-vibrator-5513758/; Jon Evans, "Bluetooth Suppositories and Other Teledildonics You Didn't Know You Needed," *Tech Crunch*, August 15, 2015, http://techcrunch .com/2015/08/15/bluetooth-suppositories-and-other-teledildonics-you-didnt-know-you-needed/.

79   Barss, *Erotic Engine*, 284.

80   Barss, email interview.

81   Elizabeth Mitchell, "Huggies Pregnancy Belt for Men Lets Dads Feel Their Babies Kicking,"

Adweek, June 14, 2013, http://www.adweek.com/prnewser/huggies-pregnancy-belt-for-men -lets-dads-feel-their-babies-kicking/67337.

82   Rubin, "Virtual-Reality Porn."

83   Barbara Herman, "Porn Industry Looks to Virtual Reality Technology for Next Boom," *International Business Times*, February 3, 2015, http://www.ibtimes.com/porn-industry -looks-virtual-reality-technology-next-boom-1802704; Zackary Canepari, Drea Cooper, and Emma Cott, "Sex Dolls That Talk Back," *New York Times*, June 11, 2015, http://www.nytimes .com/2015/06/12/technology/robotica-sex-robot-realdoll.html; Carrie Weisman, "$51,000 for a Sex Doll? Why the Industry Is Booming and Its Future Is Bright," *AlterNet*, December 1, 2014, http://www.alternet.org/sex-amp-relationships/51000-sex-doll-why-industry -booming-and-its-future-bright.

84   David Levy, *Love and Sex with Robots: The Evolution of Human-Robot Relationships* (New York: Harper Perennial, 2007), 267–268.

85   Ian Yeoman and Michelle Mars, "Robots, Men, and Sex Tourism," *Futures* 44, no. 4 (2012): 365–371, doi:10.1016/j.futures.2011.11.004; Glenn Harlan Reynolds, "The Human Screwfly Solution," *USA Today*, August 17, 2014, http://www.usatoday.com/story /opinion/2014/08/17/sex-bots-sexbots-robots-vibrators-artificial-intelligence-reproduction -technology-column/14205469/; Lauren Davis, "How Would Robotic Prostitutes Change the Sex Tourism Industry?," *io9*, April 15, 2012, http://io9.gizmodo.com/5902113/how-would -robotic-prostitutes-change-the-sex-tourism-industry.

86   Frederick Lane, email interview, February 14, 2016.

87   Cade Metz, "The Porn Business Isn't Anything Like You Think It Is," *Wired*, October, 15, 2015, https://www.wired.com/2015/10/the-porn-business-isnt-anything-like-you-think-it-is/.

88   Frederick Lane, email interview.

89   Dan Miller, interview, June 3, 2014; David Moye, "Porn Industry in Decline: Insiders Adapt to Piracy, Waning DVD Sales (NSFW)," *Huffington Post*, January 19, 2013, http://www .huffingtonpost.com/2013/01/19/porn-industry-in-decline_n_2460799.html.

90   Ross Benes, "The Porn Industry is Putting Skin Back in the Game," *Quartz*, June 24, 2014, http://qz.com/224818/the-porn-industry-is-putting-skin-back-in-the-game/.

91   Coopersmith, "Pornography, Technology, and Progress."

Chapter 7

1   PRI Staff, "Disney/Donald Duck Video on Population Control Sold by Planned Parenthood Affiliate," *Population Research Institute*, June 22, 1999, https://www.pop.org/content /disneydonald-duck-video-population-control-sold-planned-parenthood-affiliate.

2   Jeremey Laurance, "Prostitutes''People Skills' are Used to Care for Elderly," *Independent*, April 10, 2006, http://www.independent.co.uk/news/world/europe/prostitutes-people-skills -are-used-to-care-for-elderly-6104014.html; Jonathan Last, *What to Expect When No One's Expecting: America's Coming Demographic Disaster* (New York: Encounter, 2013), 99.

3   Phillip Longman, *The Empty Cradle: How Falling Birthrates Threaten World Prosperity and What to Do about It* (New York: Basic Books, 2004), 84. Footnote information in NCHS Pressroom, "Mother's Educational Level Influences Birthrate," CDC, April 24, 1997, http://www.cdc .gov/nchs/pressroom/97facts/edu2birt.htm; Mohammad Morad, "Women in Workplace and Fertility: A Study of Sylhet City, Bangladesh," *SIU Studies* 1, no. 3 (2007): 40–48, https://www .researchgate.net/publication/267334333_Women_in_Workplace_and_Fertility_A_Study _of_Sylhet_City_Bangladesh; Melanie Guldi, "Fertility Effects of Abortion and Birth Control Pill Access for Minors," *Demography* 45, no. 4 (2008): 817–824, doi:10.1353/dem.0.0026; Tadashi Yamada, "Casual Relationships Between Infant Mortality and Fertility in Developed and Less Developed Countries," *National Bureau of Economic Research*, no. 1528 (1984): doi:10.3386

/w1528; Sarah Hayford and S. Philip Morgan, "Religiosity and Fertility in the United States: The Role of Fertility Intentions," *Social Forces* 86, no. 3 (2008): 1163–1188, doi:10.1353 /sof.0.0000; Barbara Boyle Torrey, "Urbanization: An Environmental Force to Be Reckoned With," *Population Reference Bureau*, April 2004, http://www.prb.org/Publications/Articles/2004 /UrbanizationAnEnvironmentalForcetoBeReckonedWith.aspx; Mark Mather, "Fact Sheet: The Decline in U.S. Fertility," *Population Reference Bureau*, July 2012, http://www.prb.org /Publications/Datasheets/2012/world-population-data-sheet/fact-sheet-us-population.aspx.

4   Teitelbaum and Winter, *The Global Spread*, 278.

5   Teitelbaum, email interview, March 5, 2016.

6   Jonathan Last, "Make Boomsa for the Motherland!," *Slate*, April 25, 2013, http://www.slate .com/articles/life/family/2013/04/can_a_country_boost_its_low_birth_rate_examples _from_around_the_world.html.

7   Last, "Make Boomsa."

8   Rachel Nuwer, "Singapore's 'National Night' Encourages Citizens to Make Babies," *Smithsonian*, August 8, 2012, http://www.smithsonianmag.com/smart-news/singapores-national-night -encourages-citizens-to-make-babies-15402105/.

9   Tiana Norgen, *Abortion before Birth Control: The Politics of Reproduction in Postwar Japan* (Princeton, NJ: Princeton University Press, 2001), 82–88; Mariko Kato, "Abortion Still Key Birth Control," *Japan Times*, October 20, 2009, http://www.japantimes.co.jp /news/2009/10/20/reference/abortion-still-key-birth-control/#.Vs97BPkrLIU.

10   Mark Hanrahan, "Japan Population Decline: Third of Nation's Youth Have 'No Interest' in Sex," *Huffington Post*, January 30, 2012, http://www.huffingtonpost.com/2012/01/30/japan -population-decline-youth-no-sex_n_1242014.html.

11   Abigail Haworth, "Why Have Young People in Japan Stopped Having Sex?," *Observer*, October 20, 2013, http://www.theguardian.com/world/2013/oct/20/young-people-japan-stopped -having-sex.

12   Ibid.

13   Ibid. Footnote information in Teitelbaum and Witner, *The Global Spread*, 185–186; T.B., "Why the Japanese Are Having So Few Babies," *Economist*, July 23, 2014, http://www .economist.com/blogs/economist-explains/2014/07/economist-explains-16.

14   Haworth, "Why Have Young People in Japan Stopped Having Sex?" Footnote information in Teitelbaum, email interview.

15   The World Bank, "Fertility Rate, Total (Births per Woman)," accessed February 23, 2016, http://data.worldbank.org/indicator/SP.DYN.TFRT.IN.

16   Rakesh Kochhar, "10 Projections for the Global Population in 2050," Pew Research Center, February 3, 2014, http://www.pewresearch.org/fact-tank/2014/02/03/10-projections-for -the-global-population-in-2050/.

17   BBC News, "Japan Population to Shrink by One-Third by 2060," *BBC News*, January 30, 2012, http://www.bbc.com/news/world-asia-16787538.

18   Adam Pasick, "Sales of Adult Diapers to Surpass Baby Diapers in Aging Japan," *Quartz*, July 11, 2013, http://qz.com/103000/sales-of-adult-diapers-surpass-baby-diapers-in-aging-japan/.

19   Last, *What to Expect*, 142.

20   Longman, *The Empty Cradle*, 50.

21   Roger Pulvers, "Reversing Japan's Rising Sex Aversion May Depend on a Rebirth of Hope," *Japan Times*, April 29, 2012, http://www.japantimes.co.jp/opinion/2012/04/29 /commentary/reversing-japans-rising-sex-aversion-may-depend-on-a-rebirth-of-hope/# .Vs3fHfkrLIU; Alex Martin, "Young Men, Couples Shunning Sex," *Japan Times*, January 14, 2011, http://www.japantimes.co.jp/news/2011/01/14/national/young-men-couples -shunning-sex/#.Vs3gS_krLIU.

22   Daisuke Wakabayashi and Miho Inada, "Incentive for Parenthood," *Wall Street Journal*,
      October 9, 2009, http://www.wsj.com/articles/SB125495746062571927; Yukiko Asai,
      "Parental Leave Reforms and the Employment of New Mothers: Quasi-Experiment Evidence
      from Japan," *Labour Economics* 36 (2015): 72–83, doi:10.1016/j.labeco.2015.02.007;
      Minami Funakoshi, "Japan Cries Out for Daycare," *Wall Street Journal*, August 7, 2013,
      http://www.wsj.com/articles/SB10001424127887324653004578651310946954352
      ; "Government to Support Matchmaking, Men's Child-Rearing to Raise Birthrate," *Japan
      Times*, March 13, 2015, http://www.japantimes.co.jp/news/2015/03/13/national/social
      -issues/government-to-support-matchmaking-mens-child-rearing-to-raise-birthrate/#
      .Vs3plfkrLIX; "Cabinet Seeks to Raise Percentage of Men Taking Paternity Leave to 80%
      by 2020," *Japan Times*, March 20, 2015, http://www.japantimes.co.jp/news/2015/03/20
      /national/cabinet-seeks-to-raise-percentage-of-men-taking-paternity-leave-to-80
      -by-2020/#.Vs3qPPkrLIV.

23   World Economic Forum, "Global Gender Gap Index 2016," accessed September, 11, 2017,
      http://reports.weforum.org/global-gender-gap-report-2016/rankings/.

24   Chris Cooper and Yuki Hagiwara, "'Devil Wives' Vilified as Japan Mothers Seek to Keep
      Jobs," *Bloomberg*, November 1, 2012, http://www.bloomberg.com/news/articles/2012-11-01
      /japan-s-devil-wife-leads-motherhood-work-balance-tussle.

25   Ibid.

26   Michael Teitelbaum and Jay Winter, *The Global Spread of Fertility Decline: Population, Fear,
      and Uncertainty* (New Haven, CT: Yale University Press, 2013), 170. Footnote information in
      Reuters, "'Birth-Giving Machine' Gaffe Hits Nerve in Japan," *Reuters*, February 2, 2007, http
      ://www.reuters.com/article/us-japan-politics-idUST16444120070202.

27   Kirk Spitzer, "Japan Looks for a Few Good Women to Revive Economy," *USA Today*, January
      15,   2014,   http://www.usatoday.com/story/news/world/2014/01/15/japan-working
      -women/4463815/; Masamito, "Can Women Really 'Shine' Under Abe?," *Japan Times*,
      November 22, 2014, http://www.japantimes.co.jp/life/2014/11/22/lifestyle/can-women
      -really-shine-abe/#.Vs3txPkrLIU.

28   William Pesek, "Sexism Stands in the Way of 'Abenomics' Saving Japan," *Bloomberg*, May
      26,   2013,   http://www.bloombergview.com/articles/2013-05-26/sexism-stands-in-way
      -of-abenomics-saving-japan; Kwan Weng Kin, "Japanese Women Trash 'Notebook' Idea for
      Having Babies," *Straits Times*, May 20, 2013, http://news.asiaone.com/News/Latest+News
      /Diva/Story/A1Story20130518-423685.html.

29   Last, *What to Expect*, 150–160.

30   The World Bank, "Fertility Rate." Footnote information in Laurent Toulemon, "Fertility among
      Immigrant Women in France: New Data, a New Approach," Lecture, Population Association
      of America, Los Angeles, March 30, 2006, http://paa2006.princeton.edu/papers/61103.

31   Anne Chemin, "France's Baby Boom Secret: Get Women into Work and Ditch Rigid Family
      Norms," *Guardian*, March 21, 2015, http://www.theguardian.com/world/2015/mar/21
      /france-population-europe-fertility-rate.

32   Jon Henley, "France Plans to Pay Cash for More Babies," *Guardian*, September 21, 2005,
      http://www.theguardian.com/world/2005/sep/22/france.jonhenley1.

33   Last, *What to Expect*, 149; Last, "Make Boomsa." Footnote information in The Connexion,
      "Parental Leave Rules Explained," *Connexion*, December 2010, http://www.connexionfrance
      .com/maternity-paternity-leave-parental-rules-france-11284-news-article.html.

34   Kevin Milligan, "Quebec's Baby Bonus: Can Public Policy Raise Fertility?," C.D. Howe
      Institute, January 24, 2002, http://cdhowe.org/pdf/milligan_backgrounder.pdf.

35   Last, *What to Expect*, 161.

36   Last, *What to Expect*, 160–161; Gunnar Andersson, "Family Policies and Fertility in Sweden,"

presented at CESifo Conference Centre, Munich, February 1–2, 2008, https://www.cesifo
-group.de/portal/pls/portal/!PORTAL.wwpob_page.show?_docname=1007992.PDF.
Footnote information in Last, *What to Expect*, 161; Anne Gauthier and Jan Hatzius, "Family
Benefits and Fertility: An Econometric Analysis," *Population Studies* 51, no. 3 (1997): 295–306,
doi:10.1080/0032472031000150066.

37 Rafael Lalive and Josef Zweimuller, "How Does Parental Leave Affect Fertility and Return to
Work?: Evidence from Two Natural Experiments," *Quarterly Journal of Economics* 124, no. 3
(2009): 1363–1402, doi:10.1162/qjec.2009.124.3.1363.

38 Steven Landsburg, *More Sex Is Safer Sex: The Unconventional Wisdom of Economics* (New York:
Free Press, 2008), 33–34.

39 Ibid., 33–34.

40 Lalive and Zweimuller, "How Does Parental Leave."

41 Chemin, "France's Baby Boom."

42 Jay Winter, email interview, February 28, 2016.

43 Michael Teitelbaum and Jay Winter, "Bye-Bye Baby," *The New York Times*, April 4, 2014,
http://www.nytimes.com/2014/04/05/opinion/sunday/bye-bye-baby.html?mtrref=undefined
&gwh=354CEDF70673E8A10A9309FCD48DEAF1&gwt=pay&assetType=opinion&
_r=0. Footnote information in Rebecca Traister, *All the Single Ladies: Unmarried Women and
the Rise of an Independent Nation* (New York: Simon & Schuster, 2016).

44 Longman, *The Empty Cradle*, 17; John Bongaarts and Steve Sinding, "Population Policy in
Transition in the Developing World," *Science* 333, no. 6042 (2011): 574–576, doi:10.1126
/science.1207558.

45 June Kronholz and John Lyons, "Smaller Families in Mexico May Stir U.S. Job Market," *Wall
Street Journal*, April 28, 2006, http://www.wsj.com/articles/SB114618828786138329; Sam
Dillon, "Smaller Families to Bring Big Change in Mexico," *New York Times*, June 8, 1999,
http://www.nytimes.com/1999/06/08/world/smaller-families-to-bring-big-change-in
-mexico.html?pagewanted=all.

46 The World Bank, "Fertility Rate."

47 China Daily, "Total Population, CBR, CDR, NIR and TFR of China (1949–2000)," *China
Daily*, October 20, 2010, http://www.chinadaily.com.cn/china/2010census/2010-08/20
/content_11182379.htm; Shuai Zhang, "China to Dramatically Ease 'One-Child' Policy," *CBS
News*, November 15, 2013, http://www.cbsnews.com/news/china-to-dramatically-ease-one
-child-policy/.

48 Therese Hesketh and Zhu Wei Xing, "The Effect of China's One-Child Family Policy after 25
Years," *New England Journal of Medicine* 353, no. 11 (2005): doi:10.1056/NEJMhpr051833.

49 Ibid.

50 Mara Hvistendahl, *Unnatural Selection: Choosing Boys over Girls, and the Consequences of a
World Full of Men* (New York: PublicAffairs, 2011), 142. Footnote information in Demick,
"Judging China's One-Child Policy."

51 The World Bank, "Fertility Rate"; Teitelbaum and Winter, *The Global Spread*, 119–121.

52 Teitelbaum and Winter, *The Global Spread*, 119–121.

53 Barbara Demick, "Judging China's One-Child Policy," *New Yorker*, October 30, 2015, http
://www.newyorker.com/news/news-desk/chinas-new-two-child-policy.

54 Therese Hesketh, "The Consequences of Son Preference and Sex-Selective Abortion in
China and Other Asian Countries," *CMAJ* 183, no. 12 (2011): 1374–1377, doi:10.1503/
cmaj.101368.

55 Hvistendahl, *Unnatural Selection*, 233.

56 Dan Levin, "Many in China Can Now Have a Second Child, but Say No," *New York Times*,
February 25, 2014, http://www.nytimes.com/2014/02/26/world/asia/many-couples-in

-china-will-pass-on-a-new-chance-for-a-second-child.html?_r=0; Chris Buckley, "China Ends One-Child Policy, Allowing for Two Children," *New York Times*, October 29, 2015, http ://www.nytimes.com/2015/10/30/world/asia/china-end-one-child-policy.html?_r=0.

57   Gretchen Livingstone, "Without One-Child Policy, China Still Might Not See Baby Boom, Gender Balance," Pew Research Center, November 20, 2015, http://www.pewresearch.org /fact-tank/2015/11/20/will-the-end-of-chinas-one-child-policy-shift-its-boy-girl-ratio/. Footnote information in Fong, *One Child*, 66.

58   Lily Kuo, "Why China's Hoped-for Baby Boom Is Turning Out to Be a Bust," *Quartz*, January 13, 2015, http://qz.com/325571/why-chinas-hoped-for-baby-boom-is-turning-out-to-be-a-bust/.

59   Mark Hanrahan and Eric Baculinao, "China population crisis: New two-child policy fails to yield major gains," CNBC, January 28, 2017, https://www.cnbc.com/2017/01/28/china -population-crisis-new-two-child-policy-fails-to-yield-major-gains.html.

60   Simon Denyer, "'One Is Enough': Chinese Families Lukewarm over Easing of One-Child Policy," *The Washington Post*, January 25, 2015, https://www.washingtonpost.com /world/asia_pacific/one-is-enough-chinese-families-lukewarm-over-easing-of-one-child -policy/2015/01/22/bdfeff1e-9d7e-11e4-86a3-1b56f64925f6_story.html.

61   Jing-Bao Nie, *Behind the Silence: Chinese Voices on Abortion* (New York: Rowman & Littlefield, 2005), 98.

62   Nie, *Behind the Silence*, 105–117; Hvistendahl, *Unnatural Selection*, 148–149.

63   Christina Larson, "In China, More Girls Are on the Way," *Bloomberg*, July 31, 2014, http ://www.bloomberg.com/bw/articles/2014-07-31/chinas-girl-births-ratio-improves-as -country-gets-more-educated.

64   Ibid.

65   Ibid.

66   Ibid.

67   Elizabeth Winkler, "China's One-Child Policy May Be Making the Country More Violent," *New Republic*, June 27, 2014, https://newrepublic.com/article/118439/chinas-one-child -policy-may-be-making-country-more-violent#footnote-118439-1.

68   Douglas Almond and Lena Edlund, "Son-Biased Sex Ratios in the 2000 United States Census," *Proceedings of the National Academy of Sciences* 105, no. 15 (2008): 5681–5682, doi:10.1073/ pnas.0800703105.

69   Helen Fisher, *Anatomy of Love: The Natural History of Monogamy, Adultery and Divorce* (New York: W. W. Norton, 1992), 108; Mark Regnerus and Jeremy Uecker, *Premarital Sex in America: How Young Americans Meet, Mate, and Think about Marrying* (New York: Oxford University Press, 2010), 122, 245.

70   Hvistendahl, *Unnatural Selection*, 167.

71   Ibid., 163.

72   Ibid., 160–168; Norimitsu Onishi, "Korean Men Use Brokers to Find Brides in Vietnam," *New York Times*, February 22, 2007, http://www.nytimes.com/2007/02/22/world/asia/22brides .html?_r=0.

73   Hvistendahl, *Unnatural Selection*, 184; Nam You-Sun, "N. Korean Women Up for Sale in China: Activist," *Agence France-Presse*, May 13, 2010, http://reliefweb.int/report/democratic -peoples-republic-korea/nkorean-women-sale-china-activist.

74   Hvistendahl, *Unnatural Selection*, 185; Lee Tae-hoon, "Female North Korean Defectors Priced at $1,500," *Korea Times*, May 5, 2010, http://www.koreatimes.co.kr/www/news /nation/2010/09/120_65400.html.

75   Hvistendahl, *Unnatural Selection*, 172; VietNamNet Bridge, "Vietnam's Per Capita Income Reaches Nearly $2,200," *VietNamNet Bridge*, July 15, 2015, http://english.vietnamnet.vn/fms /business/136071/vietnam-s-per-capita-income-reaches-nearly—2-200.html.

76   Hvistendahl, *Unnatural Selection*, 168.

77   China Daily, "S. Koreans Buying Wives in Cambodia," *China Daily*, March 26, 2008, http
        ://www.chinadaily.com.cn/cndy/2008-03/26/content_6565536.htm.

78   Hvistendahl, *Unnatural Selection*, 177.

79   Ibid, 185–192.

80   Louise Brown, *Sex Slaves: The Trafficking of Women in Asia* (London: Virago Press, 2000), 41.

81   Ibid., 63.

82   Hvistendahl, *Unnatural Selection*, 165–166.

83   Ibid., 209.

84   Ibid., 177 178; Lena Edlund, "Son Preference, Sex Ratios, and Marriage Patters," *Journal of
        Political Economy* 107, no. 6 (1999): 1275–1304, doi:10.1086/250097. Footnot information in
        I Ivistendahl, *Unnatural Selection*, 172.

85   Census and Statistics Department Hong Kong Special Administrative Region, "Women
        and Men in Hong Kong: Key Statistics," July 2016, http://www.statistics.gov.hk/pub
        /B11303032016AN16B0100.pdf.

86   David Cox, "Hong Kong's Troubling Shortage of Men," *Atlantic*, December 2, 2013,
        http://www.theatlantic.com/china/archive/2013/12/hong-kongs-troubling-shortage-of
        -men/281942/.

87   Sushma Subramanian and Deborah Jian Lee, "For China's Educated Single Ladies, Finding Love
        Is Often a Struggle," *Atlantic*, October 19, 2011, http://www.theatlantic.com/international/
        archive/2011/10/for-chinas-educated-single-ladies-finding-love-is-often-a-struggle/246892/.

88   Cox, "Hong Kong's Troubling Shortage of Men."

89   Ibid.

90   Winkler, "China's One-Child Policy."

91   Lena Edlund et al., "More Men, More Crime: Evidence from China's One-Child Policy," *IZA
        Working Paper*, no. 3214, doi:10.1111/j.0042–7092.2007.00700.x.

92   Winkler, "China's One-Child Policy."

93   Jane Golley and Rod Tyers, "Gender 'Rebalancing' in China," *Asian Population Studies* 10, no. 2
        (2014): 125–143, doi:10.1080/17441730.2014.902159.

94   Joseph Henrich, Robert Boyd, and Peter Richerson, "The Puzzle of Monogamous Marriage,"
        Philosophical Transactions of the Royal Society B: Biological Sciences, 367, no. 1589 (2012): 657–
        669, doi:10.1098/rstb.2011.0290.

95   Hvistendahl, *Unnatural Selection*, 234; Anjani Trivedi and Heather Thomas, "India's Man
        Problem," *New York Times*, January 16, 2013, http://india.blogs.nytimes.com/2013/01/16
        /indias-man-problem/?_r=0.

96   Winkler, "China's One-Child Policy."

97   Valerie Hudson and Andrea Den Boer, *Bare Branches: The Security Implications of Asia's Surplus
        Male Population* (Cambridge MA: MIT Press, 2005); The Week Staff, "China's Looming
        Woman Shortage: 5 Possible Consequences," *The Week*, April 12, 2010, http://theweek.com
        /articles/495327/chinas-looming-woman-shortage-5-possible-consequences; Niall Ferguson,
        "The Rise of Asia's Bachelor Generation," *Newsweek*, March 6, 2011, http://www.newsweek
        .com/ferguson-rise-asias-bachelor-generation-66103.

98   Bill Powell, "Gender Imbalance: How China's One-Child Law Backfired on Men," *Newsweek*,
        May 28, 2015, http://www.newsweek.com/2015/06/05/gender-imbalance-china-one-child
        -law-backfired-men-336435.html.

99   Adam Miller, "China Needs Millions of Brides ASAP," *Bloomberg*, December 25, 2014, http
        ://www.bloombergview.com/articles/2014-12-25/china-needs-millions-of-brides-asap;
        Charles Clover, "The Mystery of China's Missing Brides," *Financial Times*, December 18, 2015,
        http://www.ft.com/intl/cms/s/0/d44122c0-a435-11e5-873f-68411a84f346.html.

100   Shang-Jin Wei and Xiaobo Zhang, "The Competitive Saving Motive: Evidence from Rising Sex Ratios and Savings Rates in China," *National Bureau of Economic Research*, no. 15093 (2009): doi:10.3386/w15093.

101   Shang-Jin Wei, "Why Do the Chinese Save So Much?," *Forbes*, February 2, 2010, http://www.forbes.com/2010/02/02/china-saving-marriage-markets-economy-trade.html.

102   Powell, "Gender Imbalance."

103   Nick Stockton, "The Biggest Threat to the Earth? We Have Too Many Kids," *Wired*, April 22, 2015, http://www.wired.com/2015/04/biggest-threat-earth-many-kids/.

104   Connelly, *Fatal Misconception*, 378.

105   Ibid., 23.

106   Mei Fong, *One Child: The Story of China's Most Radical Experiment* (New York: Houghton Mifflin Harcourt, 2016), 210.

107   Last, *What to Expect*, 160.

108   Ibid., 162.

Chapter 8

1   Adee Braun, "Looking to Quell Sexual Urges? Consider the Graham Cracker," *Atlantic*, January 15, 2014, http://www.theatlantic.com/health/archive/2014/01/looking-to-quell-sexual-urges-consider-the-graham-cracker/282769/.

2   John Money, *The Destroying Angel: Sex, Fitness & Food in the Legacy of Degeneracy Theory, Graham Crackers, Kellogg's Corn Flakes & American's Health History* (New York: Prometheus, 1985), 20.

3   Braum, "Looking to Quell."

4   Money, *Destroying Angel*, 66.

5   Ibid., 17.

6   Ibid.

7   Ibid, 19–20.

8   Ibid.

9   Jack Cashill, *Hoodwinked: How Intellectual Hucksters Have Hijacked American Culture* (Nashville: Nelson Current, 2005); Andrew Greeley, *Sexual Intimacy: Love and Play* (New York: Grand Central Publishing, 1988), 354.

10   Elof Carlson, "Scientific Origins of Eugenics," Image Archive on the American Eugenics Movement, accessed March 14, 2016, http://www.eugenicsarchive.org/html/eugenics/essay2text.html.

11   Braum, "Looking to Quell."

12   Ibid.

13   Money, *Destroying Angel*, 24.

14   Elizabeth Fee and Theodore Brown, "John Harvey Kellogg, MD: Health Reformer and Antismoking Crusader," *American Journal of Public Health* 92, no. 6 (2002): 935, doi:10.2105/AJPH.92.6.935.

15   Money, *Destroying Angel*, 84.

16   Ibid., 84.

17   Ibid.

18   Money, *Destroying Angel*, 99; Therese Oneill, "John Harvey Kellogg's Legacy of Cereal, Sociopathy, and Sexual Mutilation," *Jezebel*, May 24, 2016, http://pictorial.jezebel.com/john-harvey-kelloggs-legacy-of-cereal-sociopathy-and-1777402050.

19   Money, *Destroying Angel*, 25.

20   Ibid., 25.

21   Ibid.

22   Ibid., 25–26.

23   Ibid.

24   Ibid., 26.

25   Ibid.

26   Evelyne Ender, *Sexing the Mind: Nineteenth-Century Fictions of Hysteria* (Ithaca NY: Cornell University Press, 1995), 37.

27   Rachel Maines, *The Technology of Orgasm: "Hysteria," the Vibrator, and Women's Sexual Satisfaction* (Baltimore: The Johns Hopkins University Press, 1999), 23.

28   Cecilia Tasca et al., "Women and Hysteria in the History of Mental Health," *Clinical Practice & Epidemiology in Mental Health* 8 (2012): 110–119, doi:10.2174/17450179012080101 10; Mara Hvistendahl, "The Vibrator," *Scientific American*, September 1, 2009, http://www .scientificamerican.com/article/the-vibrator/.

29   Maines, *Technology of Orgasm*, 3.

30   Ibid, 89.

31   Ibid.; Maya Dusenberg, "Timeline: Female Hysteria and the Sex Toys Used to Treat It," *Mother Jones*, June 1, 2012, http://www.motherjones.com/media/2012/05/hysteria-sex-toy-history-timeline.

32   Maines, *Technology of Orgasm*, 23, 114.

33   Ibid., 67.

34   Ibid.

35   Ibid., 67–68.

36   Marlow Stern, "'Hysteria' and the Long, Strange History of the Vibrator," *Daily Beast*, April 27, 2012, http://www.thedailybeast.com/articles/2012/04/27/hysteria-and-the-long-strange -history-of-the-vibrator-vertical.html.

37   Adam Frucci, "The Steam-Powered Vibrator and Other Terrifying Early Sex Machines NSFW," *Gizmodo*, February 2, 2010, http://gizmodo.com/5466997/the-steam-powered -vibrator-and-other-terrifying-early-sex-machines-nsfw.

38   Tanja Laden, "Fucking Hysterical: A Timeline of Vintage Vibrators," *Vice*, April 11, 2013, http://www.vice.com/read/fucking-hysterical-a-timeline-of-vintage-vibrators.

39   Rachel Maines, "The Steam-Powered, Coal-Fired Vibrator," *Big Think*, 6:59, April 23, 2012, https://www.youtube.com/watch?v=f4sDGIAcUN8.

40   Laden, "Fucking Hysterical."

41   Maines, "The Steam-Powered."

42   Maines, *Technology of Orgasm*, 4. Footnote information in Rachel Maines, email interview, March 25, 2016.

43   Ibid., 19.

44   Stern, "'Hysteria' and the Long, Strange History of the Vibrator." Footnote information in Kelly Bourdet, "Vibrators Cured Hysteria But We Are Still Hysterical," *Vice*, May 21, 2012, http ://motherboard.vice.com/blog/vibrators-cured-so-called-hysteria-but-is-it-really-gone.

45   Maines, *The Technology of Orgasm*, 104–105.

46   Peter Jaret, "The Ins and Outs of Impotence Drugs," *New York Times*, February 29, 2008, http://www.nytimes.com/ref/health/healthguide/esn-erectiledysfunction-expert.html.

47   John Calfee, "Public Policy Issues in Direct-to-Consumer Advertising of Prescription Drugs," *Journal of Public Policy & Marketing* 2, no. 21 (2002): 174–193, doi:10.1509/ jppm.21.2.174.17580; Meika Loe. *The Rise of Viagra: How the Little Blue Pill Changed Sex in America* (New York: New York University Press, 2004), 55.

48   Loe, *Rise of Viagra*, 3.

49   Ibid., 7. Footnote information in Alison Mitchell and David Rosenbaum, "The Tax Issue: Dole and Clinton Refocus on Tax-Cut Plans as an Option," *New York Times*, June 9, 1996, http ://www.nytimes.com/1996/06/09/us/politics-the-tax-issue-dole-and-clinton-refocus-on -tax-cut-plans-as-an-option.html?pagewanted=all.

50   Loe, *Rise of Viagra*, 52.

51   Ibid, 256–257.

52   David Stipp and Robert Whitaker, "The Selling of Impotence," *Fortune*, March 16, 1998, http://archive.fortune.com/magazines/fortune/fortune_archive/1998/03/16/239307/index.htm.

53   Loe, *Rise of Viagra*, 51.

54   Edward Laumann, Anthony Paik, and Raymond Rosen, "Sexual Dysfunction in the United States: Prevalence and Predictors," *JAMA* 281, no. 6 (1999): 537–544, doi:10.1001/jama.281.6.537. Jonathan Bor, "A breakthrough for both sexes Viagra: Doctors are eager to find out whether the new male impotence pill will also help women with sexual dysfunction," *Baltimore Sun*, April 22, 1998, http://articles.baltimoresun.com/1998-04-22/news/1998112016_1_viagra-male-impotence-dysfunction-in-women; Lawrence Altman, "FDA Approves an Injection to Treat Sexual Impotence," *The New York Times*, July 8, 1995, http://www.nytimes.com/1995/07/08/us/fda-approves-an-injection-to-treat-sexual-impotence.html.

55   Loe, *Rise of Viagra*, 51.

56   Ibid., 52.

57   Ibid.

58   Jesse Bering, "Not So Fast… What's So 'Premature' About Premature Ejaculation?," *Scientific American*, November 15, 2010, http://blogs.scientificamerican.com/bering-in-mind/not-so-fast-whats-so-e2809cprematuree2809d-about-premature-ejaculation/.

59   Loe, *Rise of Viagra*, 52.

60   Brendan Koerner, "Disorders Made to Order," *Mother Jones*, July/August 2002, http://www.motherjones.com/politics/2002/07/disorders-made-order.

61   Ray Moynihan and Barbara Mintzes, *Sex, Lies & Pharmaceuticals: How Drug Companies Are Bankrolling the Next Big Condition for Women* (Vancouver: Greystone Books, 2010), 7.

62   Molly Redden, "The Controversial Doctor Behind the New 'Viagra for Women,'" *Mother Jones*, September 2, 2015, http://www.motherjones.com/politics/2015/08/irwin-goldstein-controversial-doctor-behind-new-viagra-women.

63   Koerner, "Disorders Made to Order."

64   Stipp and Whitaker, "The Selling of Impotence."

65   Ibid.

66   Mildred Cho and Lisa Bero, "The Quality of Drug Studies Published in Symposium Proceedings," *Annals of Internal Medicine* 124, no. 5 (1996): 485–489, doi:10.7326/0003-4819-124-5-199603010-00004.

67   Henry Thomas Stelfox et al., "Conflict of Interest in the Debate over Calcium-Channel Antagonists," *New England Journal of Medicine* 338, no. 2 (1998): 101–106, doi:10.1056/NEJM199801083380206.

68   Ashley Wazana, "Physicians and the Pharmaceutical Industry: Is a Gift Ever Just a Gift?," *JAMA* 283, no. 3 (2000): 373–380, doi:10.1097/00006254-200008000-0001; Mary-Margaret Chren and Charles Seth Landefeld, "Physicians' Behavior and Their Interactions with Drug Companies: A Controlled Study of Physicians Who Requested Additions to a Hospital Drug Formulary," *JAMA*, 271, no. 9 (1994): 684–689, doi:10.1001/jama.271.9.684.

69   ABC News, "Better in Bed: 'O-Shot' Claims to Boost Female Sexual Satisfaction," *ABC News*, February 6, 2014, http://abcnews.go.com/blogs/lifestyle/2014/02/better-in-bed-o-shot-claims-to-boost-female-sexual-satisfaction/.

70   Toni Clarke and Ransdell Pierson, "FDA Approves 'Female Viagra' with Strong Warning," *Reuters*, August 19, 2015, http://www.reuters.com/article/us-pink-viagra-fda-idUSKCN0QN2BH20150819; Sarah Boseley, "FDA Approval of 'Female Viagra' Leaves

Bitter Taste for Critics," *Guardian*, August 19, 2015, https://www.theguardian.com /science/2015/aug/19/fda-approval-female-viagra-critics-addyi-us-licence.

71   Andrew Pollack, "F.D.A. Approves Addyi, a Libido Pill for Women," *New York Times*, August 18, 2015, http://www.nytimes.com/2015/08/19/business/fda -approval-addyi-female -viagra.html." Footnote information in Clarke and Pierson, "FDA Approves 'Female Viagra'"; Katie Thomas and Gretchen Morgenson, "The Female Viagra, Undone by a Drug Maker's Dysfunction," *New York Times*, April 9, 2016, http://www.nytimes.com/2016/04/10 /business/female-viagra-addyi-valeant-dysfunction.html?_r=0.

72   ABC News, "Better in Bed."

73   Bloomberg, "Viagra Keeps Pfizer's China Sales Rising," *Bloomberg*, May 3, 2015, http://www .bloomberg.com/news/articles/2015-05-03/viagra-keeps-pfizer-s-china-sales-rising.

74   Didi Kirsten Tatlow, "A Closer Look at Sexual Dysfunction in China," *New York Times*, November 5, 2014, http://sinosphere.blogs.nytimes.com/2014/11/05/sex-study-spotlights -erectile-dysfunction-in-china/.

75   Bloomberg, "Viagra Keeps Pfizer's China Sales Rising."

76   Ibid.

77   Didi Kirsten Tatlow, "A Closer Look."

78   Times Wire Reports, "Viagra Sales Help Boost Pfizer Profit," *Los Angeles Times*, July 10, 1998, http://articles.latimes.com/1998/jul/10/business/fi-2327.

79   David Goetzl, "Hearts, Flowers & Viagra: Happy Valentine's Day," *Advertising Age*, January 31, 2000, http://adage.com/article/news/hearts-flowers-viagra-happy-valentine-s-day/59611/.

80   John-Manuel Andriote, "Legal Drug-Pushing: How Disease Mongers Keep Us All Doped Up," *Atlantic*, April 3, 2012, http://www.theatlantic.com/health/archive/2012/04/legal -drug-pushing-how-disease-mongers-keep-us-all-doped-up/255247/;   Allen   Frances, "Female Sexual Dysfunction and Disease Mongering," *Psychology Today*, March 4, 2013, https ://www.psychologytoday.com/blog/dsm5-in-distress/201303/female-sexual-dysfunction -and-disease-mongering.

81   Vince Parry, "The Art of Branding a Condition," *Medical Marketing and Media* 38, no. 5 (2003): 43–49, https://rws511.pbworks.com/w/file/fetch/68702371/Parry_art_branding _condition.pdf.

82   Loe, *Rise of Viagra*, 47; Julie Rovner, "Why Catholic Groups' Health Plans Say No to Contraceptives, Yes to Viagra," *NPR*, February 13, 2012, http://www.npr.org/sections/health -shots/2012/02/13/146822713/why-catholic-groups-health-plans-say-no-to-contraceptives -yes-to-viagra; Father Rocky Hoffman, "Viagra," *Catholic News Agency*, June 14, 2011, http ://www.catholicnewsagency.com/column/viagra-1604/; Bruce Handy, "The Viagra Craze," *Time*, June 24, 2001, http://content.time.com/time/magazine/article/0,9171,139084,00.html.

83   Loe, *Rise of Viagra*, 48.

84   Lauren Pastrana, "Viagra Saves Sex Lives and Children's Lives," *CBS Miami*, December 7, 2015, http://miami.cbslocal.com/2015/12/07/viagra-saves-sex-lives-and-childrens-lives/; Christopher Barnett and Roberto Machado, "Sildenafil in the Treatment of Pulmonary Hypertension," *Vascular Health and Risk Management* 2, no. 4 (2006): 411–422, doi:10.2147/vhrm.2006.2.4.411.

85   Loe, *Rise of Viagra*, 31.

86   Shereen El Feki, *Sex and the Citadel: Intimate Life in a Changing Arab World* (New York: Anchor Books, 2013), 75.

87   Mary Roach, *Bonk: The Curious Coupling of Science and Sex* (New York: W. W. Norton & Co., 2008), 142. Footnote information in Sidney Glina et al., "Nocturnal Penile Tumescence Monitoring with Stamps," *Journal of Sexual Medicine* 8, no. 5 (2011): 1296–1298, doi:10.1111/ j.17436109.2011.02272.x; Roach, *Bonk*, 142.

88   Loe, *Rise of Viagra*, 50.

89   Andrew Moore, Jayne Edwards, and Henry McQuay, "Sildenafil (Viagra) for Male Erectile Dysfunction: A Meta-Analysis of Clinical Trial Reports," *BioMed Central Urology* 2 (2002): doi:10.1186/1471-2490-2-6.

90   Loe, *Rise of Viagra*, 54.

91   Ibid, 14.

92   Deborah Baldwin, "Medicine Cabinets: Walk Right In," *New York Times*, March 18, 2004, http://www.nytimes.com/2004/03/18/garden/medicine-cabinets-walk-right-in.html.

Chapter 9

1   Kowalski, *Married Catholic Priests*, 228–229; Majorie Kaufman, "What's Wrong with This Picture?," *New York Times*, June 20, 1999, http://www.nytimes.com/1999/06/20/nyregion/in-person-what-s-wrong-with-this-picture.html?pagewanted=all.

2   Richard Sipe, *A Secret World: Sexuality and the Search for Celibacy* (New York: Routledge, 1990), 38; Anthony Kowalski, *Married Catholic Priests: Their History, Their Journeys, Their Reflections* (New York: The Crossroad Publishing Company, 2004), 12.

3   James Brundage, *Law, Sex, and Christian Society in Medieval Europe* (Chicago: University of Chicago Press, 1987), 69; Garry Wills, *Papal Sin: Structures of Deceit* (New York: Doubleday, 2000), 132–133; Roman Cholij, "Priestly Celibacy in Patristics and in the History of the Church," *Vatican*, accessed March 21, 2016, http://www.vatican.va/roman_curia/congregations/cclergy/documents/rc_con_cclergy_doc_01011993_chisto_en.html.

4   Brundage, *Law, Sex, and Christian Society*, 220.

5   Ibid., 192–217; Matthew 19:12; Catholic Answers, "Why Can't a Priest Ever Marry?," accessed March 21, 2016, http://www.catholic.com/quickquestions/why-cant-a-priest-ever-marry.

6   Brundage, *Law, Sex, and Christian Society*, 214; Wills, *Papal Sin*, 125–127.

7   Max Thurian, "The Theological Basis for Priestly Celibacy," *Vatican*, accessed March 21, 2016, http://www.vatican.va/roman_curia/congregations/cclergy/documents/rc_con_cclergy_doc_01011993_theol_en.html. Footnote information in Piotr Scholz, *Eunuchs and Castrati: A Cultural History*, trans. Shelley Frisch and John Broadwin (Princeton NJ: Markus Wiener Publishers, 2001), 272–276; Wills, *The Future of the Catholic Church*, 71; New Advent, "First Council of Nicaea (AD 325)," accessed March 18, 2016, http://www.newadvent.org/fathers/3801.htm.

8   Garry Wills, *What Paul Meant* (New York: Viking, 2006), 17. Richard McCarty, *Sexual Virtue: An Approach to Contemporary Christian Ethics* (Albany: SUNY Press, 2015), 134–136; Robert Murray, *Symbols of Church and Kingdom: A Study in Early Syriac Tradition* (London: T&T Clark, 2006), 303; Robin Scroggs, "Paul and the Eschatological Woman," *Journal of the American Academy of Religion* 40, no. 3 (1972): 283–303, http://www.jstor.org/stable/1461319.

9   1 Corinthians 7.

10   Wills, *Papal Sin*, 130.

11   John Paul II, "Familiaris Consortio," *Vatican*, November 22, 1981, http://w2.vatican.va/content/john-paul-ii/en/apost_exhortations/documents/hf_jp-ii_exh_19811122_familiaris-consortio.html#_ftn15.

12   Peter Brown, *The Body and Society: Men, Women, and Sexual Renunciation in Early Christianity* (New York: Columbia University Press, 1988), 55.

13   1 Corinthians 7:8–9.

14   Kowalski, *Married Catholic Priests*, 8–9.

15   David Barash and Judith Lipton, *The Myth of Monogamy: Fidelity and Infidelity in Animals and People* (New York: Henry Holt and Co., 2001), 182.

16   Wills, *Papal Sin*, 169; Garry Wills, "The Myth about Marriage," *New York Review of Books*, May 9, 2012, http://www.nybooks.com/daily/2012/05/09/marriage-myth/; Hillman, *Polygamy Reconsidered*, 26.

17   Edward Schillebeeckx, *Marriage: Secular Reality and Saving Mystery, Volume 2: Marriage in the History of the Church*, trans. N.D. Smith (London: Sheed and Ward, 1965), 134–138; Hillman, *Polygamy Reconsidered*, 26.

18   John Boswell, *Same-Sex Unions in Premodern Europe* (New York: Villard Books, 1994), 111.

19   Brown, *The Body and Society*, 6.

20   Ibid., 6; Hillman, *Polygamy Reconsidered*, 21.

21   John O'Malley, "Some Basics about Celibacy," *America*, October 28, 2002, http ://americamagazine.org/issue/409/article/some-basics-about-celibacy.

22   Wills, *Papal Sin*, 107–108, 132–133.

23   Brundage, *Law, Sex, and Christian Society*, 215.

24   Richard Sipe, *Sex, Priests, and Power: Anatomy of a Crisis* (New York: Brunner-Routledge, 1995), 88.

25   Brundage, *Law, Sex, and Christian Society*, 215.

26   Sipe, *Sex, Priests, and Power*, 88.

27   Brian Tierney, *The Crisis of Church and State 1050–1300* (Toronto: University of Toronto Press, 1988), 24–27, 48–49.

28   Brundage, *Law, Sex, and Christian Society*, 225–228.

29   Ibid., 225–228.

30   Tierney, *The Crisis of Church and State*, 48–49.

31   Brundage, *Law, Sex, and Christian Society*, 219.

32   Ibid., 218–220; Kowalski, *Married Catholic Priests*, 34–35.

33   Mary Malone, "The Unfinished Agenda of the Church: A Critical Look at the History of Celibacy," *The Way*, supplement 77 (1993): 66–75, http://www.theway.org.uk/Back /s077Malone.pdf. Footnote information in Peter Damian, *The Fathers of the Church Mediaeval Continuation: The Letters of Peter Damian 61–90*, trans. Owen Blum (Washington DC: The Catholic University of America Press, 1992), 10–11.

34   Brundage, *Law, Sex, and Christian Society*, 216–217. Footnote information in Kowalski, *Married Catholic Priests*, 35.

35   James Brundage, *Law, Sex, and Christian Society in Medieval Europe* (Chicago: University of Chicago Press, 1987), 221.

36   Sipe, *Sex, Priests, and Power*, 89.

37   David Greenberg, *The Construction of Homosexuality* (Chicago: University of Chicago Press, 1988), 288.

38   Jason Berry, *Lead Us Not into Temptation: Catholic Priests and the Sexual Abuse of Children* (New York: Doubleday, 1992), 180, 222.

39   Congregation for the Doctrine of the Faith, "Letter to the Bishops of the Catholic Church on the Pastoral Care of Homosexual Persons," *Vatican*, October 1, 1986.

40   Berry, *Lead Us Not into Temptation*, 222.

41   *Catechism of the Catholic Church*, no. 2359, accessed March 16, 2016, http://www.vatican.va /archive/ccc_css/archive/catechism/p3s2c2a6.htm.

42   McNeil, *The Church and the Homosexual*, 172.

43   Robert Bennett et al., "A Report on the Crisis in the Catholic Church in the United States," The National Review Board for the Protection of Children and Young People, February 27, 2004, 84, http://www.usccb.org/issues-and-action/child-and-youth-protection/upload/a-report -on-the-crisis-in-the-catholic-church-in-the-united-states-by-the-national-review-board.pdf.

44   Christopher Schiavone, "Broken Vows," *Boston Globe*, December 8, 2002, http://archive .boston.com/globe/spotlight/abuse/stories3/120802_schiavone.htm.

45   Thomas Groome, "The Free Flow of Fresh Air," *Boston Globe*, May 19, 2002, http://www .boston.com/globe/spotlight/abuse/print/051902_focus.htm.

46   Paul Wilkes, "The Hands that Would Shape Our Souls," *Atlantic*, December 1990, http
      ://www.theatlantic.com/past/docs/issues/90dec/wilkes.htm.

47   Sipe, *Sex, Priests, and Power*, 148.

48   Robert Nugent, "Priest, Celibate, and Gay: You Are Not Alone," in *A Challenge to Love: Gays
      and Lesbian Catholics in the Church* (New York: Crossroad, 1983); Berry, *Lead Us Not into
      Temptation*, 183–184.

49   James Martin, "The Church and the Homosexual Priest," *America*, November 4, 2000, http
      ://americamagazine.org/issue/387/article/church-and-homosexual-priest. Footnote information
      in Karen Lebacqz, "Lessons from Our Neighbors: An Appreciation and a Query to Mark Jordan,"
      in *Gay Catholic Priests and Clerical Sexual Misconduct: Breaking the Silence*, eds., Donald Boisvert
      and Robert Goss (New York: Harrington Park Press, 2005), 201.

50   Nugent, "Priest, Celibate, and Gay: You Are Not Alone," 263.

51   Ibid., 276.

52   Andrew Greeley, *Priests: A Calling in Crisis* (Chicago: University of Chicago Press, 2004),
      44–45. Footnote information in Richard Posner, *Sex and Reason* (Cambridge MA: Harvard
      University Press, 1992), 153.

53   Bennett et al., "A Report on the Crisis," 84.

54   Berry, *Lead Us Not into Temptation*, 260. Footnote information in Darlene Gavron Stevens,
      "Half of Catholic Clergy Sees a Gay Presence in Priesthood," *Chicago Tribune*, August 17,
      2002,   http://articles.chicagotribune.com/2002-08-17/news/0208170232_1_jacqueline
      -wenger-priests-councils-subculture.

55   Ibid., 267. Footnote information in Nugent, "Priest, Celibate, and Gay," 268.

56   John Boswell, *Christianity, Social Tolerance, and Homosexuality: Gay People in Western Europe
      from the Beginning of the Christian Era to the Fourteenth Century* (Chicago: University of
      Chicago Press, 1980), 190.

57   Jason Berry and Gerald Renner, *Vows of Silence: The Abuse of Power in the Papacy of John Paul
      II* (New York: Free Press, 2004), 9–10.

58   Cathy Lynn Grossman, "Gay Catholics Angry, Say They've Been Singled Out," *USA Today*,
      April 25, 2002, http://usatoday30.usatoday.com/news/nation/2002/04/25/gay-catholics
      .htm; Chuck Colbert, "The Spectrum of Belief," *Boston Globe*, March 31, 2002, http://www
      .boston.com/globe/spotlight/abuse/print/033102_focus.htm.

59   The Times Poll, "How the National Survey Was Taken," *Los Angeles Times*, October 20, 2002,
      http://articles.latimes.com/2002/oct/20/local/me-priestmethod20; Greeley, *Priests*, 36.

60   Larry Stammer, "15% Identify as Gay or 'On Homosexual Side," *Los Angeles Times*, October 20,
      2002; Greeley, *Priests*, 39–43.

61   Gary Gates, "How Many People are Lesbian, Gay, Bisexual, and Transgender," Williams
      Institute, April 2011, http://williamsinstitute.law.ucla.edu/wp-content/uploads/Gates-How
      -Many-People-LGBT-Apr-2011.pdf.

62   Katie Leishman, "Heterosexuals and AIDS," *Atlantic*, February 1987; Robert Lindsey, "AIDS
      among Clergy Presents Challenges to Catholic Church," *New York Times*, February 2, 1987, http
      ://www.nytimes.com/1987/02/02/us/aids-among-clergy-presents-challenges-to-catholic
      -church.html; Miles Corwin, "Priest with AIDS: 'It's Important that People Know,'" *Los
      Angeles Times*, February 16, 1987, http://articles.latimes.com/1987-02-16/news/mn-2442
      _1_priest-contracted-aids; Jean Latz Griffin and Cheryl Devall, "5 Catholic Clergy Among
      AIDS Toll," *Chicago Tribune*, February 3, 1987, http://articles.chicagotribune.com/1987-02-03
      /news/8701090265_1_aids-patients-aids-toll-national-catholic-reporter; Sandra Boodman,
      "Priests and AIDS: Will Church Minister to Its Own?," *Washington Post*, February 7,
      1987,   https://www.washingtonpost.com/archive/politics/1987/02/07/priests-and-aids
      -will-church-minister-to-its-own/1b17b3a1-3056-42bf-862c-f0dc23a37d5a/. Footnote information

in Jon Fuller, "Priests with AIDS," *America*, March 18, 2000, http://americamagazine.org/issue/280/article/priests-aids.

63   Judy Thomas, "Catholic Priests Are Dying of AIDS, Often in Silence," *Kansas City Star*, January 29, 2000, https://web.archive.org/web/20131204232729/http://kcsweb.kcstar.com/projects/priests/priest.htm.

64   Ibid.

65   Ibid; Kansas City Star, "AIDS in the Priesthood," accessed March 16, 2016, https://web.archive.org/web/20130731153221/http://kcsweb.kcstar.com/projects/priests/.

66   Danny Hughes, David Mitchell, and David Molinari, "Heeding the Call: Seminary Enrollment and the Business Cycle," *Applied Economics Letters* 18 (2011): 433–437, doi:10.1080/13504851003689668.

67   T. W. Burger, "Enrollment at Seminaries Surges During Trying Times," *Patriot-News*, March 7, 2009, http://www.pennlive.com/midstate/index.ssf/2009/03/enrollment_at_seminaries_surge.html.

68   Carl Cannon, "The Priest Scandal," *American Journalism Review*, May 2002, https://web.archive.org/web/20150414051727/http://ajrarchive.org/Article.asp?id=2516.

69   Ibid.

70   Rachel Martin, "Abuse Scandal Still Echoes through the Catholic Church," *NPR*, January 12, 2007, http://www.npr.org/templates/story/story.php?storyId=6765175.

71   Tom Roberts, "Milwaukee Eighth Diocese to File for Bankruptcy," *National Catholic Reporter*, January 5, 2011, http://ncronline.org/news/accountability/milwaukee-eighth-diocese-file-bankruptcy.

72   Greeley, *Priests*, 100.

73   John Jay College Research Team, "The Nature and Scope of Sexual Abuse of Minors by Catholic Priests and Deacons in the United States 1950-2002," *John Jay College of Criminal Justice*, February 2004.

74   Laurie Goodstein, "Church Report Cites Social Tumult in Priest Scandals," *New York Times*, May 17, 2011, http://www.nytimes.com/2011/05/18/us/18bishops.html?_r=0. Footnote information in John Jay, "Nature and Scope," 7.

75   John Jay College Research Team, "The Causes and Context of Sexual Abuse of Minors by Catholic Priests in the United States, 1950–2010," *John Jay College of Criminal Justice*, May 2011.

76   Thomas Doyle, Richard Sipe, and Patrick Wall, *Sex, Priests, and Secret Codes: The Catholic Church's 2,000-Year Paper Trail of Sexual Abuse* (Los Angeles: Volt Press, 2006), 14, 33; Donald Cozzens, *The Changing Face of the Priesthood: A Reflection on the Priest's Crisis of Soul* (Collegeville, MN: The Liturgical Press, 2000), 124; Michael Joseph Gross, "The Vatican's Secret Life," *Vanity Fair*, December 2013, http://www.vanityfair.com/culture/2013/12/gay-clergy-catholic-church-vatican.

77   Tom Roberts, "Critics Point to John Jay Study's Limitations," *National Catholic Reporter*, May 23, 2011, http://ncronline.org/news/accountability/critics-point-john-jay-studys-limitations.

78   Tom Roberts, "Bishops Were Warned of Abusive Priests," *National Catholic Reporter*, March 30, 2009, http://ncronline.org/news/accountability/bishops-were-warned-abusive-priests.

79   James Martin, "John Jay Report: On Not Blaming Homosexual Priests," *America*, May 17, 2011, http://americamagazine.org/content/all-things/john-jay-report-not-blaming-homosexual-priests.

80   Mary Gail Frawley-O'Dea, "The John Jay Study: What It Is and What It Isn't," *National Catholic Reporter*, July 19, 2011, http://ncronline.org/news/accountability/john-jay-study-what-it-and-what-it-isnt.

81   Stephan Kappler, Kristin Hancock, and Thomas Plante, "Roman Catholic Gay Priests: Internalized Homophobia, Sexual Identity, and Psychological Well-Being," *Pastoral Psychology* 62 (2013): 805–826, doi10.1007/s11089-012-0505-5.

82   Berry and Renner, *Vows of Silence*, 303–304.

83   Michelle Boorstein, "'I'm Gay and I'm a Priest, Period,'" *Washington Post*, January 31, 2016, https://www.washingtonpost.com/local/social-issues/im-gay-and-im-a-priest-period/2016 /01/31/ab09c83e-bfb6-11e5-83d4-42e3bceea902_story.html.

84   Gerard Thomas, "A Gay Priest Speaks Out," *Commonweal*, January 24, 2005, https://www .commonwealmagazine.org/gay-priest-speaks-out-1.

85   Sipe, *Sex, Priests, and Power*, 95.

86   Boorstein, "'I'm Gay and I'm a Priest, Period'"; Patsy McGarry, "'Comfortable Being Gay': A Priest Speaks," *Irish Times*, January 11, 2014, http://www.irishtimes.com/news/social-affairs /religion-and-beliefs/comfortable-being-gay-a-priest-speaks-1.1651119.

87   Jason Breslow, "Robert Mickens: From Benedict to Francis," *Frontline*, February 25, 2014, http://www.pbs.org/wgbh/frontline/article/robert-mickens-from-benedict-to-francis/.

88   "Secrets of the Vatican" *Frontline* documentary, 1:23:44, February 25, 2014, http://www.pbs .org/wgbh/frontline/film/secrets-of-the-vatican/. Footnote information in Mark Jordan, *The Silence of Sodom: Homosexuality in Modern Catholicism* (Chicago: University of Chicago Press, 2000), 177; Sipe, *Sex, Priests, and Power*, 145.

89   Richard Wagner, "Gay Catholic Priests: A Study of Cognitive and Affective Dissonance," (doctoral disssertation, Institute for Advanced Study of Human Sexuality, 1981), http://www .sexarchive.info/BIB/GCP_SCAD.htm.

90   Richard Wagner, *Secrecy, Sophistry and Gay Sex in the Catholic Church: The Systematic Destruction of an Oblate Priest* (Las Vegas: The Nazca Plains Corp., 2011), 2.

91   James Wolf, ed., *Gay Priests* (New York: Harper & Row, 1989), 26.

92   Ibid., 26.

93   Ibid., 151.

94   "Congregation for the Doctrine of the Faith," *Vatican*, accessed March 16, 2016, http://www .vatican.va/roman_curia/congregations/cfaith/documents/rc_con_cfaith_pro_14071997 _en.html.

95   Ibid.

96   Doctrine of the Faith, "On the Pastoral Care of Homosexual Persons."

97   Ibid.

98   John Thavis, *The Vatican Diaries: A Behind-the-Scenes Look at the Power, Personalities, and Politics at the Heart of the Catholic Church* (New York: Penguin, 2013), 265–266.

99   Ibid., 266; Congregation for Catholic Education, "Instruction Concerning the Criteria for the Discernment of Vocations with Regard to Persons with Homosexual Tendencies in View of Their Admission to the Seminary and to Holy Orders," *Vatican*, November 4, 2005, http://www.vatican .va/roman_curia/congregations/ccatheduc/documents/rc_con_ccatheduc_doc_20051104 _istruzione_en.html. Footnote information in Congregation for the Doctrine of the Faith, "Some Considerations Concerning the Response to Legislative Proposals on the Non-Discrimination of Homosexual Persons," *The Vatican*, July 24,1992, http://www.vatican.va/roman_curia /congregations/cfaith/documents/rc_con_cfaith_doc_19920724_homosexual-persons _en.html; United States Conference of Catholics Bishops, "Ministry to Persons with a Homosexual Inclination: Guidelines for Pastoral Care," *USCCB*, November 14, 2006, http://www.usccb.org /about/doctrine/publications/upload/ministry-to-persons-of-homosexual-iInclination.pdf.

100   Paul Vitello, "Prospective Catholic Priests Face Sexuality Hurdles," *New York Times*, May 30, 2010, http://www.nytimes.com/2010/05/31/nyregion/31gay.html?_r=0.

101   James Martin, "Weeding Out Gays from Seminaries," *America*, May 31, 2010, http ://americamagazine.org/content/all-things/weeding-out-gays-seminaries. Footnote information in Vitello, "Prospective Catholic Priests Face Sexuality Hurdles."

102   Congregation for Catholic Education, "Guidelines for the Use of Psychology in the Admission

and Formation of Candidates for the Priesthood," June 29, 2008, http://www.vatican.va
/roman_curia/congregations/ccatheduc/documents/rc_con_ccatheduc_doc_20080628
_orientamenti_en.html; John Thavis, "Homosexuality and the Priesthood Revisited," *Catholic
News Service*, October 31, 2008, https://cnsblog.wordpress.com/2008/10/31/homosexuality
-and-the-priesthood-revisited/.

103   Congregation for Religious, "Careful Selection and Training of Candidates for the States of
Perfection and Sacred Orders," *Vatican*, February 2, 1961, https://www.ewtn.com/library
/CURIA/CCL1961R.HTM. Footnote information in Melinda Henneberger, "Vatican
Weighs Reaction to Accusations of Molesting by Clergy," *New York Times*, March 3, 2002,
http://www.nytimes.com/2002/03/03/us/vatican-weighs-reaction-to-accusations-of
-molesting-by-clergy.html.

104   Sipe, *Sex, Priests, and Power*, 95.

105   Frontline, "Secrets of the Vatican."

106   John Allen, "Pope on Homosexuals: 'Who Am I to Judge?,'" *National Catholic Reporter*, July 29,
2013, http://ncronline.org/blogs/ncr-today/pope-homosexuals-who-am-i-judge.

107   Antonio Spadaro, "A Big Heart Open to God: The Exclusive Interview with Pope Francis,"
America, September 30, 2013, http://americamagazine.org/pope-interview.

108   Ibid.

109   Gerard O'Connell, "Pope Francis Says the Church Should Apologize to Gays," *America*, June
26, 2016, http://americamagazine.org/content/dispatches/pope-francis-says-church-should
-apologize-gays. Footnote information in James Martin, "Keeping Pope Francis' Comments
on the LGBT Community in Context," *America*, June 27, 2016, http://americamagazine.org
/content/all-things/keeping-pope-francis-comments-lgbt-community-context.

110   Bill Dickinson, "I Was a Gay Priest for 25 Years," *Daily Beast*, July 20, 2015, http://www
.thedailybeast.com/articles/2015/07/20/i-was-a-gay-priest-for-25-years.html.

111   Doctrine of the Faith, "On the Pastoral Care of Homosexual Persons."

112   Pope Francis, "Address of Holy Father Francis to Participants in the Pilgrimage of Catechists
on the Occasion of the Year of Faith and of the International Congress on Catechesis,"
Vatican, September 27, 2013, https://w2.vatican.va/content/francesco/en/speeches/2013
/september/documents/papa-francesco_20130927_pellegrinaggio-catechisti.html.

113   Stephanie Kirchgaessner, "Pope Urges Catholic Church to Disavow Conservatism and
Fundamentalism," *Guardian*, November 10, 2015, http://www.theguardian.com/world/2015
/nov/10/pope-francis-catholic-church-power-money-conservatism.

114   Pope Francis, "Evangelii, Gaudium," *Vatican*, November 24, 2013, http://w2.vatican.va
/content/francesco/en/apost_exhortations/documents/papa-francesco_esortazione
-ap_20131124_evangelii-gaudium.html.

115   Pope Francis, "Amoris Laetitia," *Vatican*, April 8, 2016, https://w2.vatican.va/content
/dam/francesco/pdf/apost_exhortations/documents/papa-francesco_esortazione
-ap_20160319_amoris-laetitia_en.pdf; Stephanie Kirchgaessner, "Pope Francis Defends
Church's Opposition to Artificial Contraception," *Guardian*, January 16, 2015, http://www
.theguardian.com/world/2015/jan/16/pope-francis-catholic-church-contraception; Michael
O'Loughlin, "Vatican reaffirms ban on gay priests," *America*, December 7, 2016, https://www
.americamagazine.org/faith/2016/12/07/vatican-reaffirms-ban-gay-priests.

116   Jamie Manson, "Are Francis and Parolin Playing Good Cop-Bad Cop on Same-Sex Marriage?,"
National Catholic Reporter, May 28, 2015, http://ncronline.org/blogs/grace-margins/are
-francis-and-parolin-playing-good-cop-bad-cop-same-sex-marriage.

117   Wills, *Papal Sin*, 212–215.

118   John Noonan, *A Church That Can and Cannot Change: The Development of Catholic Moral
Teaching* (Notre Dame, IN: University of Notre Dame Press, 2005).

119   Garry Wills, *The Future of the Catholic Church with Pope Francis* (New York: Viking, 2015), xiv.

120   Ibid.; Noonan, *A Church That Can and Cannot Change.*

121   Wills, *The Future of the Catholic Church*, xv.

122   Brundage, *Law, Sex, and Christian Society*, 7.

123   Ibid., 85; Boswell, *Christianity, Social Tolerance, and Homosexuality*, 164; Helen Fisher, *Anatomy of Love: The Natural History of Monogamy, Adultery, and Divorce* (New York: W. W. Norton, 1992), 84.

124   Wills, *Papal Sin*, 75; Paul Rigby, *The Theology of Augustine's Confessions* (New York: Cambridge University Press, 2015), 303; John Noonan, *Contraception: A History of Its Treatment by the Catholic Theologians and Canonists*, Enlarged Edition (Cambridge, MA: Harvard University Press, 1986), 282–283, 300.

125   Wills, *Papal Sin*, 80–81. Wills, *The Future of the Church*, 192.

126   Noonan, *Contraception*, 120.

127   Brundage, *Law, Sex, and Christian Society*, 161; Wills, *The Future of the Catholic Church*, 188.

128   Brundage, *Law, Sex, and Christian Society*, 7.

129   Boswell, *Christianity, Social Tolerance, and Homosexuality*, 319–321, 328. Footnote information in Wills, *Papal Sin*, 108; Hillman, *Polygamy Reconsidered*, 31.

130   Brundage, *Law, Sex, and Christian Society*, 580.

131   John Thavis, "Vatican Clarifies Pope's Reference to 'Male Prostitute' in Condoms Comment," *Catholic News Service*, November 23, 2010, https://cnsblog.wordpress.com/2010/11/23/vatican-clarifies-popes-reference-to-male-prostitute-in-condoms-comment/; John Allen, "Pope Takes the Classic Vatican Approach to Birth Control and Zika," *Crux*, February 10, 2016, http://www.cruxnow.com/church/2016/02/20/pope-takes-classic-vatican-approach-to-birth-control-and-zika-virus/.

132   John McNeil, *The Church and the Homosexual* (Boston: Beacon Press, 1993), 100.

133   Wojtyla, *Love and Responsibility*, 286–287.

134   Pope Francis, "Amoris Laetitia."

135   Karol Wojtyla, *Love and Responsibility* (San Francisco: Ignatius Press, 1993), 272.

136   Boswell, *Christianity, Social Tolerance, and Homosexuality*, 228.

137   Ibid.; Robert Blair Kaiser, "Cloud over Gay Priests," *The Tablet*, November 30, 2002, http://archive.thetablet.co.uk/article/30th-november-2002/9/r-obert-b-lair-k-aiser; Jason Berry and Gerald Renner, *Vows of Silence: The Abuse of Power in the Papacy of John Paul II* (New York: Free Press, 2004), 34–35.

138   Center for Applied Research in the Apostolate (CARA), "Frequently Requested Church Statistics," accessed March 17, 2016, http://cara.georgetown.edu/frequently-requested-church-statistics/.

139   Richard Schoenherr and Lawrence Young, "Quitting the Clergy: Resignations in the Roman Catholic Priesthood," *Journal for the Scientific Study of Religion* 29, no. 4 (1990): 463–481, doi:10.2307/1387312; Richard Schoenerr, "Numbers Don't Lie: A Priesthood in Irreversible Decline," *Commonweal*, April 7, 1985.

140   CARA, "Frequently Requested Church Statistics."

141   Wills, *Papal Sin*, 94. Footnote information in Malcolm Gladwell, "John Rock's Error," *New Yorker*, March 10, 2000, http://gladwell.com/john-rock-s-error/.

142   Greeley, *Priests*, 41.

143   Ibid., 42; Berry and Renner, *Vows of Silence*, 35.

144   Charles Sennott, "Pope Calls Sex Abuse Crime," *Boston Globe*, April 24, 2002, http://www.boston.com/globe/spotlight/abuse/print/042402_pope.htm.

145   Thavis, *Vatican Diaries*, 268.

146   Wills, *Papal Sin*, 190.

147   Brundage, *Law, Sex, and Christian Society*, 222.

148   Berry and Renner, *Vows of Silence.*

149   Ibid., 109.

150   Pew Research Center, "America's Changing Religious Landscape," *Pew Research Center*, May 12, 2015, http://www.pewforum.org/2015/05/12/americas-changing-religious-landscape/; Pew Research Center, "The Global Catholic Population," *Pew Research Center*, February 13, 2013, http://www.pewforum.org/2013/02/13/the-global-catholic-population/.

151   Sipe, *Sex, Priests, and Power,* xv–xvi.

152   Greeley, *Priests,* 39–42, 48–59, 115; Thomas Plante, Arianna Aldridge, and Christina Louie, "Are Successful Applicants to the Priesthood Psychologically Healthy?," *Pastoral Psychology* 54, no. 1 (2005): 81–90, doi:10.1007/s11089-005-6185-7.

153   Georgetown University, "Average Priest Age Now Nearly 20 Years Older Than 1970," accessed March 18, 2016, https://www.georgetown.edu/news/average-priest-age-now-nearly-20 -years-older.html.

154   Paul Sullins, "Empty Pews and Empty Altars," *America*, May 13, 2002, http://americamagazine .org/issue/372/article/empty-pews-and-empty-altars.

155   Congregation for the Doctrine of the Faith, "Inter Insigniores: On the Question of Women to the Ministerial Priesthood," *Vatican*, October 15, 1976, http://www.vatican.va/roman _curia/congregations/cfaith/documents/rc_con_cfaith_doc_19761015_inter-insigniores en.html.

156   Brown, *The Body and Society;* Jason Berry, "Secrets, Celibacy and the Church," *New York Times*, April 3, 2002, http://www.nytimes.com/2002/04/03/opinion/secrets-celibacy-and-the -church.html; O'Malley, "Some Basics about Celibacy."

157   Berry, *Lead Us Not into Temptation,* 184.

158   Evelyn Eaton Whitehead and James Whitehead, "The Gift of Celibacy," in *Human Sexuality in the Catholic Tradition*, eds., Kieran Scott and Harold Daly Horell (Plymouth, UK: Rowman & Littlefield Publishers, 2007), 137.

159   John 12:24; Matthew 20:16.

Chapter 10

1   Afsaneh Najmabadi, *Professing Selves: Transsexuality and Same-Sex Desire in Contemporary Iran* (Durham, NC: Duke University Press, 2013).

2   Shereen El Feki, *Sex and the Citadel: Intimate Life in a Changing Arab World* (New York: Anchor Books, 2013), 83.

3   Marcia Inhorn and Soraya Tremayne, *Islam and Assisted Reproductive Technologies: Sunni and Shia Perspectives* (New York: Berghahn Books, 2012), 3.

4   Soraya Tremayne, email interview, December 6, 2015.

5   Marcia Inhorn and Soraya Tremayne, eds., "Islam, Assisted Reproduction, and the Bioethical Aftermath," *Journal of Religion and Health* 54, no. 6 (2015): 1–9, doi:10.1007/s10943-015-0151-1.

6   Tremayne, email interview.

7   Ibid.

8   Marcia Inhorn, *Cosmopolitan Conceptions: IVF Sojourns in Global Dubai* (Durham, NC: Duke University Press, 2015), 16.

9   Marcia Inhorn, "Making Muslim Babies: IVF and Gamete Donation in Sunni Versus Shi'a Islam," *Culture, Medicine, and Psychiatry* 30, no. 4 (2006): 427–450, doi: 10.1007/s11013- 006-9027-x.

10   Marcia Inhorn, "Reproductive Disruptions and Assisted Reproductive Technologies in the Muslim World," in *Reproductive Disruptions: Gender, Technology, and Biopolitics in the New Millennium*, ed. Marcia Inhorn (New York: Berghahn Books, 2007), 195–196.

11   Inhorn, *Cosmopolitan Conceptions,* 17.

12   Inhorn, "Making Muslim Babies."

13   Marcia Inhorn, email interview, January 5, 2015.

14   El Feki, *Sex and the Citadel*, 83.

15   Ibid., 10–11.

16   Marcia Inhorn, *Local Babies, Global Science: Gender, Religion, and In Vitro Fertilization in Egypt* (New York: Routledge, 2003), ix; Tremayne, email interview.

17   Inhorn, *Local Babies*, ix.

18   Farouk Mahmoud, "Controversies in Islamic Evaluation of Assisted Reproductive Technologies," in *Islam and Assisted Reproductive Technologies*, eds. Marcia Inhorn and Soraya Tremayne (New York: Berghahn Books, 2012), 70; Inhorn, *Local Babies*, 4.

19   Inhorn and Tremayne, *Islam and Assisted Reproductive Technologies*, 4–5.

20   Inhorn, *Local Babies*, 4–7; Marcia Inhorn, "Global Infertility and the Globalization of New Reproductive Technologies: Illustrations from Egypt," *Social Science & Medicine* 56 (2003): 1837–1851, doi:10.1016/S0277–9536(02)00208–3.

21   Inhorn, *Local Babies*, 6.

22   Soraya Tremayne, "The 'Down Side' of Gamete Donation: Challenging 'Happy Family' Rhetoric in Iran," in *Islam and Assisted Reproductive Technologies*, eds. Marcia Inhorn and Soraya Tremayne (New York: Berghahn Books, 2012), 150.

23   Inhorn, *Local Babies*, 6.

24   Ibid., 217.

25   Ibid., 268.

26   Gillian Bentley and C. G. Nicholas Mascie-Taylor, eds., *Infertility in the Modern World: Present and Future Prospects* (Cambridge: Cambridge University Press, 2000), 17.

27   PBS, "18 Ways to Make a Baby," *Nova Transcripts*, October 9, 2001, http://www.pbs.org /wgbh/nova/transcripts/2811baby.html.

28   Inhorn, *Local Babies*, 268.

29   Inhorn, "Making Muslim Babies"; Tremayne, "The 'Down Side' of Gamete Donation."

30   El Feki, *Sex and the Citadel*, 43.

31   Ibid.

32   Inhorn, email interview.

33   Inhorn, "Reproductive Disruptions," 191.

34   Elizabeth Pisani, *The Wisdom of Whores: Bureaucrats, Brothels, and the Business of AIDS* (New York: W. W. Norton & Company, 2008), 201.

35   Inhorn, "Making Muslim Babies."

36   El Feki, *Sex and the Citadel*, 5.

37   Ihhorn, *Local Babies*, ix.

38   Inhorn, "Global Infertility and the Globalization of New Reproductive Technologies."

39   Isidore Singer et al, eds., *The Jewish Encyclopedia: A Descriptive Record of the History, Religion, Literature, and Customs of the Jewish People from the Earliest Times to the Present Day*, Volume 11 (New York: Funk & Wagnalls Company, 1907), 216; Raymond Apple, "Looking for a Shabbos Goy," *Jerusalem Post*, February 24, 2016, http://www.jpost.com/Opinion/Looking-for-a -Shabbos-Goy-446010.

40   Sharon Otterman, "An Orthodox, Online Version of the Deep-Freeze for Passover," *New York Times*, April 4, 2012, http://cityroom.blogs.nytimes.com/2012/04/04/an-orthodox-online -version-of-the-deep-freeze-for-passover/.

41   Gabriele Barbati, "Who Guards the Most Sacred Site in Christendom?: Two Muslims," *International Business Times*, March 29, 2013, http://www.ibtimes.com/who-guards-most -sacred-site-christendom-two-muslims-1161517; Pierre Klochendler, "And How Muslims

Hold the Key to Christ," *Inter Press Service*, July 29, 2012, http://www.ipsnews.net/2012/07/and-how-muslims-hold-the-key-to-christ/.

Afterword

1   Magnus Hirschfeld, *Women East and West: Impressions of a Sex Expert* (London: William Heinemann, 1935), 304.

2   John D'Emilio and Estelle Freedman, *Intimate Matters: A History of Sexuality in America* (Chicago: University of Chicago Press, 2012), 388.

3   Mary Roach, *Bonk: The Curious Coupling of Science and Sex* (New York: W. W. Norton & Co., 2008), 14.

4   Dean Hamer, *The Science of Desire: The Search for the Gay Gene and the Biology of Behavior* (New York: Simon & Schuster, 1994), 220–221.

5   Jean Stengers and Anne Van Neck, *Masturbation: The History of a Great Terror* (New York: St. Martin's Press, 2001), 177.

index

acknowledgments

I must first send an obligatory thanks to my family members and friends who put up with my complaints and erratic schedule throughout the past few years. Especially to my brother Troy and his wife Kristy, who allowed me to mooch like a teenager. And to my parents, who continue to love me even though they think I'm insane for choosing to move to a strange place to work in an unstable industry.

I'm very fortunate that my agent, Carly Watters, believed in the book's concept, even when it took me awhile to clearly conceptualize my intentions. Without her, this book would not have gotten published, and it's to her credit that a nobody like myself can now claim to be an author. Although I'm still very ignorant about the publishing world, she's taught me so much, and I'm very fortunate that she took a chance on me early in my career.

I want to thank Stephanie Bowen for getting Sourcebooks interested in publishing this book. And my editor Anna Michels deserves recognition for giving the book careful and thorough edits, challenging my thinking, catching my screw-ups, and helping me to repackage this thing into something more digestible and marketable than what I turned in.

Many researchers and sources have been helpful in answering questions and providing quality feedback. Thank you Helen Epstein, Edward Green, Daniel Halperin, Andrew Francis-Tan, Gabe Rotello, Michael Price, Walter Scheidel, Lynn Saxon, David Barash, Nathaniel Frank, Steve Estes, Victoria Basham, David Eisenbach, Marvin Zuckerman, Rachel Maines, Meika Loe, Marcia Inhorn, Soraya Tremayne, Jason Berry, John Thavis, Richard Wagner, Richard Sipe, James Martin, John O'Malley, Amin Ghaziani, Curtis Lipscomb, Milton Diamond, Patchen Barss, Frederick Lane, Frederick Wasser, Jay Winter, Michael Teitelbaum, Nicola Bulled, Ogi Ogas, and Mary Roach.

I also need to thank the many researchers whose work paved the way for this book. To quote Phillip Longman: "I make no pretense of having discovered or developed any new facts or data in this book. If the work has any originality, it is as an interpretive gathering of many disciplines."* Much of this book was based on secondary research, in which I connected separate ideas and topics while attempting to translate academic literature for a broader lay audience. For those wanting to learn more about the topics covered in this book, I *highly* recommend browsing through the citations and

---

* Longman, *The Empty Cradle*, xiii.

checking out some of the fantastic books that inspired and informed my writing.

To Danae Lenz, thank you for putting in so much time in the project even though you had little to gain from it. Your feedback and edits were always on point.

As a freelancer, I've been lucky to work with many great editors at *Sports on Earth*, the *Wall Street Journal*, *AdExchanger*, *Adweek*, *SB Nation*, *Rolling Stone*, and *Decider*, who supplied me enough work to stave off bankruptcy while I put this book together. I also owe a debt of gratitude to *Crain's Detroit Business* for giving me my start and to *Esquire* and *Deadspin* for letting me work in their offices and write ridiculous stuff. And I'm grateful that *Digiday* hired me after I completed this damn thing.

To my great friend Jordan Behrens: it's incredible that it was already five years ago that we started mapping out our ideas. Although life changes quickly turned this into a solo project, I really appreciate your constant interest, feedback, and willingness to listen to my bullshit. We ended up with much different lives in much different worlds, but your helpfulness and empathy never diminished, and for that I am very lucky.

I'm very blessed to have met Richard Kimbrough when I did. Richard introduced me to query letters and proposals when I first set out to obtain an agent. I had no idea what the hell I was doing, but thankfully Richard helped me understand a confusing environment.

Throughout the publishing process I've certainly had doubts, and no one has made me feel better about my situation than A. J. Jacobs, who cheered me up whenever we met and who may well be the kindest man in the universe. I am so damn lucky that A. J. replied to my shameless email to meet up a few years ago, and I'm even luckier that he allowed me to work with him on his family reunion project. Whenever you meet your idols, there's always great possibility for disappointment, especially if they turn out to be assholes. But A. J. turned out to be even funnier and nicer in person than he portrays himself in his books, which is pretty incredible. I really still can't believe he wrote the foreword for my book. If you are reading this book and you aren't related to me, chances are it's because you saw A. J.'s name on the cover.

And finally, to Rachel, my main squeeze. Whenever I've ranted about evolution and mating and discussed how women generally have a predisposition to prefer wealthy men who are also often significantly older, you've done an amazing job of showing, rather than telling, that the theory isn't universal. From an evolutionary standpoint, it makes little sense for a woman with your attractiveness, ambition, and phenomenal personality to commit to a guy like me. But I'm so grateful that you've loved this poor-ass weirdo anyway.

about the author

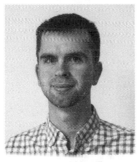

Photo credit © Matt Fraher

Ross Benes is a reporter who previously worked for *Deadspin*, *Digiday* and *Esquire*, where he wrote about sex, sports, statistics, and pop culture. His work has also appeared in *Adweek*, *Business Insider*, *Mental Floss*, *New York* magazine, *Quartz*, Refinery29, *Rolling Stone*, *Slate*, the *Wall Street Journal*, *Vice*, and *World Policy Journal*. A native of Brainard, Nebraska, he splits time between his home state and New York.